CARDIOLOGY RESEARCH AND CLINICAL DEVELOPMENTS

DRUGS IN CARDIOPULMONARY RESUSCITATION

Cardiology Research and Clinical Developments

Additional books in this series can be found on Nova's website under the Series tab.

Additional E-books in this series can be found on Nova's website under the E-books tab.

Pharmacology – Research, Safety Testing and Regulation

Additional books in this series can be found on Nova's website under the Series tab.

Additional E-books in this series can be found on Nova's website under the E-books tab.

CARDIOLOGY RESEARCH AND CLINICAL DEVELOPMENTS

DRUGS IN CARDIOPULMONARY RESUSCITATION

THEODOROS XANTHOS
EDITOR

Nova Science Publishers, Inc.
New York

Additional color graphics may be available in the e-book version of this book.

Library of Congress Cataloging-in-Publication Data

Drugs in cardiopulmonary resuscitation / editor, Theodoros Xanthos.
p. ; cm.
Includes bibliographical references and index.
ISBN 978-1-61122-512-9 (hardcover)
1. Cardiovascular emergencies--Chemotherapy. 2. CPR (First aid) 3.
Cardiovascular agents. I. Xanthos, Theodoros.
[DNLM: 1. Heart Arrest--drug therapy. 2. Acute Coronary Syndrome--drug
therapy. 3. Cardiopulmonary Resuscitation. 4. Cardiovascular
Agents--therapeutic use. WG 205]
RC675.D78 2010
616.1'025--dc22
2010038624

Published by Nova Science Publishers, Inc. † New York

Contents

Preface

Although approximately one million cardiac arrests occur every year in the USA and Europe, cardiac arrest remains a clinical condition still characterized by poor prognosis. One possible explanation may be the fact that although 70% of cardiac arrests take place in out-of-hospital settings, the majority of the victims do not receive basic life support (BLS) prior to the arrival of emergency medical services (EMS). Survival of out-of-hospital cardiac arrest victims strongly depends on prompt cardiopulmonary resuscitation (CPR). Survival rates will only improve, if delay time until initiation of CPR is kept to an absolute minimum. Good quality CPR, with an emphasis on chest compressions is a key component for the victims' survival. Drugs play a secondary role in the treatment of these patients. This book presents the latest research in drug therapy in CPR.

Capter 1 - The outcomes from cardiac arrest remain poor, in spite of advances in medical science. Since its discovery and isolation at the turn of the twentieth century, adrenaline has held primacy amongst the armamentarium of drugs used in cardiopulmonary resuscitation. Evidence supporting its use is scarce, and research has been hampered by the perception that randomised, placebo-controlled trials might be unethical. However, concerns have been raised that some of the wide-ranging effects of adrenaline may be detrimental. This chapter begins with a review of the basic physiology and pharmacology of adrenaline. It discusses the clinical data describing its use in cardiopulmonary rescuscitation, and highlights some of the obstacles to drawing positive conclusions about its efficacy.

Chapter 2 - Over the last twenty years, vasopressin has provided the closest challenge to the supremacy of adrenaline in cardiopulmonary resuscitation (CPR). The discovery of its two main physiological functions has given rise to its two names: 'vasopressin' and 'anti-diuretic hormone'. The initial successes of animal experiments have not been so clearly reflected in the human studies, to the disappointment of many who search for a means to improve outcomes from cardiac arrest. This chapter reviews the physiology of the vasopressin system, including discussions of the effects of vasopressin on various tissues. Many physiological studies give conflicting results and the differences between the trials reveal much about the complexity of the body's responses. The history of the use of vasopressin in cardiac arrest follows a similar course, with disagreements between researchers in the outcomes from animal experiments and in the interpretation of human trial data. All of this controversy is explored in the pages which follow.

Chapter 3 - Atropine antagonizes the actions of acetylcholine (Ach); therefore, it is commonly classified as an anticholinergic or parasympatholytic agent. It exerts its properties by non-selectively blocking muscarinic receptors. Atropine has various central and peripheral effects. Due to its parasympatholytic effects, atropine is currently indicated as a first-line agent for the management of symptomatic bradycardia and as a second-line agent for the treatment of bradycardic pulseless electrical activity and asystole. Furthermore, atropine is used in the treatment of organophosphate (OP) poisoning. This chapter, after a brief summary of basic pharmacology and actions of atropine, is intended to clarify the current role of the drug regarding the management of cardiac arrest; thus, it focuses on experimental and clinical data either supporting or condemning its use.

Chapter 4 - Despite the use of vasopressors in cardiopulmonary resuscitation (CPR), hospital discharge rates for both in-hospital and out-of hospital cardiac arrest (CA) remain dismal. Therefore, the use of antiarrhythmic agents with potential beneficial effects in CA such as amiodarone and magnesium, and ions with substantial effects in cardiac mechanics, such as calcium, is investigated in the international literature.

Amiodarone has been found to increase survival to hospital admission in shock-refractory ventricular fibrillation (VF). Current guidelines recommend it as the antiarrhythmic of choice in refractory VF/pulseless ventricular tachycardia (VT).

On the other hand, the routine administration of magnesium and calcium during CA failed to show any benefit and therefore it is not advocated by current guidelines. Magnesium is only recommended for the treatment of shock-refractory VF in the presence of possible hypomagnesemia or torsades de pointes.

The recommendations for calcium administration in CA are limited only to pulseless electrical activity (PEA) when specific reversible causes (hypokalemia, hypocalcemia, calcium-channel blockers overdose) need to be treated. However, these treatment recommendations are based on evidence provided by trials performed following resuscitation strategies according to previous guidelines. Data from studies implementing the 2005 International Liaison Committee on Resuscitation (ILCOR) guidelines are necessary in order to better evaluate the efficacy of these agents in CA.

Chapter 5 - A primary challenge in the development of clinical practice guidelines is keeping pace with the stream of new data upon which recommendations are based.

Management of a patient with Acute Coronary Syndromes (ACS), although tailored in specific algorithms, proves everyday to be challenging so as not only to make the diagnosis as soon as possible but also to go on establishing the appropriate therapeutic protocol.

This last one is of particular importance since the pathophysiology of ACS is not the same. Anti-ischemic therapy remains a cornerstone in the treatment of all ACS patients providing pain relief and improving the prognosis of patients with unstable angina/Non-ST-segment elevation myocardial infarction (UA/NSTEMI) and ST-segment elevation myocardial infarction (STEMI).

Chapter 6 - The goals of antithrombotic therapy for patients with ST-segment elevation myocardial infarction (STEMI) are to establish and maintain patency of the infarct-related artery, limit the consequences of myocardial ischemia, enhance myocardial healing, and reduce the likelihood of recurrent events. For patients with unstable angina/non-ST-segment elevation myocardial infarction (UA/NSTEMI), antithrombotic therapy has 2 components: 1) anticoagulant therapy, which targets the clotting cascade to prevent the deposition of fibrin strands in the clot and is categorized into i) intravenous (IV), subcutaneous (SC) and oral anticoagulants ii) direct thrombin inhibitors, iii) factor Xa inhibitors and 2) antiplatelet therapy, which reduces platelet activation and aggregation, integral steps in the formation of a thrombus after plaque disruption, which will be discussed in detail in the following chapter.

Chapter 7 - Clinical outcomes for patients with Acute Coronary Syndromes (ACS) can be optimized by revascularization coupled with aggressive medical therapy that includes, amongst others (anti-ischemic, anticoagulant, lipid-lowering) antiplatelet drugs. Antiplatelet therapy includes aspirin, clopidogrel, ticlopidine and newer $P2Y_{12}$ adenosine diphosphate (ADP) inhibitors, as well as glycoprotein (GP) IIb/IIIa inhibitors.

Since platelets play a crucial role in ACS, newer antiplatelet drugs continue to be developed with the goal of maximizing the reduction in atherothrombotic events while minimizing bleeding complications.

Chapter 8 - This chapter discusses the functions of β-adrenoreceptors in the intact and failing human heart, as well as the connection that seems to be between β-adrenergic stimulation and arrhythmiogenesis. Chronic beta-blockers usage has expanded over the last decades and indications now include hypertension, cardio-protection after myocardial infarction, angina, congestive heart failure, and rate control for arrhythmias. Beta-blockade is also independently associated with improved survival in patients with ventricular fibrillation (VF) or symptomatic ventricular tachycardia (VT). The anti-ischemic and anti-anginal actions of beta-blockers are discussed, as well as the beneficial outcomes of β-adrenergic blockade in experimental models and in human studies in the cardiopulmonary resuscitation (CPR) field.

Chapter 9 - Nitroglycerin (glyceryl trinitrate, GTN) is a representative of the organic nitrates or nitrovasodilators. Its beneficial therapeutic effect is attributed to selective vasodilation of large arteries and large conductance veins with minimal effect on the arteriolar tone. Evidence indicates that GTN and other nitrates function as prodrugs that, when bioactivated, release nitric oxide (NO). It is hypothesised that the principal mechanism of GTN-induced vasorelaxation is the activation of the soluble guanylyl cyclase (sGC), an intracellular NO receptor, and the subsequent increase in tissue levels of the second messenger cyclic 3'5'-guanosine monophosphate (cGMP). cGMP, in turn, activates cGMP-dependent protein kinase C (PKC) which induces vasorelaxation. Recently, it has been demonstrated that the mitochondrial isoform of aldehyde dehydrogenase (mtALDH or ALDH2) is responsible for the bioactivation of GTN. Tolerance develops after continuous use of GTN, leading to reduced responsiveness of blood vessels to GTN and other organic nitrates or to the requirement of higher doses of these drugs. Tolerance is attributed to the formation of the strong oxidant peroxynitrite, a potent cellular oxidant. GTN has clear benefits for the treatment of angina pectoris, congestive heart failure, unstable angina, non-ST-segment myocardial infarction, acute myocardial infarction and variant angina. During cardiopulmonary resuscitation (CPR), the co-administration of a vasodilator, such as nitroglycerin, with one or even two vasopressors has been suggested, in animal models. Still, further investigation is necessary for the administration of GTN during CPR.

Chapter 10 - This chapter discusses the broad spectrum of clinical usage, diagnostic applications, experimental challenges and future perspectives of adenosine.

Adenosine, an adenylic nucleotide metabolite, widely distributed throughout the human body, exerts a wide range of regulatory effects.

From a cardiovascular perspective, data indicate that the adenosinergic system is important in mediating protection (e.g. via pre- and post-conditioning) and in determining myocardial resistance to insult or to reperfusion-ischemia injury.

Besides, adenosine exerts its effects through currently four known adenosine receptor (AR) subtypes namely A_1R, $A_{2A}R$, $A_{2B}R$ and A_3R. In general, $A_{2A}R$ is the predominant receptor subtype responsible for coronary blood flow regulation, which dilates coronary arteries. Interestingly, adenosine exerts its cardiac electrophysiologic effects via A_1R (e.g. anti-b-adrenergic action).

Regarding the supraventricular tissues, adenosine remains as a "first line" pharmacologic agent for the treatment of supraventricular arrhythmias, due to its effect on inhibiting rapidly the atrioventricular (AV) nodal conduction.

In addition to its clinical role as an antiarrhythmic agent, adenosine has been also administered under conditions of hypoxia, ischemia, and cardiac arrest. Thus, basic research has implicated adenosine as an endogenous distress molecule with essential impact on immune response, adaptation to limited oxygen availability, anti-inflammatory action.

Specific AR agonists or antagonists in conjunction with studies in genetic models for adenosine generation have identified a rapidly expanding field of biomedical roles and potential therapeutic applications of extracellular adenosine signaling.

Chapter 11 - The post-resuscitation period should comprise a second, more complex phase of interventions which are likely to influence, significantly, the final outcome. As a critical component of post-resuscitation care, prompt optimisation of hemodynamic status by means of targeted interventions is vital in order to maximize the likelihood of a good outcome. In this setting, prompt administration of fluids and potentially vasopressors and inotropes are common treatment modalities of circulatory support after cardiac arrest. Furthermore, vasoactive agents may be required in the setting of underlying conditions complicating the post-resuscitation condition of the patient. The clinical efficacy of inotropes and vasopressors has been largely investigated through examination of their impact on hemodynamic end points, and clinical practice has been driven in part by expert opinion, extrapolation from animal studies, and physician preference. Careful and frequent monitoring of hemodynamic parameters and other measures, as required, is crucial to ensure optimal outcomes with the use of vasoactive agents. Clearly these agents are all supportive measures to stabilise the patient prior to some form of definitive therapy, and it is important to emphasise that all these pharmacological agents are associated with potentially significant side effects.

Chapter 12 - Current guidelines for neonatal resuscitation at birth stress the importance of temperature control, airway management and support of circulation for the majority of neonates who require help at birth. For the minority of neonates in which the basic steps of resuscitation fail to reverse an adverse situation, medications are justifiable. The 2005 International Liaison Committee on Resuscitation (ILCOR) guidelines state: "Medications are rarely needed in neonatal resuscitation. Those that may be used include epinephrine and fluids. Very rarely, a narcotic antagonist, sodium bicarbonate, or vasopressors may be useful after resuscitation". Even though medications have been in use in neonatal resuscitation for many years, their doses, order and route of administration have been the source of an ongoing debate among neonatologists. Existing data are mainly extrapolated from animal studies or studies on adults. This chapter will focus on the evidence behind the medications that are currently used in neonatal resuscitation.

In: Drugs in Cardiopulmonary Resuscitation
Editor: Theodoros Xanthos

ISBN: 978-1-61122-512-9

Chapter 1

Adrenaline in Cardiac Arrest

Phil Michael
Consultant Anaesthetist, North Wales NHS Trust, Glan Clwyd Hospital, Bodelwyddan, Rhyl, Denbighshire, LL18 5UJ.

Abstract

The outcomes from cardiac arrest remain poor, in spite of advances in medical science. Since its discovery and isolation at the turn of the twentieth century, adrenaline has held primacy amongst the armamentarium of drugs used in cardiopulmonary resuscitation. Evidence supporting its use is scarce, and research has been hampered by the perception that randomised, placebo-controlled trials might be unethical. However, concerns have been raised that some of the wide-ranging effects of adrenaline may be detrimental. This chapter begins with a review of the basic physiology and pharmacology of adrenaline. It discusses the clinical data describing its use in cardiopulmonary rescuscitation, and highlights some of the obstacles to drawing positive conclusions about its efficacy.

Introduction

Despite falling rates of cardiovascular disease, in most European countries around 40% of all-cause mortality is attributable to this spectrum of illness [1]. Worldwide, cardiovascular disease is the leading cause of death in both men and women [2]. Sudden cardiac arrest accounts for many of these deaths. Population-based reports of emergency medical services' experience from the United States of America give survival estimates of approximately 8% [3] for out-of-hospital cardiac arrests. In a pooled analysis of reported out-of-hospital arrests in Europe over 24 years, survival rates were about 10% [4]. In-hospital cardiac arrest yields similar results [5]. This is because although emergency management can be instigated earlier in the hospital setting, there is an increased likelihood of asystolic cardiac arrest with its overall poorer prognosis. Additionally, the fact that these are inpatients suggests that this population carries a disease process which has lessened their physiological reserve. With such dismaying results from a common medical occurrence, methods to try to improve the outcome of cardiac arrest are in desperate need. Over the past few decades, Cardiopulmonary Resuscitation (CPR) algorithms have been developed in order to establish best practice management, with some degree of congruency worldwide. CPR training for healthcare professionals as well as non-clinical staff has become commonplace; indeed, it is frequently part of the mandatory training packages that have become widespread in UK hospitals. The management of cardiac arrest is divided into the simultaneous strands of advanced life support and basic life support, the latter having become synonymous with CPR. The purpose of advanced life support is restoration of spontaneous circulation. It encompasses two main goals. The first is to treat the underlying cause of the cardiac arrest, such as with defibrillation in the case of a 'shockable' cardiac rhythm. The second is the use of additional measures designed to maximise the effectiveness of basic life support, which itself aims to maintain coronary and cerebral perfusion with external chest compression and manual ventilation. External chest compression delivers an estimated 10-20% of normal myocardial blood flow [6]. Arterial vasopressors have been incorporated into treatment algorithms for cardiac arrest with the intention of increasing coronary and cerebral perfusion pressure. Adrenaline has been utilised for this purpose for several decades. More recently, researchers have been investigating alternative vasopressors in cardiac arrest, most notably arginine vasopressin. This chapter will revise the pharmacology and physiology of adrenaline and will discuss the use of this drug in cardiac arrest and its role advanced life support algorithms. Vasopressin will be the subject of the next chapter.

Adrenaline Receptor Physiology

The sympathetic nervous system is the excitatory limb of the autonomic nervous system. It acts largely in opposition to the parasympathetic limb. The pre-ganglionic sympathetic neurones are generally shorter than their parasympathetic counterparts. The neurotransmitter for both sets of pre-ganglionic synapses is acetylcholine and the receptors are termed 'cholinergic'. The sympathetic ganglia run in chains in proximity to the thoracic and lumbar spinal cord, from whence the post-ganglionic neurones run. These are long and synapse onto end-organs. The sympathetic post-ganglionic neurotransmitter is usually noradrenaline and the receptors are therefore termed adrenergic, whereas the post-ganglionic parasympathetic receptors are cholinergic. There are two classes of adrenergic receptor, α and β, and these are G-protein linked cell-membrane receptors. Subtypes of α and β receptors have been identified and each have a wide distribution and range of functions. However, the system of sub-classification has seen several revisions over recent decades, since few drugs are specific enough as a ligand for each subtype to allow functional and binding studies to adequately separate the receptors. The advent of cloning technology has allowed the sub-classification to progress [7].

The α receptor has been classified into α_1 and α_2, and each was initially further divided into subtypes with some degree of overlap as further identification developed. The α_l adrenergic receptors, now recognised as α_{1A}, α_{1B} and α_{1D}, are concentrated around arterial and venous trees, but are also located in smooth muscle structures such as the urogenital and gastrointestinal tracts. The α_I adrenergic receptor also exists within the central nervous system, specifically around the hippocampus. Studies in genetically engineered mice have highlighted differences in the functions of the individual subtypes. The α_{IA} adrenoceptor seems to play an important role in the homeostatic maintenance of blood pressure, whereas the response to surges in catecholamines seems largely governed by α_{1B} [8]. The α_2 receptors are distributed both presynaptically and post-synaptically. Three subtypes have been identified: α_{2A}, α_{2B} and α_{2C}. The presynaptic α_{2A} receptor has been shown to inhibit secretion of noradrenaline from sympathetic neurones whereas α_{2C} is responsibie foi inhibition of adrenaline release from the chromaffin cells of the adrenal medulla [9]. The postsynaptic α_2 receptors are also distributed around the vascular tree and the central nervous system. On binding of an appropriate ligand each α receptor therefore elicits a response appropriate to its tissue localization. Stimulation of α receptors around vascular smooth muscle results in arterial and venous vasoconstriction. However, α_2 receptors within the ventrolateral medulla, notably α_{2A}, cause hypotension and bradycardia when activated by an appropriate ligand, by way of a reduction in sympathetic outflow. This is the mechanism of action of centrally acting hypotensive agents such as clonidine, dexmedetomidine and monoxidine [10]. The α_{2A} receptor is also implicated in the other actions of these drugs, such as the hypnotic and analgesic effects, as well as platelet aggregation. The opposing vasoconstrictor response seems likely to be mediated by agonists at the α_{2B} receptor, which is responsible for the pressor response to α adrenergic agonists [11]. Additionally, the α_{2B} receptor is important in the analgesic effects of nitrous oxide in the spinal cord [10, 11]. Notably, the post-synaptic α_2 receptor seems to be absent from the myocardium. However, all these receptor roles are an oversimplification and the clinical relevance must be interpreted with caution. There is considerable variation in adrenoceptor expression and distribution between species. Suffice to say that our understanding of the fine control over pressure and flow within individual vascular beds by the α adrenoceptors is still in its infancy.

The β adrenergic receptors have been subdivided into 3 classes. Traditionally, the β_1 receptor has been described in cardiac muscle cells where it mediates positive inotropic and chronotropic responses. In some animal models, stimulation of the β_1 receptor has been shown to promote apoptosis in cardiac myocytes [12]. It also controls renin secretion in the kidney and lipolysis in white adipose tissue. Within the brain, the β_1 receptor mediates melatonin secretion and is involved in mood [13]. β_2 receptors also cause positive inotropy and chronotropy within the myocardium when stimulated, though only to a lesser extent than the b_1 receptor. Additionally, the β_2 receptor appears to activate different intracellular signalling pathways, such as the stimulatory or inhibitory G-proteins (G_s or G_i), depending upon the specific agonist [12]. The β_2 receptor plays its main role outside the heart, where it is involved in the relaxation of smooth muscle, especially in the bronchial tree. It is important in the control of insulin secretion from the pancreatic islets [14]. The β_3 receptor is responsible for relaxation of other smooth muscle, such as in the gastrointestinal tract and urological system [15]. It is also expressed in adipocytes, where it is involved in the development of obesity [14]. β_3 receptors are thought to exhibit an endothelium-dependent vasodilatory effect within the coronary microcirculation, and the same work suggested an endothelium-independent coronary vasodilation mediated by β_1 and β_2 receptors [16]. These effects would go some way to mitigating against the increased myocardial oxygen consumption conferred by β adrenergic agonists. All three β adrenergic receptor subtypes are present in skin fibroblasts, where they play a role in cell proliferation and DNA synthesis [17].

Synthesis

In the late nineteenth century, the adrenal gland was known to produce a profoundly active substance and in 1901 Takamine successfully extracted the active 'adrenaline' [18].

Adrenaline is a naturally occurring catecholamine, an aromatic amine structurally based on a catechol ring. It is produced by the chromaffin cells of the adrenal medulla where it is then stored in chromaffin granules. The synthesis begins with the amino acid tyrosine, which is ingested or is produced from the hydroxylation of phenylalanine. The tyrosine is first hydroxylated within the cytosplasm of the chromaffin cells or in adrenergic neurones to dihydroxyphenylalanine or 'DOPA'. DOPA then undergoes decarboxylation to become dopamine. Further hydroxylation of the dopamine in granulated vesicles produces noradrenaline. This is the final step in catecholamine synthesis outside the adrenal medulla. However, an additional step involving methylation of the amino group occurs within the adrenal medulla to produce adrenaline [19].

Metabolism [20]

The sequence of breakdown of catecholamines (including adrenaline) into metabolites such as metanephrine and vanillylmandelic acid (VMA) has been scrutinised in recent years, and our understanding has grown considerably in this regard. The metabolic pathways vary depending upon the site of the reactions. Circulating adrenaline is taken into neuronal and extraneuronal tissues, the latter including the kidneys and liver. (Figure 1)

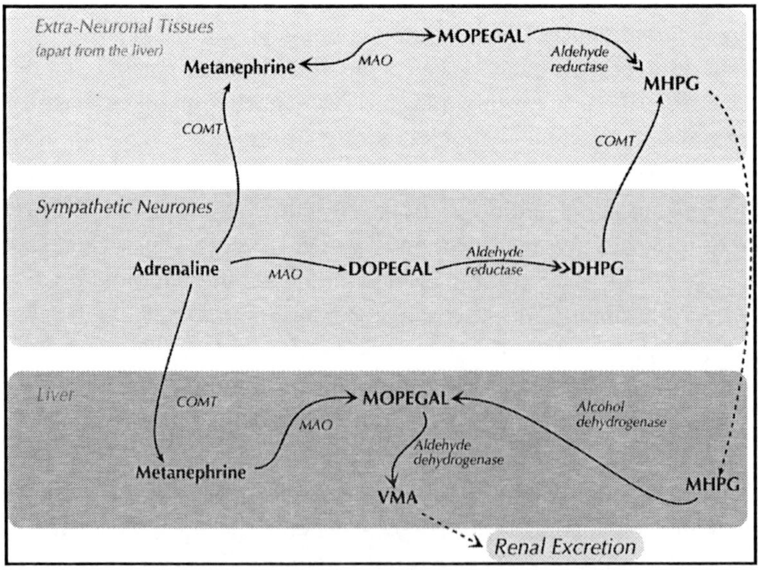

Figure 1. The metabolism of adrenaline (see text for explanation).

In sympathetic nerves, monoamine oxidase (MAO) catalyses the deamination of adrenaline to 3,4-dihydroxyphenylglycolaldehyde (DOPEGAL). This is a reactive aldehyde which is quickly reduced to the more stable 3,4-dihydroxyphenylglycol (DHPG) by aldehyde reductase, prior to release into the circulation. DHPG is then taken up by extra-neuronal tissues and is converted to 3-methoxy-4-hydroxyphenylglycol (MHPG) by the action of catechol-o-methyl transferase (COMT).

In extra-neuronal tissues, COMT catalyses the conversion of adrenaline to metanephrine. MAO, then, catalyses the oxidative deamination of metanephrine to 3-methoxy-4-hydroxyphenylglycolaldehyde (MOPEGAL). This is another reactive aldehyde, and it is rapidly reduced to MHPG by aldehyde reductase. This last step does not take place in the liver, where the opposite reaction takes place.

Within the liver, adrenaline is converted to metanephrine and then MOPEGAL as described for other extra-neuronal tissues. Circulating MHPG is taken up by the liver where it is also converted into MOPEGAL by hepatic alcohol dehydrogenase. The final step is conversion to MOPEGAL to VMA by hepatic aldehyde dehydrogenase. The VMA so produced is then excreted by the kidneys.

Action and Uses

Adrenaline is a powerful agonist at both α and β adrenergic receptors. As already described, these are extremely widespread and are involved in controlling much of the body's internal milieu. When utilised in high doses, as in a cardiac arrest, the desired increase in systemic vascular resistance is mediated by the α_1 receptor.

The profound peripheral vasoconstriction results in increased blood pressure. In low doses, such as when given by intravenous infusion in the critical care setting, the β effects predominate.

In the heart, these are manifest as positive inotropic and chronotropic effects; in other words there is an increase in the force and rate of myocardial contractions. Although these effects will also increase blood pressure, the price for this is that myocardial oxygen requirements are elevated.

Adrenaline is available as a clear, colourless solution of various concentrations. In cardiac arrest, ready-mixed syringes containing 10 millilitres of 0.1 mg/ml adrenaline are available in emergency drug boxes for intravenous administration, followed by a flush.

It can also be delivered via an endotracheal tube, if venous access has not been established. Adrenaline is available as a 1 mg/ml solution in ampoules of varying size for dilution and use in infusions in the critical care setting. It is also used in anaphylaxis and anaphylactoid reactions, where the recommended adult dose is 0.5 to 1mg delivered intramuscularly. Another popular use is in combination with local anaesthetic where adrenaline causes localised vasoconstriction and reduced redistribution of the local anaesthetic agent. This prolongs the anaesthetic effect. Indeed some practitioners infiltrate local anaesthetic agents with adrenaline with the primary aim of reducing venous bleeding as opposed to the analgesic effect, such as in surgical procedures of the head and neck. Here the concentration of adrenaline used is between 1 in 80000 and 1 in 300000, though most commonly a 1 in 200000 solution is used (5 micrograms/ml).

Effects of Adrenaline

Respiratory Effects

Adrenaline is a potent bronchodilator and causes an increase in minute volume, which may serve to aid oxygenation in and around cardiac arrest. However, this effect may be offset by its tendency to increase pulmonary vascular resistance and increase the tenacity of bronchial secretions [19].

Metabolic Effects

Adrenaline stimulates glycogenolysis, lipolysis and gluconeogenesis, whilst at the same time inhibiting insulin secretion and promoting release of glucagon [19,21,22]. This combination causes increased plasma glucose, free fatty acids and glycerol. The impact of any or all of these effects is an unknown quantity in cardiac arrest. However, glycaemic control is a significant issue in the phase of post-resuscitation care for these patients.

Effects on Platelets

Adrenaline enhances platelet aggregation, mediated by increasing cyclo-oxygenase activity and by α_2 adrenoceptor activation [23]. It also potentiates vasopressin-induced platelet aggregation [24]. At doses used in cardiac arrest, the level of platelet aggregation is of the order of 10%, though this may be significantly higher in when doses are increased [25]. Considering that the cause of most cardiac arrests is related to coronary thrombosis, this seems counterproductive.

Effects on Cerebral Circulation

Behringer *et al.* retrospectively analysed data gathered from more than four years of admissions to their emergency department [26]. In order to minimise confounding variables, they focused on patients presenting in ventricular fibrillation (VF) and specified sensible exclusion criteria. Those who recovered quickly (within 3 minutes of the first 3 defibrillation attempts) were at one end of the exclusion spectrum. At the other end were those who were known to have reduced neurological or cardiac function prior to the cardiac arrest. They also excluded any patients who had another cardiac arrest within 6 months. They defined the 'no flow' duration (the time between collapse to the time of onset of basic or advanced life support) and the 'low flow' duration (from the beginning of life support to the return of spontaneous circulation - ROSC -). They categorised 178 patients into those who had a 'no flow' time of less than or greater than two minutes. Each of these 'no flow' groups were subdivided into those whose 'low-flow' duration was less than or greater than ten minutes. This sub-classification allowed comparison within each group between the outcomes of those who received more than or less than 5 mg adrenaline. The researchers found that for each group, the proportion of patients who had a favourable neurological outcome was greater in those who received less than 5 mg adrenaline than in those who received more.

In addition, recent experimental data by Ristagno *et al.* suggest that adrenaline reduces cerebral perfusion at the level of the microcirculation, and that this is mediated by its $\square_1$ adrenergic effects [27]. In this trial, pigs were randomised into four groups before being anaesthetised, prepared for the trial, and their ventricles put into fibrillation. The pigs were prepared for the invasive monitoring of the required variables, including electrocardiography, pulmonary artery catheterisation, arterial gas analysis, and arterial pressure monitoring. The carotid arteries were exposed for flow measurements and a craniotomy was performed to allow assessment of cerebral micro-perfusion. One group received premedication with prazocin (an α_1 adrenergic antagonist) and propranolol (a non-selective β-blocker), another group received pretreatment with yohimbine (an α_2 adrenergic antagonist) and propranolol. The remaining two groups were given placebo at this stage. VF was then established and after 3 minutes, mechanical ventilation was resumed and chest compressions commenced. The two premedicated groups and one of the placebo groups were given adrenaline after one minute of CPR. The remaining placebo group received a second placebo. After another 3 minutes, defibrillation was attempted, and repeated if necessary according to a strict trial protocol. The group receiving no pre-treatment and adrenaline seemed to show a marginally improved mean arterial pressure during CPR, and slightly higher carotid blood flow than the other groups, though the prazocin/propranolol group showed similar improvements. However, in this study, cerebral microvascular blood flow (MBF) was shown to be reduced during cardiac arrest, and consequently cerebral carbon dioxide tensions increased and oxygen tensions decreased. All these figures tended towards baseline values in the post-resuscitation phase. Interestingly, both the placebo group and the prazocin group showed significantly less reduction in cerebral MBF than the adrenaline-only or the adrenaline/yohimbine groups. Also, the placebo and prazocin groups returned to baseline MBF quicker than the other groups. These results were mirrored by the measurements of cerebral oxygen and carbon dioxide tensions: the placebo and prazocin groups faired better than the other two.

Measures of serum lactate from arterial samples were significantly higher in the groups given adrenaline without prazocin than in either the placebo group or the prazocin group. This suggests that the reduction in microperfusion is not limited to the cerebral circulation.

Within the confines of this study it appears that the advantage of improved MAP conferred by adrenaline during CPR is more than offset by the reduction in micro-perfusion it causes.

Adrenaline in Cardiac Arrest

In the situation of cardiac arrest, the primary goal of treatment is early ROSC. Adrenaline has been used in cardiac resuscitation in the laboratory setting since 1906 [28]. However, its use in the clinical environment remained controversial for several decades as there were concerns about its propensity for causing VF when injected directly into a cardiac chamber [29]. The intravenous route of drug delivery was thought to lead to a delay in treatment [30].

Much of the early research into cardiac arrest was based on studies such as those of Crile and Dolley [28] and Redding and Pearson [30], where laboratory conditions and animal experiments attempted to recreate the situation of cardiac arrest. This usually took the form of asphyxia or electrically induced VF in anaesthetised animals. These were most often dogs in the early work, or pigs more recently, but some studies have used various rodents. In any case, experimental animals are often young and otherwise healthy. This raises some similarities with the paediatric setting, where cardiac arrest, mercifully rare, usually follows a respiratory arrest except in those cases of pre-exist cardiac abnormality. However, adult cardiac arrest in the clinical setting is often a vastly different pathological state. Cardiac arrest is most commonly cardiac in origin rather than secondary to asphyxia. The underlying pathology is related to atherosclerosis and plaque rupture, leading to thrombus formation and myocardial infarction.

There have been no randomised and blinded controlled trials of modern cardiac arrest scenarios comparing adrenaline with placebo in humans [31]. Such studies have been regarded in the past as ethically difficult to justify, and so the role of adrenaline is almost unassailable unless an alternative drug is presented. The few trials which have attempted this comparison have been unable to confirm a benefit with adrenaline [32].

In a retrospective analysis of 310 consecutive cardiac arrest patients [33], 30 patients survived to hospital discharge. Of these survivors, only one patient received adrenaline as part of their advanced life support resuscitation. Another six survivors received adrenaline but only as an inotrope or vasoconstrictor following ROSC. The remaining 240 patients who received adrenaline did not survive to hospital discharge. Of those patients not given adrenaline, 36.5% were eventually discharged. This is not to attribute cause and effect, however. Those patients whose clinical situation necessitated adrenaline administration were clearly in a poor risk group. The use of adrenaline did little to alter this fact.

A prospective interventional study in Seattle around the same time looked at out-of-hospital VF [34]. Over 2 years, 373 patients were allocated to receive adrenaline or lignocaine if the first defibrillation attempt was unsuccessful. 106 patients were allocated to receive lignocaine and 93 to adrenaline. Results were compared with those of similar patients in the preceding two years, when neither adrenaline nor lignocaine was used routinely and a continuous infusion of sodium bicarbonate was part of the regular treatment algorithm. Rates of survival to hospital discharge were significantly lower in those patients who received adrenaline (18%) or lignocaine (15%) than in those who received either sodium bicarbonate only or no drug (38%) during the trial period. Overall survival to discharge was 20%, compared with 24% in the preceding two year period, so the drug treatments that were introduced did not improve outcomes. However, the dose of adrenaline used in this study was only 0.5 mg, so drawing conclusions about the efficacy or otherwise of adrenaline remained difficult.

Indeed, the optimum dose of adrenaline is still a matter for debate. With such widespread and variable effects by one drug, it seems impossible to ascertain whether that drug is beneficial or harmful at any given dose within the spectrum of clinical scenarios encompassed by cardiac arrest. This is without attempting to define an ideal dose for all circumstances. The series of trials by Pearson and Redding described 1 mg doses delivered by way of intracardiac injection for dogs with a body mass of between 6 and 14 kg [35]. The same dose was used in their illustrative human case reports of a 33 year old adult male patient with cardiac arrest secondary to a pneumothorax and 17 month old boy found face-down in shallow water [30].

One prospective trial [36] randomised patients to receive either high dose adrenaline (10 mg) with placebo in both in-hospital and out-of-hospital arrests. The standard 1 mg dose, as recommended by most advanced life support algorithms, was given to those 145 patients not randomised, out of 339 who were eligible. The study groups were not matched. Out of preference of the supervising physicians, the patients in the 1 mg adrenaline group were more likely to be male, with no previous cardiac history and without significant other co-morbidity, and to have presented in VF. Those presenting in asystole were more likely to be enlisted into either the treatment arm or the placebo group. Logic would imply that the 1 mg adrenaline group therefore contained those patients who were much more likely to have a successful outcome. This was not the case. The 1 mg adrenaline group produced the only 3 patients who survived to hospital discharge of the 339 in total, and this finding was not deemed statistically significant. Rather than finding whether 10 mg of adrenaline was better than placebo, the group found no significant difference in survival regardless of adrenaline.

The picture was far from clear. Herlitz and colleagues reviewed data from out-of-hospital cardiac arrests in Göteborg, Sweden, between 1981 and 1992 [37]. All cardiac arrests attended by the emergency medical services were documented in forms which allowed subgroup analysis of large amounts of data. The researchers specifically focussed on 1203 out of 1360 patients who suffered VF arrests whose documentation was adequately detailed. The data that was collected spanned a decade in which certain changes were implemented, one of the most important of which was the authorisation to give adrenaline. During the early part of the period under scrutiny, only a few nurses were able to administer the drug, whereas during the latter stages it was given by an increasing number of paramedics. Therefore, the population provided a set of temporal control subjects: those before and those after widespread availability of adrenaline in out-of-hospital arrests. Overall results showed that although survival to hospital admission was similar whether adrenaline was given or not, those who received adrenaline were less likely to survive to hospital discharge. Furthermore, when looking at the subgroup of patients in refractory VF (i.e. those who remained in VF despite three defibrillatory shocks), patients given adrenaline were more likely to regain spontaneous circulation and survive to hospital admission, but they were not more likely to survive to hospital discharge. A similar result was found in those patients whose rhythm changed from VF to asystole or pulseless electrical activity (PEA - known at the time as electromechanical dissociation or EMD).

One the surface, such a result might seem to suggest lack of benefit from adrenaline. However the authors were quick to point out that this was not a randomised controlled trial and patients who received adrenaline were more likely to have been the complicated cases that required more protracted resuscitation and post-resuscitation efforts. Those not given adrenaline are more likely to have been those who regained spontaneous circulation within the first three shocks. It may have been the case that without adrenaline, these few survivors of complicated cardiac arrests may not have been so fortuitous. There were other changes implemented during the study period which may have been confounding variables, such as equipment changes and improvements in the interval between the time of arrest and the arrival of the paramedic team.

The idea of a registry of cardiac arrests seemed to have been popular in Sweden, as from 1990, a national registry of out-of hospital arrests has taken place there. Holmberg *et al.* reviewed the national data from 1990 to 1995, looking at 10966 cases of cardiac arrest in which resuscitation was attempted, [38]. The independent variables studied were the use of adrenaline and endotracheal intubation; the main outcome variable was survival at one month. In the subgroup of patients found in VF and who required 1-3 shocks, those given adrenaline had a significantly lower survival rate than those who were not. For patients in refractory VF, there was also a trend towards reduced survival in those who received adrenaline, though the difference was not statistically significant.

The results for patients with a non-VF arrest were slightly more complex. No significant survival difference between adrenaline and non-adrenaline patients was found in the subgroup whose cardiac arrest was either unwitnessed or witnessed by a bystander. However, in patients whose non-VF arrest was witnessed by the paramedic crew, those who received adrenaline had a significantly reduced survival rate. In a similar manner to the previous Swedish survey, this was not a randomised trial and selection bias may limit many of the inferences from the above results. The algorithm for managing VF at the time involved 3 successive attempts at defibrillation before the first administration of adrenaline. Those whose VF responded within the first three defibrillations were likely to have the better prognosis and adrenaline was not indicated. Similarly, those patients with a crew-witnessed, non-VF arrest may have had a prolonged peri-arrest period and hence the paramedic team was already present. Again, this implies a certain amount of patient selection involved in the decision to administer adrenaline. Nonetheless, the lack of a survival benefit with adrenaline in those with persistent VF was perhaps less likely to be attributable to selection bias. However, all these data are related to other factors, including the other independent variable that was studied, namely intubation. Confounding variables therefore make detailed inference difficult and unreliable. The authors conclude their paper with a sentiment echoed by many others: Randomised controlled studies are needed.

A bewildering array of confounding factors is certainly not the only reason for the difficulty in proving a positive effect of adrenaline in cardiac arrest. Several documented and suspected adverse effects legitimately raise questions about its safety in this situation [39]. It is known to increase myocardial oxygen demand, for example, and may reduce myocardial function in the post-resuscitation phase. Additionally, adrenaline is an agonist with a prolific portfolio of receptor activities. Many of its actions involve different effects from different receptor subtypes and represent a balance between vasoconstriction and vasodilatation of specific vascular beds. As a result, the haemodynamic effects are rather complicated [40]. There are reports which suggest that high doses of adrenaline may provoke coronary artery spasm [41]. The propensity for adrenaline to cause cardiac dysrythmias has already been mentioned. This is more pronounced in ischaemic states [22]. The other effects of adrenaline which have already been described may have a direct bearing on the outcome from cardiac resuscitation.

Conclusion

Despite forays into the use of other drugs, adrenaline has been the mainstay of vasopressor therapy in cardiac arrest since the inception of treatment for cardiac arrest. Its primary role is to improve mean arterial blood pressure during CPR in order to provide adequate perfusion to vital organs, including brain and heart. In theory this should minimise neurological impairment from cerebral hypoxia and maximise the chances of ROSC by improving myocardial oxygenation. Concerns about the use of adrenaline are mainly due to its -agonist effects. These increase the oxygen demand and consumption of an already ischaemic myocardium, and confer the pro-arrhythmogenic nature of adrenaline in the post-resuscitation phase. Adrenaline may cause coronary and cerebral vasoconstriction with a detrimental effect on blood flow to both these organs, despite an increase in the perfusing pressure. Adrenaline accelerates platelet aggregation and thrombus formation via its effects on cyclo-oxygenase and by α_2-mediated effects on platelets [23]. Thus, its use may be seen as counterproductive in a situation which arises primarily as a result of thromboembolic coronary artery disease.

The results from clinical trials have proved less than appealing, with long-term survival figures on average at 10% for in-hospital and out-of-hospital cardiac arrest. The requirement for adrenaline has been identified as a factor strongly associated with a poor outcome in cardiac arrest [33]. Those patients who have the best outcomes in cardiac arrest are those in VF who receive early CPR and defibrillation and achieve ROSC without the need for vasopressor drugs. When these patients are excluded from the calculation, Gueugniaud's paper suggests that the likelihood of survival of the remaining patients is of the order of 2%, at least for out-of-hospital cardiac arrest. Retrospective data showed no improvement in survival with the introduction of adrenaline and trends towards reduced survival rates with adrenaline in subgroup analyses of patients who received adrenaline compared with those who did not [37,38]. The only prospective trials comparing adrenaline with placebo in cardiac arrest showed a lack of benefit when adrenaline was used [34,36]. In all cases, any inference about adrenaline versus placebo was limited because of methodology.

Indeed, the standard 1 mg dose of adrenaline seems to be directly contraindicated in cardiac arrest in the early postoperative period following cardiac surgery [42]. In these cases, urgent re-sternotomy is indicated and small doses of 50-100 μg of adrenaline may be helpful to maintain perfusion until this can be achieved.

It can be seen that despite its prominence in algorithms for advanced life support, the use of adrenaline is not without controversy. It has been suggested that a more tempered approach would be to use adrenaline as necessary to maintain a mean perfusing pressure during resuscitation, but withhold further administration beyond that endpoint [43]. However, such a strategy would require advanced monitoring and procedures to guide resuscitation teams, and even then would require an evidence-base to define such endpoints. Alternatives to adrenaline have also been researched with some positive findings in a number of cases. The most prominent of these alternative resuscitation drugs to date is vasopressin, to which the discussion now turns.

References

[1] Sans S, Kesteloot H, Kromhout D. The burden of cardiovascular diseases mortality in Europe. Task Force of the European Society of Cardiology on Cardiovascular Mortality and Morbidity Statistics in Europe. *Eur. Heart J.* 1997;18(8):1231–1248.

[2] Mathers C, Fat DM, Boerma JT, Organization. WH. *The Global Burden of Disease: 2004 Update*. Geneva, Switzerland: World Health Organization; 2008.

[3] Rea TD, Eisenberg MS, Sinibaldi G, White RD. Incidence of EMS-treated out-of-hospital cardiac arrest in the United States. *Resuscitation*. 2004;63(1):17–24.

[4] Atwood C, Eisenberg MS, Herlitz J, Rea TD. Incidence of EMS-treated out-of-hospital cardiac arrest in Europe. *Resuscitation*. 2005;67(1):75–80.

[5] Dichtwald S, Matot I, Einav S. Improving the Outcome of In-Hospital Cardiac Arrest: The Importance of Being EARNEST. *Semin Cardiothorac Vasc Anesth*. 2009;13(1):19–30.

[6] Kern KB. Coronary perfusion pressure during cardiopulmonary resuscitation. *Best Practice and Research Clinical Anaesthesiology*. 2000/9;14(3):591–609.

[7] Civantos Calzada B, Aleixandre de Artinano A. Alpha-adrenoceptor subtypes. *Pharmacol. Res*. 2001;44(3):195–208.

[8] Tanoue A, Koshimizu T, Shibata K, Nasa Y, Takeo S, Tsujimoto G. Insights into alpha1 adrenoceptor function in health and disease from transgenic animal studies. *Trends Endocrinol. Metab*. 2003;14(3):107-13.

[9] Brede M, Nagy G, Philipp M, Sorensen JB, Lohse MJ, Hein L. Differential control of adrenal and sympathetic catecholamine release by alpha 2-adrenoceptor subtypes. *Mol. Endocrinol*. 2003;17(8):1640-6.

[10] Knaus AE, Muthig V, Schickinger S, Moura E, Beetz N, Gilsbach R, Hein L. Alpha2-adrenoceptor subtypes--unexpected functions for receptors and ligands derived from gene-targeted mouse models. *Neurochem. Int*. 2007;51(5):277-81.

[11] Kable JW, Murrin LC, Bylund DB. In vivo gene modification elucidates subtype-specific functions of alpha(2)-adrenergic receptors. *J. Pharmacol. Exp. Ther*. 2000;293(1):1–7.

[12] Brodde O, Bruck H, Leineweber K. Cardiac adrenoceptors: physiological and pathophysiological relevance. *J. Pharmacol. Sci*. 2006;100(5):323-37.

[13] Davis E, Loiacono R, Summers RJ. The rush to adrenaline: drugs in sport acting on the beta-adrenergic system. *Br. J. Pharmacol*. 2008;154(3):584-97.

[14] Philipson LH. beta-Agonists and metabolism. *J. Allergy Clin. Immunol*. 2002;110(6 Suppl):S313-7.

[15] Tanaka Y, Horinouchi T, Koike K. New insights into beta-adrenoceptors in smooth muscle: distribution of receptor subtypes and molecular mechanisms triggering muscle relaxation. *Clin. Exp. Pharmacol. Physiol*. 2005;32(7):503-14.

[16] Dessy C, Moniotte S, Ghisdal P, Havaux X, Noirhomme P, Balligand JL. Endothelial beta3-adrenoceptors mediate vasorelaxation of human coronary microarteries through nitric oxide and endothelium-dependent hyperpolarization. *Circulation*. 2004;110(8):948-54.

[17] Furlán C, Sterin-Borda L, Borda E. Activation of beta3 adrenergic receptor reases DNA synthesis in human skin fibroblasts via cyclic GMP/nitric oxide pathway. *Cell Physiol. Biochem*. 2005;16(4-6):175-82.

[18] Aronson JK. "Where name and image meet"--the argument for "adrenaline". *BMJ*. 2000;320(7233):506-9.

[19] Peck TE, Williams M. *Pharmacology for Anaesthesia and Intensive Care*. In: Pharmacology for Anaesthesia and Intensive CareLondon: Greenwich Medical Media, Ltd; 2000. p. 164-166.

[20] Eisenhofer G, Kopin IJ, Goldstein DS. Catecholamine metabolism: a contemporary view with implications for physiology and medicine. *Pharmacol. Rev*. 2004;56(3):331-49.

[21] Mycek MJ, Harvey RA, Champe PC. *Pharmacology*. In: PharmacologyPhiladelphia: Lippincott-Raven; 1997. p. 55-63.
[22] Rang HP, Dale MM, Ritter JM. *Pharmacology*. Edinburgh; New York: Churchill Livingstone; 1995.
[23] Cameron HA, Ardlie NG. The facilitating effects of adrenaline on platelet aggregation. *Prostaglandins Leukot. Med.* 1982;9(1):117-28.
[24] Bushfield M, McNicol A, MacIntyre DE. Possible mechanisms of the potentiation of blood-platelet activation by adrenaline. *Biochem. J.* 1987;241(3):671-6.
[25] Poullis DM. Repeated administration of vasopressin but not epinephrine maintains coronary perfusion pressure after early and late administration during prolonged cardiopulmonary resuscitation in pigs. *Circulation*. 2000;101(16):E174-5.
[26] Behringer W, Kittler H, Sterz F, Domanovits H, Schoerkhuber W, Holzer M, Müllner M, Laggner AN. Cumulative epinephrine dose during cardiopulmonary resuscitation and neurologic outcome. *Ann. Intern. Med.* 1998;129(6):450-6.
[27] Ristagno G, Tang W, Huang L, Fymat A, Chang Y, Sun S, Castillo C, Weil MH. Epinephrine reduces cerebral perfusion during cardiopulmonary resuscitation. *Crit. Care Med.* 2009;37(4):1408–1415.
[28] Crile G, Dolley DH. An experimental research into the resuscitation of dogs killed by anesthetics and asphyxia. *J. Exp. Med.* 1906;8(6):713-725.
[29] Dripps RD, Kirby CK, Johnson J, Erb WH. Cardiac Resuscitation. *Ann. Surg.* 1948;127(4):592-604.
[30] Pearson JW, Redding JS. Epinephrine in cardiac resuscitation. *Am. Heart J.* 1963;66:210-4.
[31] of the European Resuscitation Council ALSWG. The 1998 European Resuscitation Council guidelines for adult advanced life support. *BMJ.* 6 1998;316(7148):1863–1869.
[32] Rainer TH, Robertson CE. Adrenaline, cardiac arrest, and evidence based medicine. *J. Accid. Emerg. Med.* 1996;13(4):234-7.
[33] Roberts D, Landolfo K, Light RB, Dobson K. Early predictors of mortality for hospitalized patients suffering cardiopulmonary arrest. *Chest*. 1990;97(2):413-9.
[34] Weaver WD, Fahrenbruch CE, Johnson DD, Hallstrom AP, Cobb LA, Copass MK. Effect of epinephrine and lidocaine therapy on outcome after cardiac arrest due to ventricular fibrillation. *Circulation*. 1990;82(6):2027-34.
[35] Redding JS, Pearson JW. Evaluation of drugs for cardiac resuscitation. *Anesthesiology*. 1963;24:203-7.
[36] Woodhouse SP, Cox S, Boyd P, Case C, Weber M. High dose and standard dose adrenaline do not alter survival, compared with placebo, in cardiac arrest. *Resuscitation*. 1995;30(3):243-9.
[37] Herlitz J, Ekström L, Wennerblom B, Axelsson A, Bång A, Holmberg S. Adrenaline in out-of-hospital ventricular fibrillation. Does it make any difference? *Resuscitation*. 1995;29(3):195-201.
[38] Holmberg M, Holmberg S, Herlitz J. Low chance of survival among patients requiring adrenaline (epinephrine) or intubation after out-of-hospital cardiac arrest in Sweden. *Resuscitation*. 2002;54(1):37-45.
[39] Tang W, Weil MH, Sun S, Noc M, Yang L, Gazmuri RJ. Epinephrine increases the severity of postresuscitation myocardial dysfunction. *Circulation*. 1995;92(10):3089-93.

[40] Penson PE, Ford WR, Broadley KJ. Vasopressors for cardiopulmonary resuscitation. Does pharmacological evidence support clinical practice? *Pharmacol. Ther.* 2007;115(1):37-55.

[41] Karch SB. Coronary artery spasm induced by intravenous epinephrine overdose. *American Journal of Emergency Medicine*. 1989;7(5):485–488.

[42] Tsagkataki M, Levine A, Strang T, Dunning J. Should adrenaline be routinely used by the resuscitation team if a patient suffers a cardiac arrest shortly after cardiac surgery? *Interact Cardiovasc Thorac Surg.* 2008;7(3):457-62.

[43] Sutton RM, Berg RA, Helfaer MA. Epinephrine for resuscitation from cardiac arrest: A double-edged sword? *Crit. Care Med.* 2009;37(4):1518–1520.

In: Drugs in Cardiopulmonary Resuscitation
Editor: Theodoros Xanthos
ISBN: 978-1-61122-512-9

Chapter 2

Vasopressin in Cardiac Arrest

Phil Michael
Consultant Anaesthetist, North Wales NHS Trust, Glan Clwyd Hospital, Bodelwyddan, Rhyl, Denbighshire, LL18 5UJ

Abstract

Over the last twenty years, vasopressin has provided the closest challenge to the supremacy of adrenaline in cardiopulmonary resuscitation (CPR). The discovery of its two main physiological functions has given rise to its two names: 'vasopressin' and 'anti-diuretic hormone'. The initial successes of animal experiments have not been so clearly reflected in the human studies, to the disappointment of many who search for a means to improve outcomes from cardiac arrest. This chapter reviews the physiology of the vasopressin system, including discussions of the effects of vasopressin on various tissues. Many physiological studies give conflicting results and the differences between the trials reveal much about the complexity of the body's responses. The history of the use of vasopressin in cardiac arrest follows a similar course, with disagreements between researchers in the outcomes from animal experiments and in the interpretation of human trial data. All of this controversy is explored in the pages which follow.

Introduction

Towards the end of the nineteenth century, around the same time as extracts from the adrenal glands were investigated for their potent cardiovascular effects, similar experiments were being carried out for other glands. In 1895, Oliver and Schäfer, writing from London, described that extracts from the pituitary gland had similar cardiovascular effects to adrenaline, in that blood pressure and the force of myocardial contractions were increased. In contrast to adrenaline, though, they noted that there was no acceleration of heart rate with the pituitary extract [1]. Three years later, Howell, a professor of physiology from Johns Hopkins University, identified that the extracts of the anterior lobe of the pituitary (or *hypophysis cerebri*) had minimal effects on blood pressure, and that the powerful vasopressor effect came from extracts of the posterior lobe (the infundibular body) [2]. Eighteen years later, hypophyseal extract was noted for its antidiuretic properties and for the next few decades the pressor effects lay largely dormant in scientific research. In the 1950s, when vasopressin was isolated and synthesised, it was proved that the antidiuretic and vasopressor effects were carried out by the same hormone [3]. Since the early 1990s, there has been a significant body of work suggesting that vasopressin may be an additional or alternative vasopressor in cardiac arrest.

Synthesis and Release of Vasopressin

Vasopressin is synthesised as a prohormone in the hypothalamus by the magnocellular and parvocellular neurones of the supraoptic and paraventricular nuclei. From there it is transported to the posterior lobe of the pituitary gland and stored in secretory granules. During transport, the prohormone is cleaved to produce the polypeptide hormone vasopressin, which consists of nine amino acid residues. These nine vary slightly between mammalian species, and for this reason, the human form is often referred to as arginine vasopressin (AVP - *Figure 1*).

AVP is released into the circulation in response to a variety of stimuli, the most important of which relate to states of reduced circulating blood volume. These are raised plasma osmolality, hypotension (detected by arterial baroreceptors), and hypovolaemia (detected by ventricular baroreceptors). These stimuli become part of the negative feedback-loop which helps to regulate the release of AVP. Other stimuli for the release of AVP include pain, hypoxia, nausea, and hypoglcaemia [4].

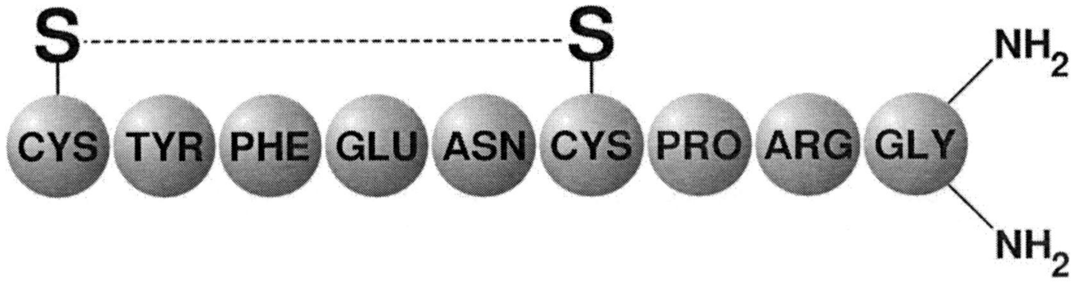

Figure 1. The amino acd structure of arginine vasopressin, depicting the disulphide bond between the cysteine residues.

Vasopressin Receptors

The main actions of vasopressin are mediated through specific vasopressin receptors, of which three subtypes have been identified. Although initially named V_{1a}, V_{1b} and V_2, a change in the nomenclature has yielded V_1 (from V_{1a}), V_2 and V_3 (from V_{1b}). Like the adrenoceptors, vasopressin receptors are transmembrane receptors linked to G-proteins. They are distributed according to subtype and function. The V_1 receptor is expressed at a number of sites, the most important of which is vascular smooth muscle. Here, binding of vasopressin causes vasoconstriction mediated via phosphopholipase C. Other sites for the V_1 receptor include platelets (where vasopressin facilitates platelet aggregation), the liver, testes and brain. The V_1 receptor is involved in the modulation of social behaviour [5].

The V_2 receptor is mainly found in the collecting ducts of the kidneys, and it is responsible for the antidiuretic properties of AVP. Stimulation of V_2 receptors causes the insertion of aquaporins into the luminal surface of the collecting ducts which leads to increased renal water reabsorption. This effect is mediated by the adenylate cyclase/cyclic AMP second-messenger system [6].

The V_3 receptor is located in the central nervous system, where it is involved in thermoregulation, modulation of corticotrophin secretion and the maintenance of circadian rhythms [7,8]. Like the V_1 receptor, V_3 functions are also mediated by the phospholipase second messenger system, and it is also thought to be important in behavioural functions such as social memory and anxiety [5].

Due to the structural similarities between vasopressin and oxytocin, the other hormone of the posterior pituitary, vasopressin it is known to act on oxytocin receptors. It produces vasodilatation within the uterus and within certain vascular endothelium. In cardiac endothelium, it is also thought to act at the P_2 purinergic receptors, a family of cell-surface receptors which bind to adenosine triphosphate but not to adenosine [9].

Metabolism of Vasopressin

In health, most of the circulating AVP is bound to platelets, and the unbound 10% retains its vasoactivity [10]. Thus the action of vasopressin can be significantly influenced by thrombocytopaenia. The plasma half-life of intravenously administered AVP is estimated to be 24 minutes [11], though various reviews have described a range from 4 to 35 minutes [4,8,12,13]. There is also some evidence that the endobronchial route of administration for vasopressin is equally as effective as when the intravenous route [14]. Unlike its synthetic analogue desmopressin, vasopressin is broken down by trypsin and is therefore not administered enterally. Metabolism is mainly splanchnic and renal, though other sites of vasopressin metabolism, such as the amniotic sac in sheep and the brain, have been noted experimentally [15]. There is some suggestion that vasopressin metabolites may have some physiological function within the brain. Additionally, increased clearance of vasopressin has been described in pregnancy, and the placenta is thought to release vasopressinase into the maternal circulation [16]. Experiments in anaesthetised dogs [17] identified that the liver was responsible for approximately half of the splanchnic extraction of vasopressin, and that the spleen did not contribute to the prehepatic clearance. This suggested that the liver and intestines are almost equally responsible for splanchnic metabolism of vasopressin. The hepatic extraction of vasopressin has a high capacity with no evidence of saturation at high concentrations [15].

The renal clearance of vasopressin is by both filtration (up to 75%) and enzymatic degradation (25%). A proportion of the renal metabolism of vasopressin occurs by hydrolysis in the proximal tubule, that is after filtration. A physiological role for this metabolic function has yet to be clarified [15].

Actions of Vasopressin

With such a wide array of receptor activities, it is perhaps unsurprising that vasopressin has numerous physiological actions. These have been outlined briefly with the appropriate vasopressin receptor, above. In the following section, some of the effects of vasopressin will be dealt with in more detail.

Vasopressin and Regulation oF Blood Pressure

Vasopressin is not released from the pituitary gland in hypovolaemia until its severity gives rise to unloading of the arterial baroreceptors located in the carotid sinus and aorta. Holmes *et al.* (2004) describe the four main mechanisms by which arginine vasopressin is involved in the regulation of blood pressure, via control of blood vessel diameter [18].

First, AVP is thought to close potassium-ATP (K_{ATP}) channels. When activated (opened), these K_{ATP} channels hyperpolarise the smooth muscle cell by allowing potassium efflux, thereby preventing voltage-gated calcium channels from opening. Smooth muscle contraction is thus inhibited, leading to vasodilation. By closing these K_{ATP} channels, AVP produces vasoconstriction.

Second AVP, acting via V_1 receptors, inhibits the production of nitric oxide synthase (NOS) and reduces the action of nitric oxide. Nitric oxide causes vasodilation by activating K_{ATP} channels and, via increasing levels of cyclic guanosine monophosphate (cGMP), activates myosin light chain phosphatase.

Third, the actions of noradrenaline and angiotensin II are potentiated by AVP. The process for this is thought to involve inhibition of G-protein coupled receptor down-regulation, but the precise mechanism has yet to be elucidated.

Vasopressin and Vasodilation

Despite the fact that the main effect of vasopressin on blood vessels is vasoconstriction, the nonapeptide is known to cause a degree of vasodilation in various systems. An in vitro study in rats showed that with increasing doses of vasopressin, cerebral arterioles initially vasodilated, then constricted, and then dilated back to their initial diameter [19]. One canine study used cerebral angiography to show a significant vasodilating action of vasopressin in vivo up to a maximum of 1 nmol dose, beyond which there was no further increase in vessel diameter [20]. They also found a regional selectivity in that the arteries of the Circle of Willis exhibited more of a response than those outside the circle. It was suggested that the in vivo results are due to the net effect of vasopressin acting via both an endothelium-dependent increase in nitric oxide activity (vasodilation) and the V_1 receptor action within the smooth muscle (vasoconstriction). A similar result was found in pulmonary vasculature in an in vitro canine study, with low dose AVP producing endothelium-dependent dilatation and higher doses causing constriction [21]. Another in vivo study, this time in arteries of human forearms, gave slightly different results, with vasoconstriction at low doses and vasodilation at high doses of vasopressin [22]. The reasons for this difference are not clear, but it may again reflect the balance between the effects of vasopressin on nitric oxide release and the actions at the V_1 receptor. The mechanism for the augmented release of endothelial nitric oxide has been attributed to oxytocin receptor activation [18]. The oxytocin receptor has been found to be expressed by human vascular endothelial cells [23], and it is known that vasopressin has agonist activity at the oxytocin receptor [24]. Incidentally, this may also explain the systemic vasodilation which takes place secondary to intravenous administration of oxytocin or its synthetic analogue syntocinon.

Actions of Vasopressin on Coronary Arteries

Similarly, studies looking at coronary arteries have had mixed results from the effects of vasopressin. In 1976, Heyndrickx *et al.* published experiments to show that vasopressin increased coronary resistance in conscious dogs [25]. Of note however, was their finding that this reduction in coronary flow was not reduced after AVP administration when the heart rate was maintained by pacing. A 1984 study showed that vasopressin dilated coronary arteries and described the V_1 receptor as the mediator [26]. Two years later, a study in isolated rats' hearts showed a reduction in coronary blood flow with increasing doses of arginine vasopressin [27]. The AVP was added to the coronary perfusate and thus directly into the coronary arteries.

In another study, also using isolated rat hearts, coronary vasoconstriction increased with increasing AVP concentration. With the coronary perfusion pressure held constant, AVP caused an increase in myocardial contractility at low doses, followed by a decrease in contractility at higher doses [28]. Again, the V_1 receptor was identified as the mediator. Then in 1990, Boyle and Segel published another study using rats' hearts with a rather interesting finding. The vasoconstriction caused by AVP was attenuated when the heart was in a state of reduced oxygenation, as in the case of hypoxia or hypotension [29]. This would appear to suggest that whilst coronary vasoconstriction might be an adverse side-effect of vasopressin administration in a normal physiological state, the effect would be less problematic in cases of poor myocardial oxygenation, as in a cardiac arrest. Nevertheless, in 1991, a study was published with data to show that not only did vasopressin cause coronary vasoconstriction, but the vasoconstriction was significant enough to cause myocardial ischaemia [30]. This was evidenced by left ventricular dysfunction, reduced myocardial pH and reduced regional myocyte shortening at constant oxygen consumption. This was an animal study using anaesthetised dogs with no known coronary artery disease. The vasopressin was infused directly into the coronary arteries.

Despite the seemingly mounting evidence of adverse coronary effects of vasopressin, its proponents were simultaneously demonstrating its potential effectiveness in CPR and comparing its actions favourably against adrenaline [31,32].

The debate continued and experiments carried out on isolated segments of human epicardial coronary arteries demonstrated vasoconstriction when bathed in solution containing vasopressin [33]. The maximum vasoconstriction was 11.8% of the contractile response to a high-concentration potassium solution and no vasodilatation occurred in response to low doses of vasopressin as was suggested by the early experiments.

Further evidence that AVP could induce coronary vasoconstriction was published in 1998 [34]. The experiments were divided into two parts, the first of which involved intracoronary injections of AVP in anaesthetised goats. Similar to other experiments, coronary blood flow was reduced with increasing doses of vasopressin. The second part of the study used isolated coronary artery segments taken from goats. The segments were suspended in organ baths and AVP was added to the bathing solution. Tension measurements indicated that the addition of AVP yielded dose-dependent contractions, and that the maximal contractions increased with removal of the endothelium (a statistically insignificant finding) and with the addition of L-NAME (a nitric oxide synthase inhibitor - a statistically significant finding). By this time, clinical trials of vasopressin in cardiac arrest had already taken place [35,36].

However, in 1999 Okamura *et al.* published data from experiments on isolated segments taken from the coronary arteries of monkeys [37]. A concentration-related relaxation was identified when AVP was added to the bathing solution. This was abolished when the endothelium was removed from the segments or when nitric oxide synthase was inhibited. This action of vasopressin seems to be in keeping with the studies on pulmonary vasculature [21] and cerebral arteries [20] mentioned earlier. However, unlike the previous studies, Okamura *et al.* identified the V_1 receptor as responsible for the vasodilatation.

Several studies have been published by Lindner and Wenzel *et al.* demonstrating improved organ perfusion, including coronary vasodilation, with vasopressin during various models of cardiac arrest [31,32,38-41]. More recently, perhaps in order to counter the belief that AVP induces coronary vasoconstriction, this group explored the haemodynamic effects of vasopressin in sinus rhythm [42].

Again, their experimental model used anaesthetised pigs. After the experimental preparations, an intravenous dose of 0.4 U/kg of arginine vasopressin was administered. They found an increase in both the mean arterial pressure and in the cross sectional area of the left anterior descending (LAD) coronary artery. The latter was measured using an intra-arterial ultrasound device. During the second part of their study, they used L-NAME to block nitric oxide synthase and found the same degree of LAD vasodilation with AVP. This suggested that the vasodilation was not dependent on endothelial nitric oxide, contrary to what had previously been described.

To summarise then, many studies show conflicting data to describe whether vasopressin causes coronary vasoconstriction or coronary vasodilatation. The reasons for this discrepancy must be multifactorial. It is possible that significant inter-species variation exists between the different animal models used in the experiments.

For example, it is known that the precise make-up of vasopressin varies between the bovine, porcine and human forms - hence 'arginine vasopressin' is used to specify the human form. There may also be receptor variation between species [42] which may partly explain the differences in the study outcomes but also may hinder extrapolation to human pharmacotherapy. Other differences between the studies exist. For example some studies used live or anaesthetised animal models whilst other studies used isolated segments of arterial tissue. Some used intravenous injection of AVP, others used intracoronary infusions. There is also a discrepancy between the dosage administered, with some authors describing a fixed intravenous dose roughly equating to that recommended by the American Heart Association resuscitation guidelines, whilst other authors describe administering known volumes of solution containing different concentrations of AVP.

To further complicate matters, the authors also use different units of measurement such as micrograms versus micromoles per kilogram, versus international units (IU). At present, the precise effects and mechanisms of action of AVP on the coronary circulation are still the subject of debate, and studies describing vasoconstriction and vasodilation will no doubt continue to be published. It is important to ask, therefore, how relevant is this delineation in the situation of cardiac arrest? Other factors may outweigh these possible risks.

Vasopressin and Heart Rate

From the time of Oliver and Schäfer's 1895 article, the effects of vasopressin on heart rate have been documented. Specifically, vasopressin reduces the heart rate as might be expected from the baroreceptor reflex after augmentation of blood pressure.

In their experiments on conscious dogs however, Heyndrickx *et al.* also found a reduction in heart rate with AVP after denervation of the arterial baroreceptors [25]. They were in agreement with the findings of previous studies that there must be a component of the bradycardia which is a result of a direct action of vasopressin on the heart [43-45].

Additionally, it is thought that central V_1 vasopressin receptors may modulate sympathetic tone directly and hence affect the baroreceptor reflex [46].

Vasopressin and Cardiac Function

Heyndrickx *et al.* also looked at cardiac output changes after administration of AVP. The increased afterload caused by systemic vasoconstriction understandably reduced myocardial contractility [25]. This, coupled with the reduction of heart rate, means that vasopressin reduces cardiac output. Most studies seem to agree with this finding [10,27,42,47].

It is also thought that activation of V_1 receptors leads to impaired myocardial relaxation, which outweighs the positive inotropic effect of increased intracellular calcium it also causes [13].

Vasopressin and Platelet Aggregation

As previously mentioned, platelets express the V_1 receptor, and their activation by vasopressin leads to platelet aggregation via release of thromboxane [10]. This effect acts synergistically with that of adrenaline on platelet aggregation [48].

Additionally, stimulation of V_2 receptors increases the release of von Willebrand factor, facilitating platelet adhesion. Laboratory data confirms that vasopressin induces a weakly procoagulant response [49]. The clinical implications of this are uncertain, as vasopressin has been associated with a reduction in platelet count when used as an infusion in the treatment of vasodilatory shock [50].

Despite this, during a low-flow state such as cardiac arrest, on the background of a likely thrombo-embolic primary cause and with thrombolysis as a distinctly possible therapeutic option, the potential for vasopressin to alter the state of coagulation must not be ignored.

Miscellaneous Actions of Vasopressin

The actions of vasopressin on other systems may influence patient management and outcomes in the critical care setting [51]. The recent review article by Dunser *et al.* summarises the effects neatly. These include effects on metabolism of glucose, amino acids and proteins. Additionally, vasopressin modulates immune function, mitochondrial function and thermoregulation. As yet, there have been no clinical studies demonstrating the impact of these effects on patient outcomes.

Vasopressin in Cardiac Arrest

The interest in the potential usefulness of vasopressin as a pressor drug in cardiac arrest arose after research into the stress hormone response during CPR was published in 1992 [52]. In a series of 34 patients suffering out-of-hospital cardiac arrest, the researchers sought differences in the stress response between those in whom return of spontaneous circulation (ROSC) was achieved compared with those in whom it was not. ROSC was achieved in twenty patients, of whom only five survived to hospital discharge without major neurological impairment. Blood was sampled from an external jugular vein between one and two minutes following the first administration of adrenaline and thereafter at 5, 15, 30 and 60 minutes after ROSC. The main findings were that adrenocorticotropic hormone (ACTH) and vasopressin levels were markedly raised during and after CPR. Additionally the median plasma concentrations of these hormones were significantly higher in those patients in whom ROSC was achieved than in those in whom it was not. However, there were no further differences in the levels in those five who survived to discharge. Lindner *et al.* raised the question as to whether administration of ACTH or vasopressin might usefully potentiate the effects of catecholamines in cardiac arrest.

Almost a year later a study, also featuring Dr. Lindner, explored the haemodynamic effects of vasopressin during and after CPR. This was a randomised, blinded experiment using anaesthetised pigs that compared single doses of 0.8 U/kg AVP to 0.045 mg/kg adrenaline in an open-chest model of ventricular fibrillation (VF). The adrenaline dose here equates to 3.15 mg in a 70 kg man, much higher than the 1 mg currently recommended in resuscitation guidelines. The authors referred to previous work, published only in abstract form, in which they had explored different dosages of adrenaline and found that this dose had given optimum values of coronary perfusion.

Lindner *et al.* found that those pigs receiving vasopressin had higher mean arterial pressures, a significantly increased systemic vascular resistance and better myocardial blood flow in both endocardial and vessels epicardial compared with those receiving adrenaline. Additionally, although there was a higher myocardial oxygen consumption in the vasopressin group, this was outweighed by the fact that there was a much greater increase in myocardial oxygen delivery. At the same time, there was a greater diversion of blood flow away from nonessential tissues and organs such as intestines, skin, fat and skeletal muscle towards the brain and heart in the vasopressin group than in the adrenaline group. Despite a reduction in arterial oxygen tension in the post-resuscitation phase in the vasopressin group, possibly reflecting altered lung perfusion, this group had a reduction in indices of acidaemia, such as pH, base deficit and serum lactate, suggesting better tissue oxygenation.

Lindner followed this in 1995 with another study of VF in pigs, this time a closed chest model of resuscitation [32]. They compared an even higher dose of adrenaline (0.2 mg/kg - equivalent to 14 mg in a 70 kg man) to three different doses of vasopressin (0.2, 0.4 and 0.8 U/kg) and found an increasing left ventricular myocardial blood flow and coronary and cerebral perfusion pressures with increasing doses of vasopressin. It could be argued that both these sets of experiments did not compare vasopressin with the standard 1 mg dose of adrenaline used clinically. However, the ideal dose of adrenaline was still being debated and Lindner had already compared adrenaline doses in pig models. Around this time, several authors had published or were in the process of publishing review articles suggesting that on balance, high dose adrenaline did not improve and possibly worsened outcomes in resuscitation [53-55]

In 1996, Lindner's group published a case series of eight adults who had suffered cardiac arrest whilst in hospital [56]. Though CPR and advanced life support (ALS), including adrenaline and defibrillation when appropriate, had been initiated within 1 minute of cardiac arrest, resuscitation of these patients had failed to achieve ROSC thus far. After at least 12 minutes of CPR in all cases, 40 IU of AVP was administered via a central vein. ROSC was achieved in all eight patients and three of these survived to hospital discharge with good neurology.

In the following year, the Lindner group then published a randomised clinical trial, comparing 1 mg adrenaline to 40 IU vasopressin in forty patients with out-of-hospital VF arrest [35]. The study ran from July 1994 to December 1995 and excluded patients who were less than 18 years of age, pregnant, or whose cardiac arrest was secondary to trauma or terminal illness. They also excluded those patients in whom had adrenaline had been administered via the endotracheal route. Patients received the randomly allocated trial drug if the VF was resistant to defibrillation. If ROSC was not immediately restored, standard protocol ALS continued, and therefore the patients would receive adrenaline when next indicated. The vasopressin group was more likely to achieve ROSC, and had a greater survival to hospital admission (70% vs 35%), 24-hour survival (60% vs 20%) and survival to hospital discharge (40% vs 15%) than the adrenaline group. There was no significant difference in neurology in those surviving to hospital discharge between groups.

Also in 1997, Morris *et al.* measured the effect of 1 U/kg of vasopressin on coronary perfusion pressure in a study of 10 patients in whom resuscitation from cardiac arrest was deemed unsuccessful [36]. All patients received a bolus dose of 1 mg adrenaline, five minutes prior to sampling of blood for arterial blood gases, haemoglobin, osmolality, sodium, vasopressin and adrenaline levels. The vasopressin dose was administered and CPR and pressure measurements continued for a further five minutes until repeat blood samples were taken. In four patients, coronary perfusion pressure was significantly increased after vasopressin (the responders), with no difference found in the remaining six (the non-responders). The findings were then analysed. It was noted that the mean levels of vasopressin prior to the vasopressin bolus administration were higher in the group of responders than in the non-responders. The responders also had a lower mean adrenaline level. However, whether there was a causal relationship between the plasma levels of endogenous pressors and the increase in coronary perfusion pressure in response to vasopressin is not certain.

Wenzel and Lindner published results from another experiment in 1999, again comparing adrenaline to vasopressin [40]. Whilst Lindner's earlier experiments had compared only single doses, this trial attempted to mimic the clinical situation by administering repeated doses of vasopressin and adrenaline. The study was designed in two halves, again using anaesthetised pigs and a closed-chest model of resuscitation from induced VF. The first part of the study looked at early CPR and administration of vasopressors in 12 pigs. After four minutes of untreated VF, basic life support (BLS) was established for three minutes. Half of the animals were then randomised to receive either three doses vasopressin at 0.4, 0.4 and 0.8 U/kg or three doses of adrenaline at 45, 45, and 200 μg/kg every five minutes. These doses represented optimum and maximally effective doses of each drug in this pig model. Up to five attempts at defibrillation were attempted at 22 minutes after the onset of BLS. Haemodynamic measurements were made before arrest, after three minutes of BLS and after drug administration. If resuscitation was successful, the measurements continued for an hour into the post-resuscitation phase. In the vasopressin group, each dose of vasopressin raised the mean coronary perfusion pressure, which remained above 30 mmHg, and all six animals achieved ROSC. In the adrenaline group, however, only the first dose of adrenaline raised the mean coronary perfusion pressure to above 30 mmHg and this was temporary. The remainder of resuscitation continued with a coronary perfusion pressure less than 20 mmHg and all six pigs receiving adrenaline failed to achieve ROSC. Other work has suggested that adequate coronary perfusion pressure during CPR is an important determinant and predictor of successful outcome [57,58]. The second part of Wenzel's study looked at later administration of drugs. In 12 anaesthetised pigs VF was left untreated for four minutes followed by BLS for eight minutes prior to drug administration. This time, only two doses were administered (0.4 and 0.8 U/kg for vasopressin, and 45 and 200 μg/kg for adrenaline). Again, in the vasopressin group, coronary perfusion pressure was maintained above 30 mmHg throughout most of the resuscitation attempt, and despite falling towards the last few minutes before defibrillation, remained above the crucial 20 mmHg. In the adrenaline group, coronary perfusion pressure was only transiently increased above 20 mmHg after the first administration and ROSC was not achieved in any of this group.

Despite the seemingly unequivocal data obtained from this trial, the authors identified some important limitations. Apart from the differences between laboratory experiments on healthy animals and the clinical situation of cardiac arrest in humans, these surviving pigs were sacrificed and autopsies were carried out. The post-resuscitation phase was only 60 minutes, so outcome data regarding long-term survival and neurological state remain unknown.

In the same month, results from another study of the haemodynamic effects of vasopressin in resuscitation were published by Wenzel and Lindner *et al.* Using their model of anaesthetised pigs, 0.8 U/kg of vasopressin was compared with 200 μg/kg of adrenaline in the setting of prolonged pulseless electrical activity (PEA). The vasopressin group had better myocardial and cerebral blood flow during CPR and significantly greater likelihood of achieving ROSC [39]. Again, this did not give information about the longer term.

Babar and Berg *et al.* attempted to address this question with their own experiment using a swine model of resuscitation, published later that year [59]. In this trial, 35 pigs were anaesthetised and VF was electrically induced after the appropriate monitoring paraphernalia were sited. After a two minute cardiac arrest period, chest compressions were initiated without ventilatory support for six minutes. This was followed by administration of either 0.8

U/kg vasopressin (18 pigs) or 0.02 mg/kg adrenaline (17 pigs). Chest compressions (with ventilation) were continued for ten minutes in all animals after the drug administration. The adrenaline group received two further doses of 0.02 mg/kg adrenaline at five and ten minutes after the initial dose. After 18 minutes of VF, defibrillation was attempted. Twelve of the 18 pigs from the vasopressin group achieved ROSC and 11 of these survived for 24 hours. Neurology was intact in all 11 pigs. In the adrenaline group, eight of the 17 pigs achieved ROSC all of which survived for 24 hours. Of these eight, only one had mildly impaired neurology at that stage. The difference in survival with intact neurology did not reach statistical significance. The vasopressin group was more likely to be successfully defibrillated at first attempt than the adrenaline group. Haemodynamic data agreed with other studies, namely that aortic diastolic and coronary perfusion pressure were significantly improved with vasopressin compared with adrenaline.

The inability to show an improvement in long term outcome with vasopressin seems disheartening after the dramatic results of previous studies. However, in this study several differences may have been important. Firstly, the interval between onset of VF and the start of CPR was only two minutes compared with, for example, four minutes in Wenzel's study of the same year [40]. The lack of ventilatory support prior to drug administration may not be as important as once thought, with recent data to suggest that allowing passive ventilation or agonal breathing during CPR may be more beneficial than interrupting chest compressions for intubation and mechanical ventilation [60]. Additionally, Babar's swine were anaesthetised using isoflurane for induction and maintenance, whereas intravenous agents were used in Wenzel and Lindner's model. Isoflurane has been shown to have beneficial effects in terms of myocardial preconditioning, an effect which may or may not be important in this case [61]. Additionally, in this trial one dose of vasopressin was compared with repeated doses of adrenaline.

Voeckel *et al.* explored the use of vasopressin and adrenaline in a swine model of hypovolaemic shock and cardiac arrest, in a group also featuring Drs Wenzel and Lindner [62]. The experiment was carried out on 18 young, healthy and anaesthetised pigs. The pigs were rendered hypovolaemic by removing 35% of their calculated total blood volume over 15 minutes via an arterial cannula. VF was then induced and left untreated for four minutes. This was followed by four minutes of CPR, after which the pigs received either adrenaline 200 µg/kg, vasopressin 0.8 U/kg or saline placebo. Two and a half minutes later defibrillation was attempted. If unsuccessful, a further dose of the chosen drug was given, and defibrillation tried again. All seven vasopressin animals achieved ROSC as did six of the seven adrenaline pigs, though none given the placebo reached the next stage. Over the next 15 minutes of monitoring, however, all the surviving pigs in the adrenaline group developed profound metabolic acidosis and died within 60 minutes, despite having significantly better blood flow to the cerebrum and myocardium in the early post-resuscitation phase. All the pigs in the vasopressin group survived the duration of the post-resuscitation phase.

This is further evidence that the immediate results of CPR are better with vasopressin than adrenaline. However, whether this translates into a meaningful clinical difference in long term outcome is still an unanswered question. The authors did not study the pigs for longer than the 60 minute post-resuscitation phase and the outcomes beyond this time are not known. This model was a modification of the previously used VF models of resuscitation. Further variation from these experimental protocols may yield different results, and this was shown in another study by the same group, published three months later [63].

This time, cardiac arrest was induced by asphyxia in eighteen anaesthetised piglets. There were three groups of piglets, and the study compared the use of 200 μg/kg adrenaline versus 0.8 U/kg vasopressin and a combination of 0.8 U/kg vasopressin with 45 μg/kg adrenaline. The cardiac arrest rhythms in this study varied, and asystole, PEA and VF were present. In some piglets more than one arrest rhythm was demonstrated. In the vasopressin-only group, left ventricular blood flow was significantly reduced compared with both the other two groups, and there was a trend towards higher cerebral blood flow during CPR in the combination group compared with the adrenaline group. In terms of survival, only one out of six piglets in the vasopressin group achieved ROSC compared with six out of six in the adrenaline group and four out of six in the combination therapy group. This suggested that vasopressin was not beneficial as the sole vasopressor in a paediatric porcine model of asphyxial cardiac arrest.

The importance of endogenous vasopressin in cardiac arrest was the focus of another study using this swine model [64]. The experimenters found that when a V_1 receptor antagonist was administered ten minutes prior to induction of VF, no pigs achieved ROSC. By comparison, the pigs who received exogenous vasopressin 0.8U/kg all survived, as did those pigs which received only saline placebo and were therefore relying upon endogenous vasopressors only. The inference was that activation of V_1 receptors by an endogenous substrate was essential for ROSC in this study.

Despite this apparent importance of vasopressin for survival from cardiac arrest, a blinded randomised controlled trial of in-hospital cardiac arrest was published in the same year in The Lancet which showed no benefit with vasopressin over adrenaline [65]. Two hundred patients were included in the trial which randomised 104 patients to receive 40 IU vasopressin and 96 patients to receive 1 mg adrenaline as their first vasopressor in cardiac arrest. The design of the study was such that failure to respond to the initial vasopressor led to the use of standard therapy including adrenaline. Stiell *et al.* found no difference in survival to 1 hour or to hospital discharge, and nor could they demonstrate a difference in neurology in survivors from either group. In addition to the usual exclusion criteria, such as age less than 16 years, or the diagnosis of a terminal illness, Stiell *et al.* also excluded those patients who suffered cardiac arrest within 24 hours of admission with life-threatening trauma and those whose cardiac arrest was secondary to exsanguination, such as from a ruptured aortic aneurysm. Whilst it has already been noted that laboratory work suggested an improved outcome with vasopressin in hypovolaemic cardiac arrest [62], it is difficult to suppose that this was the only reason for the failure to show a survival benefit with vasopressin in this trial. An editorial within the same journal commented upon the subgroup analysis and suggested that the survival characteristics could be delineated by age [66]. In Stiell's study, those aged 70 years or less were more likely to survive if their initial vasopressor was adrenaline, whereas those patients who were more than 70 years old were more likely to survive if they were in the vasopressin group. This adds complexity to the analysis, as the younger inpatients may have a different pathophysiology, which may alter their responses to either drug, as well as affecting the primary cause of cardiac arrest.

An important difference in this trial compared with that of Lindner [35] was the use of the in-patient population. Lindner's trial studied out-of-hospital cardiac arrests. Stiell *et al.* looked at a population with not only different pathology, but also a different mechanism of treatment, as the duration of cardiac arrest before attempted resuscitation would be much shorter in the hospital setting. The differing findings between these two human trials of vasopressin in cardiac arrest hints at the scale of the problem: the substantial variability between individual cases of cardiac arrest would require a study with a much bigger sample size.

It was three years before the results of a large, multi-centre, randomised controlled trial were published [67]. Among out-of-hospital cardiac arrests in 33 communities across Germany, France and Switzerland, they compared up to two doses each of vasopressin 40 IU versus 1 mg adrenaline in 589 patients and 597 patients, respectively. The investigators and resuscitators were blinded as to which drug they were using. Additionally, if resuscitation was unsuccessful, the attending physician had the option of administering 1 mg of open-label adrenaline.

Following the experimental data and the few clinical trials which highlighted the promise of vasopressin, the results from this trial were somewhat unexpected. The first finding was that when looking at all patients, there was no significant difference between rates of ROSC for the adrenaline and vasopressin groups: 28% vs 24.6%, respectively, achieved ROSC with the initial study drugs. Rates of survival to hospital admission were slightly, though not significantly, better with vasopressin than adrenaline at 36.3% vs 31.2%, respectively. Similarly, survival to hospital discharge was almost identical between the two groups (9.9%).

Indeed, when analysed according to cardiac arrest rhythm, those found in VF fared slightly better if they were in the adrenaline group, though survival to hospital discharge was not statistically better at 19.2% for adrenaline vs 17.8% for vasopressin.

Among those presenting in asystole, though the vasopressin group were no more likely to regain spontaneous circulation, they were more likely to survive to hospital admission and hospital discharge than the adrenaline group (29% and 4.7% respectively for vasopressin vs 20.3% and 1.5% for adrenaline).

Another outcome measure was the cerebral performance of those who survived to hospital discharge. This was graded using a four point scale borrowed from the work of a separate research group [68]. The scale ranged from good cerebral performance at one extreme, through moderate and severe cerebral disability, to coma or vegetative state at the other.

The numbers of patients for comparison were not statistically significant, and there was a similar number of patients from the vasopressin and adrenaline groups with good cerebral performance. However, there was a trend in the adrenaline group to produce slighter more patients in the moderate disability category and fewer in the category of coma or vegetative state compared with vasopressin group, from whom the opposite was true. Because the numbers of patients surviving to hospital discharge was so small, these trends in neurological outcome are very difficult to interpret with any degree of accuracy. However, the implications may be dramatic if further data could corroborate this finding. The idea that a novel treatment may improve numerical survival figures, yet simultaneously increase the likelihood of coma as an outcome would provoke much ethical debate as to the actual merits of use.

Another part of the analysis looked at patients who did not achieve ROSC with the study drugs but then received a dose of adrenaline. As could be expected from the pharmacology, and from the earlier trials of vasopressin in failed resuscitation, there were marked differences between the adrenaline group and the vasopressin group in these patients. Among those randomised to receive adrenaline, out of 359 patients who did not regain spontaneous circulation with the first two doses, 93 patients (26%) benefited from an additional dose. Of 373 patients who did not regain spontaneous circulation with vasopressin, the addition of adrenaline allowed 137 patients to achieve ROSC (36.7%). In those patients for whom two doses of adrenaline were inadequate, it is perhaps unsurprising that a further dose of the same drug would provide a successful result. This suggests that an approach of combination therapy may improve resuscitation. The question is unanswered because to complete this data set, a further trial in which patients randomised to receive adrenaline or vasopressin initially would be required to then allow the clinicians to add in a second vasopressor, which again should be either vasopressin or adrenaline but from a second randomisation. This would allow researchers to examine if those patients who initially received adrenaline but failed to achieve ROSC would fare better with the addition of a dose of vasopressin.

The subgroup analysis here showed that the outcome difference with the addition of adrenaline was most marked in those patients whose initial rhythm was VF or asystole, with a somewhat lesser difference in those presenting in PEA. These data understandably translated into improved rates of survival to hospital admission. However, as these patients were initially the poor responders to therapy, there were few who survived to hospital discharge. Out of the 137 patients in the vasopressin group who had ROSC after adrenaline, only 23 survived to hospital discharge (6.2%). Three were lost to follow-up, eight had good neurology and eight were in a coma. Of the 93 patients in the adrenaline group who regained spontaneous circulation after additional adrenaline, only 6 patients survived to hospital discharge (1.7%), one of whom was lost to follow-up. Of the remaining five, two had good cerebral performance, two were moderately impaired and one had a severe disability. None of the survivors in this group were in a coma or vegetative state.

An additional finding of the study was that those patients who, at the discretion of the attending physician, received amiodarone or a fibrinolytic agent during the resuscitation process had improved rates of survival to hospital admission. Whilst this may be as a result of a generic therapeutic benefit of these agents in CPR, it is more likely that the patients who received these drugs were in a category of patients with specific indications for these treatment protocols. Further work is needed, therefore, in order to identify the relevant issues here.

In their conclusion, the authors of the paper highlighted some of the limitations of there study. Among the more important problems was this issue of survival to hospital admission. As this largely reflects ROSC, the benefit of using this as an outcome measure is unclear. The authors also mentioned that in-hospital management of cardiac arrest patients could not be standardised and this would affect outcomes. This is a seemingly unavoidable problem because of the wide variation in individual treatment requirements as well as availability of these treatments in this multi-centre study. Some examples would be the availability of facilities for therapeutic hypothermia and emergency coronary angioplasty.

This important study was not without its critics, who agreed with Wenzel *et al.* about its limitations, and urged caution in the recommendation of vasopressin in asystolic cardiac arrest [69-72]. The main criticisms were that the use of vasopressin was associated with poor neurological outcome in more patients than adrenaline. As Wenzel and McIntyre pointed out, in those groups where neurology was poor with vasopressin, the patients who did not receive vasopressin did not survive at all [73]. It therefore seems unlikely that vasopressin was the cause of the neurological impairment in these patients. In his reply to the commentary, McIntyre points out that if this was the case, then those patients in VF who received vasopressin would have worse neurological outcomes than those in the adrenaline group, which they did not [73]. A more likely explanation is that in the patients who responded to vasopressin, this treatment allowed ROSC by the time that irreversible brain injury had already occurred. This might have been because of an extended period of unsuccessful resuscitation prior to ROSC, or because of other individual patient factors, such as pre-existing cerebrovascular disease. Another criticism was the inference of evidence from post hoc subgroup analysis, but the authors suggested that this simply highlights the requirement for further research in these areas.

In September 2004, Lindner and Wenzel's group published a summary of their findings in the context of the other work which had been published up to that point, in their progress report [74]. Within the very same supplement was another laboratory trial of vasopressin and CPR in anaesthetised pigs with electrically-induced VF [75]. This American study focussed on the potential adverse effects of vasopressin in the post-resuscitation period, singling out left ventricular dysfunction as an endpoint. Their abstract conclusions were simply that vasopressin causes worse post-resuscitation ventricular dysfunction early but 'did not compromise 24-hour outcome'. They also commented that reversal with a V_1 receptor antagonist 'did not improve survival' [75]. A casual glance at this abstract might seem that the study provided evidence against the use of vasopressin in cardiac arrest. Further scrutiny of the work would reveal that this was not the case.

In this trial, 48 pigs were randomly allocated to three groups of 16. Details of the anaesthesia were incomplete, only that isoflurane was used. If this was indeed the only anaesthetic agent involved, then comparisons with other trials in pigs are limited. Isoflurane is known to have a pungent and irritant odour and has a slow onset of action. Thus, its use as a sole agent in the induction of anaesthesia is likely to cause significant distress on the part of the subject animals. Consequently the levels of circulating catecholamines and other stress hormones may be affected.

The first group of pigs received up to two doses of adrenaline (approximately 0.02 mg/kg) as part of their resuscitation algorithm. The second and third groups received up to two doses of 0.2 U/Kg vasopressin. The third group additionally received a V_1 receptor antagonist five minutes after ROSC, whereas the other groups received only a placebo at this point. The time between onset of VF and the start of CPR was 12.5 minutes.

The endpoints for this trial were left ventricular dysfunction, measured by ejection fraction, at 30 minutes and six hours after resuscitation. Additionally survival at 24 hours was also examined. What Kern *et al.* found was that at 30 minutes the vasopressin group had significantly reduced left ventricular ejection fractions compared with either the adrenaline or V_1 antagonsist groups (23% versus 33% and 33%, respectively). However, by six hours there was no difference in the mean left ventricular ejection fractions (32%, 31% and 31% for Groups 1, 2, and 3, respectively). Additionally, the survival data for the vasopressin group was significantly better than for the other groups, with ten out of 16 pigs surviving to 24 hours in the vasopressin group compared with four out of 16 in the adrenaline group and three out of 16 in the V_1 antagonist group. The demonstrated improvement in survival with vasopressin was very different from the abstract conclusion, which suggested only that vasopressin did not compromise outcome. The conclusions of the article, as opposed to the abstract, simply suggested caution in trying to reverse the effects of vasopressin to improve post-resuscitation left ventricular dysfunction.

Similar findings to Wenzel's study were reported by another group working in the USA [76]. They retrospectively analysed out-of-hospital cardiac arrests in which paramedics treated 298 patients whilst a physician was on scene. The physician retained the option of administering vasopressin in addition to adrenaline. Thirty seven patients received both drugs, and survival to hospital admission was 41% in this group compared with 18% in the adrenaline-only group (231 patients). Subgroup analysis revealed that the difference was most marked in those patients whose initial cardiac arrest rhythm was asystole. However, the selection of patients to receive vasopressin was left to the discretion of the attending physician and, therefore, the groups were not randomised. Therefore, the main addition by this study is that of support for Wenzel's data and the idea that combination therapy with vasopressin and adrenaline in cardiac arrest may prove important and needs further research.

In January 2005, a systematic review and meta-analysis could find no strong evidence in favour or against the use of vasopressin in cardiac arrest [77]. This was unsurprising, considering that only five randomised controlled trials met the inclusion criteria for the analysis. All the studies were all widely different in structure, three of which have already been discussed in detail here. Of the remaining two, one only included ten patients and was only published in abstract form, with a large number of details therefore unavailable. The other study included 83 patients, but is only available in Chinese. This study compared low- and high-dose vasopressin with low- and high-dose adrenaline, and favoured high-dose vasopressin (1 U/kg) with significant increases in rates of ROSC and survival. This was in comparison to 1 mg or 5 mg doses of adrenaline. This was the only study in the meta-analysis in which the 95% confidence interval did not include unity.

Despite this lack of strong evidence, interest in vasopressin for cardiac arrest was not extinguished. In 2006 an observational cohort study was published, examining of out-of-hospital, non-traumatic, VF/ventricular tachycardia (VT) cardiac arrests in Slovenia [78]. It seemed to show an improvement in outcome when vasopressin was combined with adrenaline compared to adrenaline alone. However, this small study was not randomised and the control cohort, who received only adrenaline as the vasopressor in CPR, was retrospectively analysed. Also, confounding variables may have had additional weight because the study groups did not run concurrently. The outcome which improved in the vasopressin groups was again that of survival to 24 hours. Rates of survival to hospital discharge and neurological function at discharge was not different among the three groups.

A laboratory study published later that year reached similar conclusions [79]. This trial used coronary perfusion pressure as the primary outcome measure and employed an adult swine model of PEA arrest. To achieve this, VF was electrically induced in the anaesthetised pigs. This was followed by a seven minute period of no CPR and no ventilation. Then CPR was instituted followed three minutes later by up to three attempts at defibrillation. Pilot studies had demonstrated PEA in this fashion, so the investigators had planned this technique to allow their therapeutic trial. They compared 0.8 U/kg vasopressin with 0.02 mg/kg adrenaline and combination therapy using half doses (0.4 U/kg vasopressin and 0.01 mg/kg adrenaline). The drugs were given at 10.5 minutes following onset of cardiac arrest. If ROSC was not achieved at 20 minutes, the animal was crossed-over by administration of the alternative drug, or a second dose of the same if the pig had received the combination. Out of 16 pigs, 15 developed PEA and 14 of these achieved ROSC after drug administration. There was therefore no significant difference in rates of ROSC between groups. However, this was not the main outcome measure. There was an improvement in coronary perfusion in those pigs that received vasopressin. Conversely, in the group which only received adrenaline, there was no increase in coronary perfusion pressure following drug administration.

Opposing results were found in a clinical study from Pennsylvania, USA [80]. Three hundred and twenty five patients who suffered an out-of-hospital cardiac arrest were randomised to receive either 40 IU of vasopressin or placebo in addition to a dose of 1 mg adrenaline. The groups were matched, and the resuscitators were blinded as to whether the second drug was vasopressin or placebo. The rates of ROSC were not different between the two groups, regardless of cardiac arrest rhythm. There was also no difference in 30 day survival, or neurological outcome. They concluded that there was no benefit gained from combining vasopressin with adrenaline in out-of-hospital cardiac arrest.

This was not the conclusion found in another study from Slovenia [81]. They prospectively analysed data from 598 patients in an observational cohort study running from 2000 to 2006, and compared data from patients who received vasopressin with or without adrenaline in CPR with data from those who received adrenaline alone. The vasopressin group had higher rates of ROSC and survival to 24 hours. Only in the subgroup of patients in asystole was there any significant improvement in survival to hospital discharge (22.7% in the vasopressin group, compared with 9.3% in the adrenaline group). However, the cohorts were separated temporally, and it is likely that there were other confounding variables in the selection of patients for each group. Nevertheless, the researchers found that patients who received vasopressin had higher values of end-tidal carbon dioxide and mean arterial pressures during CPR than those who did not. These surrogates were shown as prognostic factors for survival in cardiac arrest.

Further interest in the use of combined adrenaline and vasopressin was mounting, and in 2007 another laboratory study was published using Wenzel and Lindner's anaesthetised swine model of VF arrest [82]. This study applied the algorithm changes of the 2005 resuscitation guidelines, using a compression to ventilation ratio of 30:2 and a single defibrillatory shock with a biphasic defibrillator. After four minutes of untreated VF, BLS commenced and continued for six minutes before the first attempt at defibrillation. The 16 pigs were subsequently randomised to receive either 45 μg/kg adrenaline or alternating adrenaline at the same dose with vasopressin 0.4 U/kg, and the cycle of drug administration began three minutes after the first shock. The results of the experiment showed that the vasopressin/adrenaline group had improved coronary and cerebral perfusion pressures and cortical cerebral blood flow compared with the adrenaline-only group. However, the study did not show, as it was not powered to show, a statistically significant difference in the rates of ROSC.

This is in contrast with a study by Stroumpoulis *et al.*, who also compared adrenaline to a combination of vasopressin and adrenaline in VF arrest [83]. They, too, used a swine model of electrically-induced VF, using piglets whose anaesthesia was maintained with a propofol infusion. There were, however, several differences in the protocol: the duration of untreated VF was eight minutes and the study drugs were administered immediately before CPR began. Chest compressions continued for two minutes before the first attempt at defibrillation, which was delivered using a monophasic defibrillator. The 22 pigs were approximately half the weight of those in Meybohm's study, at 19 kg versus 44 kg [82] and the randomisation took place before the animals were prepared for the study. There were two groups of eleven pigs; one group would receive 0.02 mg/kg adrenaline with placebo, and the other would receive 0.02 mg/kg adrenaline with 0.4 U/kg vasopressin. As in previous trials, this study showed an improved coronary perfusion pressure in the combination group. The main outcome measure was ROSC and the adrenaline group provided four survivors, compared with ten in the combination group, which was a statistically significant difference. No longer-term outcome measures were analysed.

In 2008, the results of a large clinical trial comparing 1 mg of adrenaline to a combination of 1 mg adrenaline and 40 IU vasopressin were published [84]. The multi-centre trial was set to run using 31 emergency service groups in France and data collection took two years, beginning in May 2004. The study randomised 2956 patients, 1142 in the combination arm and 1452 in the adrenaline-only arm. Notably, randomisation took place immediately in patients with asystole or PEA, but after the first three shocks in patients with VF arrest. Patients received the study drug followed by three minutes of CPR and a repeat dose of the same study drug if ROSC was not achieved. Following another three minutes of CPR, the attending physician had the option of administering open-label adrenaline. Consent for inclusion in the trial was gained retrospectively after admission to hospital, either from the next of kin or, less frequently, from the patients themselves. In total, 26 patients were excluded from the data analysis because of consent issues. Other reasons for exclusion after randomisation included traumatic cardiac arrest in 29 patients and failure to meet the inclusion criteria in a further seven patients. The main demographic difference between the two groups was male:female ratio, with 75.4% of the patients in the combination group being male compared with 71.7% in the adrenalin-only group. This variable achieved statistical significance.

The primary endpoint for the study was survival to hospital admission, with ROSC, survival to hospital discharge, good neurological recovery (comparing Glasgow Coma Scale at admission with Cerebral Performance Category at discharge) and survival to one year as secondary endpoints.

The results of this long-awaited trial were disappointing for those looking for a pharmacological revelation in the dismal results of CPR. There were no statistically significant differences in any of the outcome measures between the two treatment arms of the study. The authors concluded that the addition of vasopressin did not improve outcomes in out-of hospital cardiac arrest. This was by no means the final word on vasopressin, however, and several letters were quick to scrutinise the published trial [85,86]. The authors themselves pointed out that the trial was very different from the previous large scale study of vasopressin in cardiac arrest in that a very high proportion of enrolled patients presented in asystole [67]. By way of an explanation, the authors describe that in France there is a prevalence of automated external defibrillators, such that 80% of patients are defibrillated during the course of BLS [84]. By the time advanced cardiac life support (ACLS) has begun, many patients will have achieved ROSC and a proportion of the remainder will now be in a non-shockable rhythm. Because randomisation took place after defibrillation was attempted in patients with VF, a large proportion of the patients who were successfully resuscitated were effectively excluded from the trial and received no drugs. This is not necessarily a detractor as all drugs carry the ability to do harm as well as good. Only 9.2% of patients enrolled in the trial presented in VF, and these patients, by definition, were in refractory VF. Also, as Morris points out, the mean time-lapse between the onset cardiac arrest to the start of ALS was 16.3 minutes, well in excess of the first crucial ten minute target [85]. However, 75% of the cardiac arrests were witnessed, bystander CPR was instigated in 27%, and the first responders (providing BLS) were present on average within seven minutes of cardiac arrest. The 16 minutes time to ACLS might reasonably represent time to randomisation and administration of drugs following a period of 'low-flow' circulation rather than 'no-flow'.

In essence then, the study by Gueugniaud *et al.* compared cardiac arrest outcomes with adrenaline to outcomes with adrenaline and vasopressin in those groups with the poorest prognosis. This was reflected in the figures for survival to hospital discharge: 1.7% in the combination group and 2.1% in the adrenaline group. With such low rates of long-term survival, any differences in the post-resuscitation care, which could not be standardised, might obfuscate the results. For example, the authors mentioned that therapeutic hypothermia was used in 17.3% of patients admitted to hospital, and this was associated with improvements in neurologically intact survival. They argued that because this therapy was not randomised, its efficacy could not be analysed. Nonetheless, they cite other research which highlights improved neurological outcomes using therapeutic hypothermia in cardiac arrest. Despite this, Gueugniaud's paper gives no data on whether hypothermia was instigated in equal proportions across the treatment arms. As an extreme example, if only one group received all those therapies in the post-resuscitation care which are thought to improve outcomes, the data becomes meaningless.

In comparison, Wenzel's study achieved an overall survival to hospital discharge rate of 9.9%, and showed somewhat better outcomes in patients presenting asystole who received vasopressin than adrenaline [67]. It might therefore be expected, that with its prevalence of asystole among study subjects, Gueugniaud's trial would show better outcomes in the combination group, as these patients received vasopressin. However, it showed no improvement in outcome from asystole in the combination group.

The quick answer is to suggest that these large, randomised, and blinded trials seemed to disagree because one was right and the other was wrong. What if this was not the case? What if the results disagreed because they were asking different questions and looking at different circumstances entirely? What if the patients presenting in asystole in the combination arm of Gueugniaud's trial fared no better than the adrenaline arm precisely because they, too, received adrenaline? The research and evidence mounting which suggest that adrenaline could be detrimental in cardiac arrest has already been summarised in the previous chapter [55,87,88]. It might not be too imaginative to suggest that had Gueugniaud's trial simply compared adrenaline to vasopressin rather than the combination of drugs, in the population under scrutiny, an entirely different set of results may have been published.

Nevertheless, the interest in therapeutic combinations using vasopressin, adrenaline and other drugs has not disappeared. One recent study randomly assigned 100 patients with in-hospital cardiac arrest to receive 1 mg adrenaline or a combination of 20 IU vasopressin and 1 mg adrenaline [89]. The combination group was additionally treated with 40 mg methylprednisolone during CPR and, if shock persisted, a tapering daily dose of hydrocortisone in the post-resuscitation period. The combination group had a significantly improved ROSC rate of 81%, compared with 52% in the control group. Similarly, survival to hospital discharge was 19% in the combination group and 4% in the control group. Additionally, for the ten days following cardiac arrest, the combination group maintained higher central venous oxygen saturations and higher mean arterial pressures than the control group. Whether the improved outcomes in this trial stems from the use of glucocorticoids and indeed whether the use of vasopressin was incidental is undecided.

Conclusion

Because of the concerns about the potentially undesirable effects of adrenaline, there has always been a certain amount of interest in alternative vasopressors in cardiac arrest. Various comparisons have been made using phenylephrine, methoxamine, noradrenaline, -methyl-noradrenaline, but all have fallen by the wayside [90-92]. Vasopressin has attracted attention because it does not act on adrenoceptors and it was found early on that endogenous levels of vasopressin were higher in survivors than non-survivors of cardiac arrest [52]. The beneficial effects of vasopressin stem from its vasoconstrictor activity, mediated by the V_1 receptor, and a vasodilatory effect on coronary, renal and cerebral arteries through its effects on endothelial nitric oxide synthesis and the V_1 receptor [19,20,37,93]. However, the balance between vasoconstriction and vasodilation has been scrutinised and is not fully understood. Some disquiet about its use originates from various studies which suggest that vasopressin causes coronary and cerebral vasoconstriction [25,27,30,33,34].

Laboratory studies for the main part compare vasopressin favourably against adrenaline in cardiac arrest. [31,32,40,94], and some have shown benefit from a combination of both drugs [79,83]. Encouraging case reports and pilot studies in human patients suggested that large-scale trials of vasopressin were needed, but the first such study showed an improvement with vasopressin over adrenaline only in the subgroup of patients with asystolic cardiac arrest [67]. No randomised controlled trials directly comparing vasopressin to adrenaline in asystole have been carried out to date. The largest randomised trial of vasopressin and adrenaline focussed on these patients only because of its patient selection. Rather than comparing the two drugs, it compared a combination of vasopressin and adrenaline to adrenaline alone and found no difference in outcome [84].

All these studies have highlighted that outcomes from cardiac arrest have improved little over the past two decades, regardless of our advancing interventions. Detecting statistically significant interventions when the survival rates are so low requires, a huge number of enrolled study subjects and an extraordinary amount of planning in order to minimise confounding variables.

Currently, ACLS algorithms differ on either side of the Atlantic. The American Heart Association indicates that a single dose of vasopressin may be substituted for the first or second dose of adrenaline in the treatment of VF or pulseless VT and that providers may consider the use of vasopressin in asystolic cardiac arrest [95]. The guidelines of the European Resuscitation Council make no such suggestion, and state that there is inadequate evidence yet to support or refute the use of vasopressin instead of, or in combination with, adrenaline [96].

Perhaps advances in post-resuscitation care will improve standardisation across treatment centres. If this were to happen, studies on therapies during cardiac arrest might allow us decide whether adrenaline or vasopressin should be used at all. It is possible that as understanding of the pathophysiology of cardiac arrests improves, more specific circumstances might show a benefit from specific vasopressor drugs. Whilst this might be scientifically sound, there is a danger that allowing for multiple modifications of the life support algorithms would overcomplicate matters for ALS providers, thus making algorithms more difficult to learn and follow.

Contemporary theorists seem to be in agreement that the future of cardiac life support is in simplification and in shifting the focus of treatment to specific key areas [60,97]. 'Cardiocerebral Resuscitation' is a recent move towards changing the outcomes of out-of-hospital cardiac arrest. It focusses on measures to improve myocardial and cerebral blood flow and early restoration of spontaneous circulation. The main messages are the importance of early, effective bystander chest compressions, uninterrupted by attempts at mouth to mouth ventilation. Emergency medical teams are encouraged to provide only passive oxygen enrichment by face-mask and to reduce interruptions in chest compressions by minimising pulse-checks and by delaying intubation. Early data is promising, but only time will tell if outcomes from cardiac arrest can ever be improved.

References

[1] Oliver G, Schäfer EA. On the Physiological Action of Extracts of Pituitary Body and certain other Glandular Organs: Preliminary Communication. *J. Physiol.* 1895;18(3):277-9.

[2] Howell WM. The physiological effects of extracts of the hypophysis cerebri and infundibular body. *J. Exp. Med.* 1898;3(2):245-258.

[3] László FA, László F Jr, De Wied D. Pharmacology and clinical perspectives of vasopressin antagonists. *Pharmacol. Rev.* 1991;43(1):73-108.

[4] Vincent J, Su F. Physiology and pathophysiology of the vasopressinergic system. *Best Pract. Res. Clin. Anaesthesiol.* 2008;22(2):243-52.

[5] Frank E, Landgraf R. The vasopressin system--from antidiuresis to psychopathology. *Eur. J. Pharmacol.* 2008;583(2-3):226-42.

[6] Birnbaumer M. Vasopressin receptors. *Trends Endocrinol. Metab.* 2000;11(10):406-10.

[7] Kam PCA, Williams S, Yoong FFY. Vasopressin and terlipressin: pharmacology and its clinical relevance. *Anaesthesia.* 2004;59(10):993–1001.

[8] Treschan TA, Peters J. The vasopressin system: physiology and clinical strategies. *Anesthesiology.* 2006;105(3):599–612.

[9] Zenteno-Savin T, Sada-Ovalle I, Ceballos G, Rubio R. Effects of arginine vasopressin in the heart are mediated by specific intravascular endothelial receptors. *Eur. J. Pharmacol.* 2000;410(1):15-23.

[10] Ertmer C, Rehberg S, Westphal M. Vasopressin analogues in the treatment of shock states: potential pitfalls. *Best Pract. Res. Clin. Anaesthesiol.* 2008;22(2):393-406.

[11] Baumann G, Dingman JF. Distribution, blood transport, and degradation of antidiuretic hormone in man. *J. Clin. Invest.* 1976;57(5):1109-16.

[12] Holmes CL, Patel BM, Russell JA, Walley KR. Physiology of vasopressin relevant to management of septic shock. *Chest.* 2001;120(3):989-1002.

[13] den Ouden DT, Meinders AE. Vasopressin: physiology and clinical use in patients with vasodilatory shock: a review. *Neth. J. Med.* 2005;63(1):4–13.

[14] Wenzel V, Lindner KH. Employing vasopressin during cardiopulmonary resuscitation and vasodilatory shock as a lifesaving vasopressor. *Cardiovasc. Res.* 2001;51(3):529–541.

[15] Claybaugh JR, Uyehara CF. Metabolism of neurohypophysial hormones. *Ann. N Y Acad. Sci.* 1993;689:250-68.

[16] Davison JM, Sheills EA, Philips PR, Barron WM, Lindheimer MD. Metabolic clearance of vasopressin and an analogue resistant to vasopressinase in human pregnancy. *Am. J. Physiol.* 1993;264(2 Pt 2):F348-53.

[17] Matsui K, Share L, Brooks DP, Crofton JT, Rockhold RW. Splanchnic clearance of plasma vasopressin in the dog: evidence for prehepatic extraction. *Am. J. Physiol.* 1983;245(6):E611-5.

[18] Holmes CL, Landry DW, Granton JT. Science Review: Vasopressin and the cardiovascular system part 2 - clinical physiology. *Crit. Care*. 2004;8(1):15-23.

[19] Takayasu M, Kajita Y, Suzuki Y, Shibuya M, Sugita K, Ishikawa T, Hidaka H. Triphasic response of rat intracerebral arterioles to increasing concentrations of vasopressin in vitro. *J. Cereb. Blood Flow Metab.* 1993;13(2):304-9.

[20] Suzuki Y, Satoh S, Oyama H, Takayasu M, Shibuya M. Regional differences in the vasodilator response to vasopressin in canine cerebral arteries in vivo. *Stroke*. 1993;24(7):1049-53; discussion 1053-4.

[21] Evora PR, Pearson PJ, Schaff HV. Arginine vasopressin induces endothelium-dependent vasodilatation of the pulmonary artery. V1-receptor-mediated production of nitric oxide. *Chest*. 1993;103(4):1241-5.

[22] Tagawa T, Imaizumi T, Endo T, Shiramoto M, Hirooka Y, Ando S, Takeshita A. Vasodilatory effect of arginine vasopressin is mediated by nitric oxide in human forearm vessels. *J. Clin. Invest.* 1993;92(3):1483-90.

[23] Thibonnier M, Conarty DM, Preston JA, Plesnicher CL, Dweik RA, Erzurum SC. Human vascular endothelial cells express oxytocin receptors. *Endocrinology*. 1999;140(3):1301-9.

[24] Maybauer MO, Maybauer DM, Enkhbaatar P, Traber DL. Physiology of the vasopressin receptors. *Best Pract. Res. Clin. Anaesthesiol.* 2008;22(2):253-63.

[25] Heyndrickx G, Boettcher D, Vatner S. Effects of angiotensin, vasopressin, and methoxamine on cardiac function and blood flow distribution in conscious dogs. *AJP - Legacy*. 11 1976;231(5):1579–1587.

[26] Vanhoutte PM, Katusi ZS, Shepherd JT. Vasopressin induces endothelium-dependent relaxations of cerebral and coronary, but not of systemic arteries. *J. Hypertens. Suppl.* 1984;2(3):S421-2.

[27] Boyle WA 3rd, Segel LD. Direct cardiac effects of vasopressin and their reversal by a vascular antagonist. *Am. J. Physiol.* 1986;251(4 Pt 2):H734-41.

[28] Walker BR, Childs ME, Adams EM. Direct cardiac effects of vasopressin: role of V1- and V2-vasopressinergic receptors. *Am. J. Physiol.* 1988;255(2 Pt 2):H261-5.

[29] Boyle WA 3rd, Segel LD. Attenuation of vasopressin-mediated coronary constriction and myocardial depression in the hypoxic heart. *Circ. Res.* 1990;66(3):710-21.

[30] Maturi MF, Martin SE, Markle D, Maxwell M, Burruss CR, Speir E, Greene R, Ro YM, Vitale D, Green MV. Coronary vasoconstriction induced by vasopressin. Production of myocardial ischemia in dogs by constriction of nondiseased small vessels. *Circulation*. 1991;83(6):2111-21.

[31] Lindner KH, Brinkmann A, Pfenninger EG, Lurie KG, Goertz A, Lindner IM. Effect of vasopressin on hemodynamic variables, organ blood flow, and acid-base status in a pig model of cardiopulmonary resuscitation. *Anesth. Analg.* 1993;77(3):427-35.

[32] Lindner KH, Prengel AW, Pfenninger EG, Lindner IM, Strohmenger H, Georgieff M, Lurie KG. Vasopressin Improves Vital Organ Blood Flow During Closed-Chest Cardiopulmonary Resuscitation in Pigs. *Circulation*. 1 1995;91(1):215–221.

[33] Bax WA, Van der Graaf PH, Stam WB, Bos E, Nisato D, Saxena PR. [Arg8]vasopressin-induced responses of the human isolated coronary artery: effects of non-peptide receptor antagonists. *Eur. J. Pharmacol.* 1995;285(2):199-202.

[34] Fernández N, García JL, García-Villalón AL, Monge L, Gómez B, Diéguez G. Coronary vasoconstriction produced by vasopressin in anesthetized goats. Role of vasopressin V1 and V2 receptors and nitric oxide. *Eur. J. Pharmacol.* 1998;342(2-3):225-33.

[35] Lindner KH, Dirks B, Strohmenger HU, Prengel AW, Lindner IM, Lurie KG. Randomised comparison of epinephrine and vasopressin in patients with out-of-hospital ventricular fibrillation. *Lancet*. 1997;349(9051):535–537.

[36] Morris DC, Dereczyk BE, Grzybowski M, Martin GB, Rivers EP, Wortsman J, Amico JA. Vasopressin can increase coronary perfusion pressure during human cardiopulmonary resuscitation. *Acad. Emerg. Med.* 1997;4(9):878–883.

[37] Okamura T, Ayajiki K, Fujioka H, Toda N. Mechanisms underlying arginine vasopressin-induced relaxation in monkey isolated coronary arteries. *J. Hypertens.* 1999;17(5):673-8.

[38] Prengel AW, Lindner KH, Wenzel V, Tugtekin I, Anhaupl T. Splanchnic and renal blood flow after cardiopulmonary resuscitation with epinephrine and vasopressin in pigs. *Resuscitation*. 1998;38(1):19–24.

[39] Wenzel V, Lindner KH, Prengel AW, Maier C, Voelckel W, Lurie KG, Strohmenger HU. Vasopressin improves vital organ blood flow after prolonged cardiac arrest with postcountershock pulseless electrical activity in pigs. *Crit. Care Med.* 1999;27(3):486–492.

[40] Wenzel V, Lindner KH, Krismer AC, Miller EA, Voelckel WG, Lingnau W. Repeated administration of vasopressin but not epinephrine maintains coronary perfusion pressure after early and late administration during prolonged cardiopulmonary resuscitation in pigs. *Circulation*. 1999;99(10):1379–1384.

[41] Voelckel WG, Lindner KH, Wenzel V, Bonatti J, Hangler H, Frimmel C, Kunszberg E, Lingnau W. Effects of vasopressin and epinephrine on splanchnic blood flow and renal function during and after cardiopulmonary resuscitation in pigs. *Crit. Care Med.* 2000;28(4):1083–1088.

[42] Mayr VD, Wenzel V, Wagner-Berger HG, Stadlbauer KH, Cavus E, Raab H, Muller THD, Jochberger S, Dunser MW, Krismer AC, Schwarzacher S, Lindner KH. Arginine vasopressin during sinus rhythm: effects on haemodynamic variables, left anterior descending coronary artery cross sectional area and cardiac index, before and after inhibition of NO-synthase, in pigs. *Resuscitation*. 2007;74(2):366–371.

[43] Resnik WH, Geiling EM. The action of pituitary extract on the heart of the unanesthetized dog. *J. Clin. Invest.* 1925;1(3):217-38.

[44] Youmans WB, Good HV, Hewitt AF. Inhibitory effect of vasopressin on cardioaccelerator mechanism after sino-aortic denervation. *Am. J. Physiol.* 1952;168(1):182-8.

[45] Varma S, Jaju BP, Bhargava KP. Mechanism of vasopressin-induced bradycardia in dogs. *Circ. Res.* 1969;24(6):787-92.

[46] Zhang X, Abdel-Rahman AR, Wooles WR. Vasopressin receptors in the area postrema differentially modulate baroreceptor responses in rats. *Eur. J. Pharmacol.* 1992;222(1):81-91.

[47] Walker BR, Haynes J Jr, Wang HL, Voelkel NF. Vasopressin-induced pulmonary vasodilation in rats. *Am. J. Physiol.* 1989;257(2 Pt 2):H415-22.

[48] Bushfield M, McNicol A, MacIntyre DE. Possible mechanisms of the potentiation of blood-platelet activation by adrenaline. *Biochem. J.* 1987;241(3):671-6.

[49] Tomasiak M, Stelmach H, Rusak T, Ciborowski M, Radziwon P. Vasopressin acts on platelets to generate procoagulant activity. *Blood Coagul. Fibrinolysis.* 2008;19(7):615-24.

[50] Dünser MW, Fries DR, Schobersberger W, Ulmer H, Wenzel V, Friesenecker B, Hasibeder WR, Mayr AJ. Does arginine vasopressin influence the coagulation system in advanced vasodilatory shock with severe multiorgan dysfunction syndrome. *Anesth. Analg.* 2004;99(1):201-6.

[51] Dünser MW, Westphal M. Arginine vasopressin in vasodilatory shock: effects on metabolism and beyond. *Curr. Opin. Anaesthesiol.* 2008;21(2):122-7.

[52] Lindner KH, Strohmenger HU, Ensinger H, Hetzel WD, Ahnefeld FW, Georgieff M. Stress hormone response during and after cardiopulmonary resuscitation. *Anesthesiology.* 1992;77(4):662-8.

[53] Hubloue I, Lauwaert I, Corne L. Adrenaline dosage during cardiopulmonary resuscitation: a critical review. *Eur. J. Emerg. Med.* 1994;1(3):149-53.

[54] Woodhouse SP, Cox S, Boyd P, Case C, Weber M. High dose and standard dose adrenaline do not alter survival, compared with placebo, in cardiac arrest. *Resuscitation.* 1995;30(3):243-9.

[55] Rainer TH, Robertson CE. Adrenaline, cardiac arrest, and evidence based medicine. *J. Accid. Emerg. Med.* 1996;13(4):234-7.

[56] Lindner KH, Prengel AW, Brinkmann A, Strohmenger HU, Lindner IM, Lurie KG. Vasopressin administration in refractory cardiac arrest. *Ann. Intern. Med.* 1996;124(12):1061-4.

[57] Paradis NA, Martin GB, Rivers EP, Goetting MG, Appleton TJ, Feingold M, Nowak RM. Coronary perfusion pressure and the return of spontaneous circulation in human cardiopulmonary resuscitation. *JAMA.* 1990;263(8):1106–1113.

[58] Kern KB. Coronary perfusion pressure during cardiopulmonary resuscitation. *Best Pract. Res. Clin. Anaesthesiol.* 2000/9;14(3):591–609.

[59] Babar SI, Berg RA, Hilwig RW, Kern KB, Ewy GA. Vasopressin versus epinephrine during cardiopulmonary resuscitation: a randomized swine outcome study. *Resuscitation.* 1999;41(2):185–192.

[60] Carabini L, Tamul P, Afifi S. Cardiopulmonary to cardiocerebral resuscitation: current challenges and future directions. *Int. Anesthesiol. Clin.* Winter 2009;47(1):1–13.

[61] Agnew NM, Pennefather SH, Russell GN. Isoflurane and coronary heart disease. *Anaesthesia.* 2002;57(4):338-47.

[62] Voelckel WG, Lurie KG, Lindner KH, Zielinski T, McKnite S, Krismer AC, Wenzel V. Vasopressin improves survival after cardiac arrest in hypovolemic shock. *Anesth. Analg.* 2000;91(3):627–634.

[63] Voelckel WG, Lurie KG, McKnite S, Zielinski T, Lindstrom P, Peterson C, Krismer AC, Lindner KH, Wenzel V. Comparison of epinephrine and vasopressin in a pediatric porcine model of asphyxial cardiac arrest. *Crit. Care Med.* 2000;28(12):3777–3783.
[64] Krismer AC, Lindner KH, Wenzel V, Mayr VD, Voelckel WG, Lurie KG, Strohmenger HU. The effects of endogenous and exogenous vasopressin during experimental cardiopulmonary resuscitation. *Anesth. Analg.* 2001;92(6):1499–1504.
[65] Stiell IG, Hebert PC, Wells GA, Vandemheen KL, Tang AS, Higginson LA, Dreyer JF, Clement C, Battram E, Watpool I, Mason S, Klassen T, Weitzman BN. Vasopressin versus epinephrine for inhospital cardiac arrest: a randomised controlled trial. *Lancet.* 2001;358(9276):105–109.
[66] Morley P. Vasopressin or epinephrine: which initial vasopressor for cardiac arrests. *Lancet.* 2001;358(9276):85–86.
[67] Wenzel V, Krismer AC, Arntz HR, Sitter H, Stadlbauer KH, Lindner KH. A comparison of vasopressin and epinephrine for out-of-hospital cardiopulmonary resuscitation. *N. Engl. J. Med.* 2004;350(2):105–113.
[68] Kelsey SF, Sutton-Tyrrell K, Abramson NS, Detre KM, Reinmuth O, Safar P, Snyder JV, Schinagl E. A randomized clinical trial of calcium entry blocker administration to comatose survivors of cardiac arrest. Design, methods, and patient characteristics. The Brain Resuscitation Clinical Trial II Study Group. *Control Clin. Trials.* 1991;12(4):525-45.
[69] Nolan JP, Nadkarni V, Montgomery WH. Vasopressin versus epinephrine for cardiopulmonary resuscitation. *N. Engl. J. Med.* 2004;350(21):2206–2209.
[70] Aberegg SK. Vasopressin versus epinephrine for cardiopulmonary resuscitation. *N. Engl. J. Med.* 2004;350(21):2206–2209.
[71] Ballew KA. Vasopressin versus epinephrine for cardiopulmonary resuscitation. *N. Engl. J. Med.* 2004;350(21):2206–2209.
[72] Alvarez GF, Bihari D. Vasopressin versus epinephrine for cardiopulmonary resuscitation. *N. Engl. J. Med.* 2004;350(21):2206–2209.
[73] Nolan JP, Nadkarni V, Montgomery WH, Alvarez GF, Bihari D, Ballew KA, Aberegg SK, Wenzel V, Arntz HR, Lindner KH, Sharma GVRK, McIntyre KM. Vasopressin versus Epinephrine for Cardiopulmonary Resuscitation. *N. Engl. J. Med.* 5 2004;350(21):2206–2209.
[74] Krismer AC, Wenzel V, Stadlbauer KH, Mayr VD, Lienhart HG, Arntz HR, Lindner KH. Vasopressin during cardiopulmonary resuscitation: a progress report. *Crit. Care Med.* 2004;32(9 Suppl):S432-5.
[75] Kern KB, Heidenreich JH, Higdon TA, Berg RA, Hilwig RW, Sanders AB, Anavy N, Ewy GA. Effect of vasopressin on postresuscitation ventricular function: unknown consequences of the recent Guidelines 2000 for Cardiopulmonary Resuscitation and Emergency Cardiovascular Care. *Crit. Care Med.* 2004;32(9 Suppl):S393-7.
[76] Guyette FX, Guimond GE, Hostler D, Callaway CW. Vasopressin administered with epinephrine is associated with a return of a pulse in out-of-hospital cardiac arrest. *Resuscitation.* 2004;63(3):277–282.
[77] Aung K, Htay T. Vasopressin for cardiac arrest: a systematic review and meta-analysis. *Arch. Intern. Med.* 2005;165(1):17–24.

[78] Grmec S, Mally S. Vasopressin improves outcome in out-of-hospital cardiopulmonary resuscitation of ventricular fibrillation and pulseless ventricular tachycardia: a observational cohort study. *Crit. Care*. 2006;10(1):R13.

[79] Little CM, Marietta MH, Peng K, Heard K, Fragoso M, Severyn FA, Bebarta VS, Paradis NA. Vasopressin alone or with epinephrine may be superior to epinephrine in a clinically relevant porcine model of pulseless electrical activity cardiac arrest. *Am. J. Emerg. Med.* 2006;24(7):810–814.

[80] Callaway CW, Hostler D, Doshi AA, Pinchalk M, Roth RN, Lubin J, Newman DH, Kelly LJ. Usefulness of vasopressin administered with epinephrine during out-of-hospital cardiac arrest. *Am. J. Cardiol.* 2006;98(10):1316–1321.

[81] Mally S, Jelatancev A, Grmec S. Effects of epinephrine and vasopressin on end-tidal carbon dioxide tension and mean arterial blood pressure in out-of-hospital cardiopulmonary resuscitation: an observational study. *Crit. Care*. 2007;11(2):R39.

[82] Meybohm P, Cavus E, Dorges V, Steinfath M, Sibbert L, Wenzel V, Scholz J, Bein B. Revised resuscitation guidelines: adrenaline versus adrenaline/vasopressin in a pig model of cardiopulmonary resuscitation--a randomised, controlled trial. *Resuscitation*. 2007;75(2):380–388.

[83] Stroumpoulis K, Xanthos T, Rokas G, Kitsou V, Papadimitriou D, Serpetinis I, Perrea D, Papadimitriou L, Kouskouni E. Vasopressin and epinephrine in the treatment of cardiac arrest: an experimental study. *Crit. Care*. 2008;12(2):R40.

[84] Gueugniaud P, David J, Chanzy E, Hubert H, Dubien P, Mauriaucourt P, Braganca C, Billeres X, Clotteau-Lambert M, Fuster P, Thiercelin D, Debaty G, Ricard-Hibon A, Roux P, Espesson C, Querellou E, Ducros L, Ecollan P, Halbout L, Savary D, Guillaumee F, Maupoint R, Capelle P, Bracq C, Dreyfus P, Nouguier P, Gache A, Meurisse C, Boulanger B, Lae C, Metzger J, Raphael V, Beruben A, Wenzel V, Guinhouya C, Vilhelm C, Marret E. Vasopressin and epinephrine vs. epinephrine alone in cardiopulmonary resuscitation. *N. Engl. J. Med.* 2008 3;359(1):21–30.

[85] Morris DC. Vasopressors in cardiopulmonary resuscitation. *N. Engl. J. Med.* 2008;359(15):1624; author reply 1625.

[86] Spohr FA, Teschendorf P, Bottiger BW. Vasopressors in cardiopulmonary resuscitation. *N. Engl. J. Med.* 2008;359(15):1624–1625.

[87] Holmberg M, Holmberg S, Herlitz J. Low chance of survival among patients requiring adrenaline (epinephrine) or intubation after out-of-hospital cardiac arrest in Sweden. *Resuscitation*. 2002;54(1):37-45.

[88] Ristagno G, Tang W, Huang L, Fymat A, Chang Y, Sun S, Castillo C, Weil MH. Epinephrine reduces cerebral perfusion during cardiopulmonary resuscitation. *Crit. Care Med.* 2009;37(4):1408–1415.

[89] Mentzelopoulos SD, Zakynthinos SG, Tzoufi M, Katsios N, Papastylianou A, Gkisioti S, Stathopoulos A, Kollintza A, Stamataki E, Roussos C. Vasopressin, epinephrine, and corticosteroids for in-hospital cardiac arrest. *Arch. Intern. Med.* 2009;169(1):15–24.

[90] Redding JS, Pearson JW. Evaluation of drugs for cardiac resuscitation. *Anesthesiology*. 1963;24:203-7.

[91] Callaham M, Madsen CD, Barton CW, Saunders CE, Pointer J. A randomized clinical trial of high-dose epinephrine and norepinephrine vs standard-dose epinephrine in prehospital cardiac arrest. *JAMA*. 1992;268(19):2667-72.

[92] Klouche K, Weil MH, Sun S, Tang W, Zhao DH. A comparison of alpha-methylnorepinephrine, vasopressin and epinephrine for cardiac resuscitation. *Resuscitation*. 2003;57(1):93–100.

[93] García-Villalón AL, Garcia JL, Fernández N, Monge L, Gómez B, Diéguez G. Regional differences in the arterial response to vasopressin: role of endothelial nitric oxide. *Br. J. Pharmacol.* 1996;118(7):1848-54.

[94] Schwarz B, Mair P, Raedler C, Deckert D, Wenzel V, Lindner KH. Vasopressin improves survival in a pig model of hypothermic cardiopulmonary resuscitation. *Crit. Care Med.* 2002;30(6):1311–1314.

[95] Part 7.2: Management of Cardiac Arrest. *Circulation*. 2005;112(Suppl 1):IV-58-66.

[96] Nolan JP, Deakin CD, Soar J, Böttiger BW, Smith G, European Resuscitation Council. European Resuscitation Council guidelines for resuscitation 2005. Section 4. Adult advanced life support. *Resuscitation*. 2005;67 Suppl 1:S39-86.

[97] Ewy GA, Kern KB. Recent advances in cardiopulmonary resuscitation: cardiocerebral resuscitation. *J. Am. Coll. Cardiol.* 2009;53(2):149-57.

In: Drugs in Cardiopulmonary Resuscitation
Editor: Theodoros Xanthos
ISBN: 978-1-61122-512-9

Chapter 3

Atropine in Cardiac Arrest

Panagiotis V.S. Vasileiou, Evaggelia Kouskouni and Theodoros Xanthos

Abstract

Atropine antagonizes the actions of acetylcholine (Ach); therefore, it is commonly classified as an anticholinergic or parasympatholytic agent. It exerts its properties by non-selectively blocking muscarinic receptors. Atropine has various central and peripheral effects. Due to its parasympatholytic effects, atropine is currently indicated as a first-line agent for the management of symptomatic bradycardia and as a second-line agent for the treatment of bradycardic pulseless electrical activity and asystole. Furthermore, atropine is used in the treatment of organophosphate (OP) poisoning. This chapter, after a brief summary of basic pharmacology and actions of atropine, is intended to clarify the current role of the drug regarding the management of cardiac arrest; thus, it focuses on experimental and clinical data either supporting or condemning its use.

Introduction

Atropine is an alkaloid of the tropane group, extracted from the plant *Atropa belladonna* (deadly nightshade) and other members of the Solanaceae family, such as the *Datura stramonium* (jimsonweed) and the *Mandragora officinarum* [1-4]. These plants` roots, stems, and seeds when burned release a smoke of potent alkaloids, one of which is the antimuscarinic compound atropine. According to Gandevia, the alkaloid daturine, extracted from the *Datura stramonium* plant, was identified as atropine in 1833 and was the first agent used in treating asthma in the West [3,5].

Due to its dangerous and potentially deadly properties the term "Atropa" derives from the Greek word "Atropos". In Greek mythology, Atropos was the eldest of the three fates. The fates used to visit the newborn child and Atropos, armed with a huge pair of shears, determined when to cut the thread of life [6-7]. The origin of the term "belladonna", however, is uncertain. In Italian the term "belladonna" is typically translated as "beautiful lady" [8] so the most possible explanation has to do with the usage of this plant as a cosmetic and mydriatic agent due to its property to induce pupillary dilation [8-10]. A different theory was proposed by the botanist Bodaeus in 1644. The plant received its name because when it was administered internally it aroused the sexual fantasies of beautiful women [8,11].

Pharmacology

Atropine is a tertiary amine consisting of an aromatic acid (tropic acid) and an organic base (tropine) [12]. The ester linkage is essential for effective binding of the agent to the Ach receptors. The naturally occurring atropine is *l*(-) – hyoscyamine, but the compound readily racemizes. The commercial material is the racemic mixture of *d* and *l* hyoscyamine. The naturally occuring levorotary form [*l*(-) – hyoscyamine] is active, while *d*-hyoscyamine has little or no potency. As a result, atropine is one half as potent as its *l* isomer [12-17].

Enzymatic hydrolysis by serum atropine esterase, plasma proteins-binding, metabolism in the liver, and excretion through the kidneys compose the four main pathways of atropine's inactivation. Approximately 50% of the amount transported in the blood is loosely bound to protein [18]. About one-fourth to one-third of the dose is excreted unchanged in the urine within 24 hours of injection; accordingly, 35% of the injected atropine is excreted in the urine after metabolic alteration [19,20].

Currently, the synthesis of atropine can be achieved by means of chemical methods and different synthesis pathways in the laboratory setting [21]. Gill *et al.* studied the effects of wide temperature variations on the stability of atropine and other advanced life support (ALS) drugs under field conditions in ALS paramedic units. According to their findings atropine can be stored at temperatures of up to 84.1 ^{o}F (28.9 C^{o}) for up to 45 days and tolerate temperature spikes of up to 125 ^{o}F (51.7 C^{o}) for a cumulative time of 13.25 hours without undergoing degradation [22].

Although the grade of absorption varies widely with the route of administration, in general atropine is absorbed from the vast majority of mucous membranes except for the stomach; poor absorption of the stomach is attributable to the fact that atropine is ionized at the low pH in the gastrointestinal tube [23-24]. It can be administered intravenously (IV), intramuscularly (IM), or intraosseously (IO), and it has also been shown to be clinically effective when given by the endotracheal route (ET). These four routes of administration are used in the emergency setting. Rectal administration has been used as premedication in children [25-27].

When atropine is administered IV it disappears very quickly from the circulation [25]. Clinical studies from Kanto and Klotz in the late 80's showed that both the distribution and elimination half-life periods of atropine, when administered IV, were fast, i.e. 1-1.7 min and 2.2-4.3 h respectively. In the same study, age appeared to have a clear effect on atropine's kinetics, explaining the higher sensitivity of children and elderly to this antimuscarinic agent [25]. It has been reported that after a single 1 mg IV dose of atropine, the maximal increase in pulse rate was observed 12-16 minutes after the dose with an average half-life of 4.125 h [28]. In an experimental animal study using adolescent pigs, 0.25 mg of atropine injected IV caused significant changes in heart rate after 12-15 min, a first increase within 1 min, and the maximum increase 12 min after IV medication [29]. However, during cardiac arrest, there is no cardiac function, so effective chest compressions must be performed in order to circulate the drug. Atropine, when injected peripherally during cardiac arrest, must be followed by a flush of at least 20 ml fluid in order to facilitate drug delivery to the central circulation [30-32].

IO route is an alternative to the IV administration of atropine, when IV cannulation is difficult or impossible. Then atropine is given in the same dosage and exerts the same time effects compared to its IV administration [31-33]. IO infusion methods have been used for infants and children in the emergency setting for years [34-36]. Currently, according to the American Heart Association (AHA) and the European Resuscitation Council (ERC) guidelines, the IO route is acceptable and effective in adult resuscitation [31,32,37,38], even if extravasation, compartment syndrome, and osteomyelitis have been reported as rare complications [38-41].

The ET route can be used as a last alternative when IV or IO accesses are unobtainable [32]. Numerous animal and human studies have taken place with conflicting results concerning the optimal dose or the efficacy of this method [42]. ET administration influences the pattern of drug absorption; as a result, plasma concentrations achieved, are variable and lower compared to those achieved when the drug is given by the IV or IO routes [32]. Howard and Bingham, in 1989, compared the ET and IV administration of atropine in two groups of children and they concluded that the two methods did not differ regarding the effect on heart rate and the speed of onset of the effect [43]. Earlier studies also supported that ET and IV atropine are equally effective [44,45]. However, in one historic non-randomized cohort study in adults who suffered out-of-hospital cardiac arrest (OHCA), the rate of return of spontaneous circulation (ROSC) and rate of survival to hospital admission were significantly higher when the drugs (atropine and adrenaline) were administered IV [46]. The dose of atropine for ET administration is largely unknown, but the agent should be diluted in 10-20 ml of water and injected through a catheter or tube that extends just beyond the end of ET tube [47]. Prete *et al.* examined the time to peak plasma concentration of atropine following IV, ET, and IO administration in anesthetized monkeys. According to their findings, the time to peak plasma concentration of atropine was significantly shorter in the IV route. When compared to ET or IO route, the IV route provided higher peak plasma concentrations. In addition, the time to peak plasma concentration was faster in the IO than the ET route [48].

Mechanisms of Action

The main neurotransmitters of the peripheral nervous system are Ach and nor-epinephrine. In particular, Ach is the basic neurotransmitter of the parasympathetic nervous system; however there are parasympathetic post-gaglionic neurons which utilize nitric oxide (NO) or peptides for transmission. Ach acts on two types of receptors: the muscarinic and nicotinic cholinergic receptors. As far as atropine is concerned, muscarinic receptors are its target. Muscarinic Ach receptors (mAchRs) are members of the G-protein coupled receptors (G-PCR) superfamily [49]. This group of receptors has seven trans-membrane segments which use G-proteins as their signaling mechanism. At present, five distinct receptor genes (CHRM1-CHRM5) have been identified and each of them encodes for a separate muscarinic receptor protein resulting to five receptor subtypes (M1-M5) [49-53]. The muscarinic receptor subtypes are widely distributed throughout the central and peripheral nervous system. They are present in neurons, cardiac and smooth muscles, a variety of exocrine glands, and many other cell types [51]. However, several studies have mentioned tissue-specific subtype expression patterns [54-56]. In particular, M_1 receptors are localized throughout the parasympathetic ganglia and exocrine glands regulating cholinergic transmission [1,5]. M_2 receptors are located prejunctionally acting as feedback inhibitors of acetylocholine release from the nerve [57-61]. In the heart, the M_2 receptor subtypes are considered to be the predominant subtypes of cardiac mAchR; they are mainly involved in the repolarization phase of the action potential and modulate the duration of peak contraction [62]. Heart M_2 muscarinic receptors mediate the cardio-depressant effect of parasympathetic activation leading to bradycardia. Ventricular cells also express M_1 receptors; their role seems to be the modulation of cardiac plateau and therefore the magnitude of the peak contraction [62-66]. The M_2 and M_3 receptors are commonly co-expressed in smooth muscles in various tissues such as airway or intestinal smooth muscles [67]; for example, in airway smooth muscle, M_3 muscarinic receptors initiate contraction and M_2 muscarinic receptors inhibit relaxation [68]. M_4 receptors are found in heart where they may activate potassium (K^+) currents [62]. M_5 receptors are mostly found in the brain. According to functional criteria, muscarinic receptor subtypes can be classified into two broad categories. M_1, M_3 and M_5, in the one hand which preferentially couple to the Gq family of G-proteins. They activate phospholipase C (PLC), using pertussis toxin-insensitive G-proteins of the Gq family, but do not inhibit adenylyl cyclase. In general, they have a stimulatory effect on the target tissue. On the other hand, M_2 and M_4 receptors preferentially couple to the Gi family of G-proteins. Using pertussis toxin-sensitive G-proteins of the Gi/Go family, they inhibit adenylyl cyclase but do not activate PLC and consequently they can be characterized as inhibitory [51,53, 69]. However, the above classification is not absolute. For example, if M_2 and M_4 receptors are expressed at high levels they do activate PLC in certain cell types [70-72]. In addition, muscarinic receptors regulate ion channels through several pathways: 1) activation of second messengers, 2) direct regulation by G-protein subunits activation, 3) endocytosis or insertion into the surface membrane [73-78].

Effects of Atropine

Generally, atropine lowers the "rest and digest" activity of all muscles and glands regulated by the parasympathetic nervous system. Atropine has widespread central and peripheral actions; knowledge of the range of organ systems affected by atropine is essential to maximize its benefits while minimizing side effects.

Heart Effects

The best known cardiac effect of atropine is its ability to increase heart rate due to its vagolytic action on the sinus node (positive chronotropic action) [79-81]. In other words, atropine enhances sinus node automaticity because it accelerates the discharge rate of the sinoatrial (SA) node [82]. Atropine has also proved to be an efficacious agent in facilitation of conduction through the atria and atrioventricular node (AV). Atropine exerts a direct effect on the function of the AV junctional tissue and the subjunctional components of the cardiac conducting system [82-83]. Several groups of researchers demonstrated a shortening of the SA conduction time after administration of atropine not only to subjects with normal SA node function, but also in patients with sinus bradycardia [84-86]. Therefore, atropine is a potentially useful adjunct in situations with excessive parasympathetic tone, such as asystole, and its use in the management of bradycardic conditions, such as unstable bradycardia or slow Pulseless Electrical Activity (PEA), appears reasonable.

However, this is only the one side of the coin. Heart rate is a primary determinant of myocardial oxygen demand; thus, the positive chronotropic effect of atropine can cause an imbalance between oxygen supply and demand in the myocardium [87,88]. Furthermore, varying degrees of AV block, occasional ventricular premature contractions or even ventricular fibrillation (VF) have been reported after the administration of atropine; in any case, these effects which are applicable to the beating heart may be of little significance during cardiac arrest [89-91].

Atropine given in small doses or given slowly and not rapidly can produce a sustained bradycardia or, less frequently, may produce a biphasic effect [92-94]. The term "biphasic" refers to a response which is characterized by initial slowing of the heart rate usually followed within 2-3 minutes by a positive chronotropic effect [95]. This dose-dependent biphasic heart rate response to atropine is a well-recognized phenomenon in humans. Originally thought to be due to central activation of vagal efferent outflow, this negative chronotropic response to low-dose atropine is now known to be caused through muscarinic receptors in the central parasympathetic system [92,94,96]. In particular, the decrease in heart rate results from blockade of the M_1 receptors on the inhibitory prejunctional (or presynaptic) neurons, thus permitting increased Ach release. Higher doses of atropine block the M_2 receptors on the SA node resulting to a modest increase in cardiac rate. In summary, the exact dosage in which this phenomenon is caused is not absolutely clear, however it seems that smaller doses than 0.5 mg in adults may cause paradoxical bradycardia. Note that Chamberlain *et al.* demonstrated that in fit young adults a dose of 3 mg atropine was sufficient to completely block parasympathetic activity [97]. The clinical value of this knowledge is that during cardiac arrest the maximum dose of atropine that one can administer is 3 mg; in any case, atropine must be given rapidly via IV push. Slow infusions or individual doses less than 0.5 mg should be avoided.

Effects on Other Organs

Atropine reduces salivary and bronchial secretions. Anesthesiologists used to take advantage of this anticholinergic action of atropine during premedication in order to decrease secretions that accompany anesthesia and prevent vagal stimulation while intubating. In addition, the vagal blockade with atropine is associated with an increase in physiological and anatomic dead space and a fall in airway resistance [98,99]. This bronchodilatory effect may have additional validity regarding oxygenation during cardiac arrest.

Atropine has many other non-cardiac effects; nevertheless, the vast majority of them are not important when the drug is administered parenterally in the emergency management of cardiac arrest patients. For example, atropine by blocking all cholinergic activity on the eye exerts both mydriatic and cycloplegic effects. Toxic amounts of atropine usually, and therapeutic doses occasionally, result to "atropine flush": a term that is used to describe the dilation of cutaneous blood vessels, especially those in the blush area [100]. Clinically effective doses of atropine are, essentially, without central nervous system (CNS) effects [100]. However, atropine is capable of crossing the blood-brain barrier to some extent [101], as it has been shown in both experimental and clinical conditions[102-103]; for that reason, doses far above the therapeutic level will produce CNS effects (confusion, excitement, hallucinations); obviously this has no clinical value for the cardiac arrest patient.

Atropine in Cardiac Arrest

Although pharmacotherapy is not the cornerstone of cardiopulmonary resuscitation (CPR), atropine is recommended for, and used in, the management of asystole and slow PEA which both are non-shockable cardiac arrest rhythms. As far as asystole and PEA are concerned, drug administration is vitally important to be combined with a quick search for the underlying factor (Table 1), which, if possible, should be rapidly dealt with. The reported incidence of asystole as the first documented rhythm of cardiac arrest in adults is approximately 20-40% [104]. A study from Goteborg, Sweden, showed that asystole was the presenting rhythm in the field in 35% of patients with cardiac arrest [105]. Previous reports also suggested that asystole can be the initial event of arrest, especially in non-diseased hearts [106,107]. Different study populations and methods of reporting the initial rhythm result in variation of reported incidence. Furthermore, it must be taken into account that asystole may be the final electrocardiographic manifestation of an unwitnessed cardiac arrest that initially presented as shockable rhythm and deteriorated to asystole as time passed [108,109]. PEA, on the other hand, accounts for approximately 20% of all cardiac arrest victims [110]. Nadkarni *et al.* reported a 32% incidence of PEA as the presenting rhythm in adults with in-hospital cardiac arrest [111]. Unfortunately, the prognosis of patients developing asystole or PEA is dismal; only 1-4% of patients with PEA survive while patients with asystole rarely survive [32,104,112,113]. In the Goteborg study, only 2% of the asystolic patients survived to hospital discharge, while, in the study by Nadkarni *et al.*, the survival to hospital discharge rate was only 11.2% of patients who initially presented with PEA (in-hospital cardiac arrest), and out of which, only 62% had good neurological outcomes. [105,111].

Table 1. The underlying causes of Cardiac Arrest (6 Hs and 6 Ts rule)

6 Hs	6 Ts
Hypovolemia	Tablets (overdose)
Hypoxia	Tamponate (cardiac)
Hydrogen ion (acidosis)	Tension pneumothorax
Hyperkalemia/hypokalemia	Thrombosis (coronary)
Hypothermia	Thrombosis (pulmonary)
Hypoglycemia	Trauma

Asystole represents cardiac standstill with a total absence of any mechanical or electrical activity in the myocardium. Therefore, no cardiac output (no detectable pulse) and no ventricular depolarization occur during asystole. On the other hand, the term "Pulseless Electrical Activity" is used to include a broad group of situations (idioventricular rhythms, ventricular escape rhythms, brady-asystolic rhythms) in which a rhythm on the cardiac monitor is not accompanied by a detectable pulse. PEA represents a condition in which electrical activity in the heart is detected but myocardial mechanical activity is impeded. [30,104] Paradis *et al.* reported that 41% of patients who presented with PEA had mechanical cardiac activity that generated a low pressure but not enough to lead to a palpable pulse [114].

The use of atropine during cardiac arrest and particularly in asystole and slow PEA is based on theoretical grounds. Sympathetic and parasympathetic divisions of the autonomic nervous system have a well-recognized role in the neuronal regulation of the heart. The rationale for the suggested efficacy of atropine is that asystolic arrests may be related to excessive or unantagonized increases in parasympathetic tone; therefore, atropine as a parasympatholytic agent finds its place to the treatment of cardiac arrested patients. Experimental data obtained from studies in animals with intact hemodynamic systems have been cited. However, little has been reported on the effect of atropine on survival.

Reviewing the literature on the use of atropine sulfate in asystole reveals conflicting data either supporting or condemning its use (Table 2).

Table 2. Summary of studies which present data on the effectiveness of atropine in asystole

Study		Population	Outcomes
Gupta et al. (1975)	Anecdotal report	4 in-hospital patients developing periods of cardiac standstill	One patient recovered
Iseri et al. (1978)	Anecdotal report	15 pre-hospital brady-asystolic patients	One patient resuscitated in the field. All patients pronounced dead on arrival at the hospital
Brown et al. (1979)	Anecdotal report	6 in-hospital and 2 pre-hospital patients (only 5 were initially in asystole)	3 patients developed rhythm but died during hospitalization. 2 patients discharged
Coon et al. (1981)	Controlled prospective study	21 pre-hospital patients developing asystole or PIVR	No benefit regarding change rhythm, resumption of a palpable pulse, admission to the hospital and discharge alive
Stueven et al. (1984)	Retrospective controlled study	84 patients with out-of-hospital cardiac arrest.	Atropine administration had a beneficial effect on the successful resuscitation but did not improved long-term survival

PIVR = Pulseless Idioventricular Rhythms

Nevertheless, it was Brown *et al.*, in 1979, which suggested that "atropine may be of value in the treatment of ventricular asystole" and led AHA to include atropine sulfate in its guidelines for the management of cardiac asystole [115]. In their study, they included eight patients in cardiac arrest with asystole electrocardiographically documented and defined as no spontaneous electrical activity for at least five seconds either as the initial rhythm or as a result of defibrillation. Three of five patients that had asystole as the initial cardiac arrest rhythm received catecholamines and then atropine, and developed a rhythm but died during their hospitalization. Additionally two of the patients developed asystole during cardiac catheterization, they were treated only with atropine (no catecholamines), responded with a normal sinus rhythm, and were eventually discharged from the hospital.

A few years earlier, in 1975, Gupta and coworkers cited the cases of four patients with cardiac standstill for a period of time ranging from 2 to 22.5 seconds [116]. All patients were administered atropine and responded successfully, although three of them were not in asystole at the time of administration. The fourth one, however, received IV atropine and isoproterenol hydrochloride drip and recovered from a "long period of complete cardiac standstill". These studies unfortunately were not controlled and involved only in-hospital patients.

In 1978, Iseri and colleagues, in a study about the management of cardiac arrest patients in a paramedic system, reported a successfully resuscitated in the field patient who presented in ventricular asystole and received epinephrine and atropine [108]. Unfortunately, this patient was pronounced dead on arrival at the hospital. A second patient presenting in ventricular arrest was administered atropine, developed a junctional rhythm, but turned into ventricular asystole and was also pronounced dead on arrival at the hospital.

Trying to further clarify the clouded situation regarding the efficacy of atropine in pre-hospital cardiac arrest patients, Coon *et al.*, in 1981, studied a series of twenty-one pre-hospital cardiac-arrested patients with asystole or slow pulseless idioventricular rhythms (PIVR), either as the presenting rhythm or on the process of the resuscitation efforts [117]. Patients were divided into a control group who received other but atropine agents as first line treatment and an atropine-treated group. Atropine-treated patients received 1 mg atropine IV. In case of developing a rhythm other than asystole or PIVR, further therapy appropriate for the generated rhythm was instituted. If no change rhythm occurred within 1 minute of atropine administration, a second dose of 1 mg was given. If the initial brady-asystolic rhythm persisted, the same therapy as the control group was administered. Change in rhythm, resumption of a palpable pulse, admission to the hospital, and discharge alive from the hospital were the four parameters measured as an index of therapeutic efficacy. However, no differences were observed; approximately half the patients in both groups developed a palpable spontaneous pulse during resuscitation attempts, only two patients in each group were admitted to the hospital, and only one patient (from the control group) was discharged alive from the hospital but had severe central nervous system dysfunction. This controlled, prospective study failed to demonstrate any benefit from the administration of atropine in cardiac arrest population in the pre-hospital setting. The authors concluded that "atropine may not affect the outcome of prehospital bradyasystolic cardiac arrest of primary cardiac etiology".

In a retrospective review for a four-year period, eighty-four patients with OHCA due to refractory asystole were studied [118]. These patients presented with an initial arrest rhythm of asystole. Forty-three of them received atropine (atropine group) and forty-one did not (control group). Successful resuscitation was defined as the conveyance of a patient with a rhythm and a pulse to the emergency department. The successful resuscitation rate in the group who received atropine was 14% (6 out of 43), compared to 0% in the control group. Unfortunately, no patient who received atropine for refractory asystole was discharged alive. According to this study, atropine's use in refractory asystole had a beneficial effect on the successful resuscitation, although it did not improved long-term survival.

Lastly, a study from Rials and Tse in 1982, showed that a massive dose of 1mg/kg of atropine could prevent the development of asystole produced by b-blocking agents in digitoxin-intoxicated dogs [119].

As far as PEA is concerned, the potentially beneficial effects of atropine administration during resuscitation have not been clearly demonstrated and sufficiently investigated (Table 3).

In 1985, Kasten and Martin reported the beneficial effects of a combination of atropine and epinephrine in PEA or asystole due to bupivacaine overdose [120]. Blecic *et al.* compared the effects of high doses of atropine in combination with epinephrine with those of epinephrine alone on a closed-chest dog model of PEA [121]. After 5 minutes of chest compressions using a CPR thumper, an injection of either 0.5 mg of atropine sulfate or 5 ml of D/W 5% was given. The same injection was repeated every 5 minutes in alternant with 1 mg of adrenaline until recovery was obtained.

Table 3. Summary of studies which present data on the effectiveness of atropine in PEA

Study		Population	Outcomes
Redding et al. (1983)	Experimental control study	40 mongrel dogs. Methoxamine, CaCl2, atropine and saline were given in each group of ten dogs while being in PEA arrest asphyxially induced	Atropine was not significantly more effective than saline regarding resuscitation
Vanags et al. (1988)	Prospective comparative control study	503 out-of-hospital patients in cardiac arrest with the initial rhythm of PEA	Atropine appeared to be as effective as either epinephrine or bicarbonate in the development and generation of pulses, and in successfully resuscitating patients from PEA
Blecic et al. (1992)	Experimental control study	15 mongrel dogs in PEA arrest induced by VF. The effects of high doses of atropine in combination with epinephrine were compared with those of epinephrine alone	High doses of atropine together with epinephrine enhances the recovery from PEA and results in a better cardiac function during recovery
Engdahl et al. (2001)	Retrospective analysis of data collected prospectively	1069 patients with out-of-hospital cardiac arrest presenting as PEA	Survival among patients suffering from OHCA and PEA was poor. Treatment with atropine was associated with worse outcome

PEA: pulseless electrical activity; VF: ventricular fibrillation; OHCA: out-of-hospital cardiac arrest

Each animal was submitted to two successive cycles of CPR, one including repeated injections of atropine and one including repeated injections of D/W 5%, in a randomized order. Recovery was obtained in 10 of 11 dogs in the atropine group compared to 8 of 12 in the D/W 5% group. Even if no statistical significant difference was shown in ROSC, the use of atropine significantly reduced the duration of cardiac arrest.

Table 4. Levels of Evidence

Level of Evidence 1	Randomised clinical trials or meta-analyses of multiple clinical trials with substantial treatment effects
Level of Evidence 2	Randomised clinical trials with smaller or less significant treatment effects
Level of Evidence 3	Prospective, controlled, non-randomised cohort studies
Level of Evidence 4	Historic, non-randomised cohort or case control studies
Level of Evidence 5	Case series; patients compiled in serial fashion, control group lacking
Level of Evidence 6	Animal studies or mechanical model studies
Level of Evidence 7	Extrapolations from existing data collected for other purposes, theoretical analyses
Level of Evidence 8	Rational conjecture (common sense); common practices accepted before evidence-based guidelines

Earlier reports have also involved atropine in the treatment of patients with cardiac arrest presenting as PEA in the pre-hospital setting. During a six-year period, Vanags *et al.* evaluated the use and possible efficacy of selected pharmacological and non-pharmacological interventions in 503 patients presented in cardiac arrest with PEA [122]. Atropine was demonstrated to be as effective as either epinephrine or bicarbonate in the development and generation of a pulse and in successfully resuscitating patients. On the contrary, Redding and colleagues failed to demonstrate any beneficial effect of the administration of atropine as compared with controls (saline, calcium chloride, and methoxamine) on a dog model of hypoxia-induced PEA [123]. More recently, four prospective controlled nonrandomized cohort studies in adults with Level of Evidence (LOE) 3 (Table 4) [124-127] and one LOE 4 study [106] showed that treatment with atropine was not associated with any consistent benefits after in-hospital or OHCA. Dumot *et al.*, based on the hypothesis that a variety of factors affect survival following in-hospital cardiac arrest, examined the medical records of all hospitalized patients who underwent CPR [127]. Primary outcomes for this study were survival immediately after resuscitation, at 24 hours, at 48 hours, and at hospital discharge. According to the results, medical therapy with atropine decreased the odds of surviving to hospital discharge, representing an independent predictor of a poor outcome; the administration of any atropine during the resuscitation lowered the survival rate in half, and additional atropine doses resulted in survival to hospital discharge of less than 5%.

Atropine carries a class IIa recommendation (Table 5) for symptomatic bradycardia. The recommended dose is 0.5 mg atropine via rapid IV push. If the patient does not respond to the initial dose, repeated doses of 0.5 mg can be given every 3-5 minutes to a total of 3 mg.

Atropine is one of the mainstays of medical treatment in organophosphate (OP) poisoning. As an antimuscarinic agent, atropine blocks the muscarinic cholinergic receptors found in gastrointestinal tract, pulmonary smooth muscles, exocrine glands, heart, and eye;

however, it does not affect nicotinic receptors. The dose for adults is 1-2 mg IV bolus repeated every 1-5 minutes as needed to decrease muscarinic symptoms. Generally speaking, atropine in case of OP toxicity should be administered in large amounts in order to reverse the cholinergic symptoms. Furthermore, immediate aggressive use of atropine may eliminate the need for intubation. It has been recommended by some authors that atropine should be given until the appearance of atropinization signs (warm, dry, flushed skin, dilated pupils, increased heart rate). Nevertheless, the minimum duration of atropine administration is 24 hours which represents the time for the OP to be metabolized.

Table 5. Classes of recommendations

Class I	Evidence and/or general agreement that a given diagnostic procedure/treatment is beneficial, useful and effective
Class II	Conflicting evidence and/or divergence of opinion about the usefulness/efficacy of the treatment
Class IIa	Weight of evidence/opinion is in favour of usefulness/efficacy
Class IIb	Usefulness/efficacy is less well established by evidence/opinion
Class III	Evidence or general agreement that the treatment is not useful/effective and in some cases may be harmful

Precautions

In the face of life-threatening circumstances (e.g. asystole) there are no absolute contraindications for the use of atropine; in such situations atropine is unlikely to be harmful [32]. Patients with acute coronary syndromes represent a group in which atropine should be used cautiously [31]. This does not mean that atropine is contraindicated; on the contrary, atropine is a first line drug for compromising bradyarrhythmia caused by acute coronary ischemia [82], and it seems that atropine is most effective in treating ischemic bradyarrhythmias than non-ischemic [83,128-135].

Note that sinus bradycardia represents the 30% to 40% of AMI (Acute Myocardial Infarction)-associated arrhythmias and it is especially frequent within the first hour of inferior STEMI (ST-Elevation Myocardial Infarction) and with reperfusion of the right coronary artery (Bezold-Jarisch reflex) due to increased parasympathetic activity (vagal tone) [136].

However, the administration of atropine in patients with ischemic cardiac events has been associated with adverse reactions [135,137,138], such as worsening of second degree type II and third degree AV block (see below), pro-arrhythmic effect, and potentiation of AMI [137,138].

The latter reaction refers to patients who are in the process of an ischemic event and atropine results to "the conversion of acute ischemia to AMI" [82]. A possible mechanism may be the increased heart rate that increases oxygen demands and impedes the perfusion of the coronary arteries during the diastolic phase of cardiac cycle. Nevertheless, without precluding the use of atropine, what is for sure is the need for careful medical supervision.

Atropine is possible to be ineffective in treating high-grade AV blocks. Atropine due to its parasympatholytic properties enhances AV conduction and "exerts a direct influence on the function of the AV junctional tissue and subjunctional components of the cardiac conduction system" [83]; however, when an infranodal block exists, atropine may increase the sinus rate without affecting infranodal conduction resulting to a decrease of the effective ratio of conduction and, subsequently, to a decrease of the ventricular rate [136].

Atropine is contraindicated in patients with glaucoma as it may precipitate acute glaucoma, even with therapeutic doses due to pupillary dilation, patients with tachycardia and patients with denervated hearts (e.g. after transplantation) [30].

Conclusion

Atropine has been a commonly used medication for decades and, generally speaking, it's a safe drug. In the era of evidence-based medicine, atropine continues to have its place in the setting of cardiac arrest or elsewhere indicated; however one cannot assume *a priori* for its efficacy. The antimuscarinic properties of atropine offers a strong theoretical basis for its use, but conflicting reports make the situation foggy (Table 6). Small study sizes, different patient populations (out-of-hospital versus in-hospital cardiac arrest patients) and different study methods (retrospective versus prospective) may possibly provoke these opposite results. Nevertheless, conflicting reports raise the subject for the necessity of data from randomized trials in order to determine the efficacy of atropine in survival rates.

Table 6. Other studies regarding the effectiveness of atropine in cardiac arrest

Study		Methods	Outcomes
Ohshige et al. (2004)	Prospective comparative study	Areas where out-of-hospital CPR was performed with resuscitative drugs were compared to areas where resuscitative drugs were not administered outside the hospital	Use of resuscitative drugs (epinephrine, atropine, lidocaine) appeared to be effective in terms of resuscitation rates and 1-month survival rates
Dumot et al. (2001)	Prospective study	445 patients who experienced in-hospital cardiac arrest and received ACLS resuscitation	Increasing doses of atropine were associated with lower survival rates at 24h and 48h after resuscitation, and until hospital discharge

CPR: cardiopulmonary resuscitation; ACLS: advanced cardiac life support

In all cases, what must be highlighted is that the role of atropine, as happens for any medication used in cardiac arrest, is secondary. As far as asystole and PEA are concerned, the primary goal of treatment is to identify and treat the reversible cause. From this point of view, we have the ability to use atropine even if its validation in the complex environment of resuscitation remains in dispute.

References

[1] Scullion JE. The development of anticholinergics in the management of COPD. *Int. J. Chron. Obstruct. Pulmon. Dis.* 2007;2:33-40.

[2] Chapman KR, Mannino DM, Soriano JB, et al. Epidemiology and costs of chronic obstructive pulmonary disease. *Eur. Resp. J.* 2006;27:188-207.

[3] Gandevia B. Historical review of the use of parasympatholytic agents in the treatment of respiratory disorders. *Postgrad. Med. J.* 1975;51:213-228.

[4] Piccillo GA, Miele L, Mondati E, et al. Anticholinergic syndrome due to "Devil's Herb": When risks come from the ancient time. *Int .J. Clin. Pract.* 2006 2006;60:492-494.

[5] Restrepo RD. Use of inhaled anticholinergic agents in obstructive airway disease. *Respir. Care* 2007;52:833-847.

[6] Holzman RS. The legacy of Atropos, the fate who cut the thread of life. *Anesthesiology* 1998;89:241-249.

[7] Lai DC. More on the legacy of Atropos, with special reference to Datura stramonium. *Anesthesiology* 1999;90:1794-1795.

[8] Thomas R. Forbes : Why is it called "Beautiful Lady"? A note on Belladona. *Bull. NY Acad. Med.* 1977;53:403-406.

[9] Pepper OHP. *Medical etymology*. Philadelphia: Saunders; 1957, p.100.

[10] Wootton AC. *Chronicles of Pharnacy.* London: Macmillan; 1910, pp.24-25.

[11] Bodaeus, I. *Theophrastus De historia plantarum.* Amstelodami : Laurentius ; 1644, lib. VI, pp. 586, 1078.

[12] Eger EI. Atropine, Scopolamine, and related compounds. *Anesthesiology* 1962;23:365-383.

[13] Cushny AR. On optical isomers: the tropeines. *J. Pharmacol. Exp. Ther.* 1920;15:105-127

[14] Cushny AR. Atropine and the hyoscyamines-a study of the action of optical isomers. *J. Physiol.* 1904;30:176-194.

[15] Cushny AR, Peebles AR. Action of optical isomers; hyoscines. *J. Physiol.* 1905;32:501-510.

[16] Domino EF, Hudson RD. Observations on pharmacological actions of the isomers of atropine. *J. Pharmacol. Exp. Ther.* 1959;127: 305-312

[17] Gyermek L. Studies on the cholinergic blocking substances. I. Sites of action of compounds of the atropine group. *Acta Physiol. Acad. Shi. Hung.* 1951;2:511-517.

[18] Tonnesen M. On the absorption of atropine to the plasma proteins. *Acta Pharmacol. (Copenh)* 1956;12:247-250.

[19] Kalser SC. The fate of atropine in man. *Ann. New York Acad. Sc.* 1971;179:667-683

[20] Tonnesen M. Excretion of atropine and allied alkaloids in urine. *Acta Pharmacol. et. Toxicol.* 1950;6:147-164

[21] Kirchhoff C, Bitar Y, Ebel S, Holzgrabe U. Analysis of atropine, its degradation products and related substances of natural origin by means of reversed-phase high-performance liquid chromatography. *J. Chromatogr. A.* 2004;10456:115-120

[22] Gill MA, Kislik AZ, Gore L, Chandna A. Stability of Advanced Life Support drugs in the field. *A. J. Health Syst. Pharm.* 2004;61:597-602.

[23] Tonndorf J, Hyde RW, Chinn HI, Lett JE. Absorption from nasal mucous membrane: systemic effect of hyoscine following intranasal administration. *Ann. Otol. Rhinol. Laryngol.* 1953;62:630-641.

[24] Tonnesen M. Absorption and distribution of atropine in rats. *Acta Pharmacol. (Copenh)* 1948;4:367-378

[25] Kanto J, Klotz U. Pharmacokinetic implications for the clinical use of atropine, scopolamine and glycopyrrolate. *Acta Anaesthesiol. Scand.* 1988; 32:69-78.

[26] Bejersten A, Olsson GL, Palmer L. The influence of body weight on plasma concentration of atropine after rectal administration. *Acta Anaesthesiol. Scand.* 1985;29:782-784.

[27] Olsson GL, Bejersten A, Feychting H, Palmer L, Petterson BM. Plasma concentrations of atropine after rectal administration. *Anaesthesia* 1983;38:1179-1182.

[28] Adams RG, Verma P, Jackson AJ, Miller RL. Plasma pharmacokinetics of intravenously administered atropine in normal human subjects. *J. Clin. Pharmacol.* 1982;22:477-481.

[29] Hornchen U, Schuttler J, Stoeckel H, Ensing K, de Zeeuw RA, Eichelkraut W. Comparison of intravenous and endobronchial atropine: a pharmacokinetic and – dynamic study in pigs. *Eur. J. Anaesthesiol.* 1989;6:95-101.

[30] Rahm SJ. eACLS Study Guide, 2nd edition. Sudbury, Massachusetts. Jones and Bartletti Publishers.

[31] American Heart Association in collaboration with the International Liaison Committee on Resuscitation, guidelines for cardiopulmonary resuscitation and emergency cardiovascular care: Management of cardiac arrest. *Circulation* 2005;112:58-66.

[32] European Resuscitation Council guidelines for resuscitation 2005: Adult advanced life support. *Resuscitation* 2005;67:S39-S86.

[33] Leidel BA, Kirchhoff C, Bogner V, et al. Is the intraosseous access route fast and efficacious compared to conventional central venous catheterization in adult patients under resuscitation in the emergency department? A prospective observational pilot study. *Patient Saf. Surg.* 2009;3:24.

[34] Sacchetti AD, Linkenheimer R, Lieberman M, Haviland P, Kryszczak LB. Intraosseous drug administration: successful resuscitation from asystole. *Pediatr. Emerg. Care* 1989;5:97-98.

[35] Ramet J, Clybouw C, Benetar A, Hachimi-Idrissi S, Corne L. Successful use of an intraosseous infusion in an 800 grams preterm infant. *Eur. J. Emerg. Med.* 1998;5:327-328.

[36] Tibballs J. Endotracheal and intraosseous drug administration for paediatric CPR. *Aust. Fam. Physician* .1992;21:1477-1480.

[37] Leidel BA, Kirchhoff C. Intraosseous infusion for adults. *Chirurg* 2008;79: 315-326.

[38] Glaeser Pw, Hellmich TR, Szewczuga D, Losek JD, Smith DS. Five-year experience in prehospital intraosseous infusions in children and adults. *Ann. Emerg. Med.* 1993;22:1119-1124.

[39] Wright R, Reynolds SL, Nachtsheim B. Compartment syndrome secondary to prolonged intraosseous infusion. *Pediatr. Emerg. Care* 1994;10:157-159.

[40] Rosovsky M, FitzPatrick M, Goldfarb CR, Finestone H. Bilateral osteomyelitis due to intraosseous infusion: Case report and review of the English-language literature. *Pediatr. Radiol.* 1994;24:72-73.

[41] Donati F, Guay J. No substitute for the intravenous route. *Anesthesiology* 2001;95:1-2.
[42] Paret G, Mazkereth R, Sella R, et al. Atropine pharmacokinetics and pharmacodynamics following endotracheal versus endobronchial administration in dogs. *Resuscitation* 1999;41:57-62.
[43] Howard RF, Bingman RM. Endotracheal compared with intravenous administration of atropine. *Arch. Dis. Child* 1990;65:449-450.
[44] Bray BM, Jones HM, Grundy EM. Tracheal versus intravenous atropine. A comparison of the effects on heart rate. *Anaesthesia* 1987;42:1188-1190.
[45] Greenberg MI, Mayeda DV, Chrzanowski R, Brumwell D, Baskin SI, Roberts JR. Endotracheal administration of atropine sulphate. *Ann. Emerg. Med.* 1982;11:546-548.
[46] Niemann JT, Stratton SJ, Cruz B, Lewis RJ. Endotracheal drug administration during out-of-hospital resuscitation: where are the survivors? *Resuscitation* 2002;53:153-157.
[47] Gonzalez ER. Pharmacologic controversies in CPR. *Ann. Emerg. Med.* 1993;22:317-323.
[48] Prete MR, Hannan CJ, Burkle FM. Plasma atropine concentrations via intravenous, endotracheal, and intraosseous administration. *Am. J. Emerg. Med.* 1987;5:101-104.
[49] Mc Brien NA, Jobling AI, Truong HT, Cottriall CL, Gentle A. Expression of muscarinic receptor subtypes in three shrew ocular tissues and their regulation during the development of myopia. *Mol. Vis.* 2009;15:464-475.
[50] Wess J. Molecular biology of muscarinic acetylcholine receptors. *Crit. Rev. Neurobiol.* 1996;10:69-99.
[51] Nathanson NM. A multiplicity of muscarinic mechanisms: enough signalling pathways to take your breath away. *Proc. Natl. Acad. Sci.* USA 2000;97:6245-6247.
[52] Ishii M, Kurachi Y. Muscarinic acetylcholine receptors. *Curr. Pharm. Des.* 2006;12:3573-3581.
[53] Nathanson NM. Synthesis, trafficking, and localization of muscarinic acetylcholine receptors. *Pharmacol. Ther.* 2008;119:33-43.
[54] Levey AI, Kitt CA, Simonds WF, Price DL, Brann MR. Identification and localization of muscarinic acetylcholine receptor proteins in brain with subtype-specific antibodies. *J. Neurosci.* 1991;11:3218-3226.
[55] Dorje F, Levey AI, Brann MR. Immunological detection of muscarinic receptor subtype proteins (m1-m5) in rabbit peripheral tissues. *Mol. Pharmacol.* 1991;40:459-462.
[56] Racke K, Matthiesen S. The airway cholinergic system: physiology and pharmacology. *Pulm. Pharmacol. Ther.* 2004;17:181-198.
[57] Haddad el-B, Rousell J. Regulation of the expression and function of the M2 muscarinic receptor. *Trends Pharmacol. Sci.* 1998;19:322-327.
[58] Barnes PJ. The role of anticholinergics in chronic obstructive pulmonary disease. *Am. J. Med.* 2004;117 Suppl 12A:24S-32S.
[59] Gross NJ, Barnes PJ. A short tour around the muscarinic receptor. *Am. Rev. Respir. Dis.* 1988;138:765-767.
[60] Roffel AF, Elzinga CR, Zaagsma J. Muscarinic M3 receptors mediate contraction of human central and peripheral airway smooth muscle. *Pulm. Pharmacol.* 1990;3:47-51.
[61] Lefkowitz RJ, Hoffman BB, Tayler P. Neurohormonal transmission: The autonomic and somatic motor nervous system. In: Gilman AG, Rall TW, Nies AS, Taylor P, editors. *Goodman and Gilman's the pharmacological basis of therapeutics*, 8th ed. Elmsford NY: Pergamon Press; 1990, pp 84-121.

[62] Sauviat MP. Muscarinic modulation of cardiac activity. *J. Soc. Biol.* 1999;193:469-480.

[63] Tanito Y, Miwa T, Endou M, et al. Interaction of edrophonium with muscarinic acetylcholine M2 and M3 receptors. *Anesthesiology* 2002;94:804-814.

[64] Lefkowitz RJ, Hoffman BB, Tayler P. Neurotransmission: The autonomic and somatic motor nervous systems. In: *Goodman and Gilman's The Pharmacological Basis of Therapeutics*, 9th edition. Edited by Hardman JG, Limbird LE, Molinoff PB, Ruddon RW, Goodman Gilman A. New York, Mc Graw-Hill,1996, pp 105-139.

[65] Gallo MP, Alloatti G, Eva C, Oberto A, Levi RC. M1 muscarinic receptors increase calcium current and phosphoinositide turnover in guinea –pig ventricular cardiocytes. *J. Physiol. (Lond)* 1993;471:41-60.

[66] Sharma VK, Colecraft HM, Wang DX, et al. Molecular and functional identification of M1 muscarinic acetylcholine receptors in rat ventricular myocytes. *Circ. Res.* 1996;79:86-93.

[67] Maeda A, Kubo T, Mishina M, Numa S. Tissue distribution of mRNAs encoding muscarinic acetylcholine receptor subtypes. *FEBS Lett.* 1988; 239:339-342.

[68] Jooste E, Zhang Y, Emala CW. Rapacuronium preferentially antagonizes the function of M2 versus M3 muscarinic receptors in guinea-pig airway smooth muscle. *Anesthesiology* 2005;102:117-124.

[69] Joos GF. Potential usefulness of inhibiting neural mechanisms in asthma. *Monaldi. Arch. Chest Dis.* 2000;55:411-414.

[70] Ashkenazi A, Winslow JW, Peralta EG, et al. A single M2 muscarinic receptor subtype coupled to both adenylyl cyclase and phosphoinositide turnover. *Science* 1987;238:672-675.

[71] Tietje KM, Goldman PS, Nathanson NM. Cloning and functional analysis of a gene encoding a novel muscarinic acetylcholine receptor expressed in chick heart and brain. *J. Biol. Chem.* 1990;265:2828-2834.

[72] Katz A, Wu D, Simons MI. Subunits βγ of heterotrimetric G protein activate b2 isoform of phospholipase C. *Nature* 1992;360:686-689.

[73] Wickman K, Chapman DE. Ion channel regulation by G proteins. *Physiol. Rev.* 1995;75:865-885.

[74] Herlitze S, Garcia DE, Mackie K, Hille B, Scheuer T, Catterall WA. Modulation of Ca +2 channels by G protein beta gamma subunits. *Nature* 1996;380:258-262.

[75] Nemec J, Wickman K, Clapham DE. Gbetegamma binding increases the open time of IKAch: kinetic evidence for multiple Gbetagamma binding sites. *Biophys. J.* 1999;76:246-252.

[76] Nesti E, Everill B, Morielli AD. Endocytosis as a mechanism for tyrosine kinase-dependent suppression of a voltage-gated potassium channel. *Mol. Biol. Cell* 2004;15:4073-4488.

[77] Singh BB, Lockwich TP, Bandyopadhyay BC, et al. VAMP2-dependent exocytosis regulates plasma membrane insertion of TRPC3 channels and contributes to agonist-stimulated Ca+2 influx. *Mol. Cell* 2004;15:635-646.

[78] Cayouette S, Lussier MP, Mathieu EL, Bousquet SM, Boulay G. Exocytotic insertion of TRPC6 channel into the plasma membrane upon Gq protein-coupled receptor activation. *J. Biol. Chem.* 2004;279:7241-7246.

[79] Rudolf RD, Bulmer FMR. Some cardiac effects of atropine. *Am. J. Med. Sci.* 1924;168:641-653

[80] Nalefski LA, Brown CF. Action of atropine on the cardiovascular system in normal persons. *AMA Arch. Intern. Med.* 1950;86:898-907.
[81] Gravenstein JS, Ariet M, Thonby JI. Atropine on the electrocardiogram. *Clin. Pharmacol. Ther.* 1969;10:660-666.
[82] Brady WJ, Perron AD. Administration of atropine in the seting of acute myocardial infarction: potentiation of the ischemic process? *Am. J. Emerg. Med. 2001*;19:81-83.
[83] Brady WJ, Swart G, DeBehnke DJ, Ma OJ, Aufderheide TP. The efficacy of atropine in the treatment of hemodynamically unstable bradycardia and atrioventricular block: prehospital and emergency department considerations. *Resuscitation* 1999;41:47-55.
[84] Bisset JK, deSoyza N, Kane JJ, Smith NM. Improved sinus node sensing after atropine. *Am. Heart J.* 1976;91:752-756.
[85] Dhingra RC, Amat-y-Leon F, Wyndham C, Denes P, Wu D, Pouget JM, Rosen KM. Electrophysiological effects of atropine on human sinus node and atrium. *Am. J. Cardiol.* 1976;38:429-434.
[86] Dhingra RC, Amat-y-Leon F, Wyndham C, Denes P, Wu D, Miller RH, Rosen KM. Electrophysiological effects of atropine on sinus node and atrium in patients with sinus node dysfunction. *Am. J. Cardiol.* 1976;38:848-855.
[87] Knoebel SB, Mc Henry PL, Philips JF, et al. Atropine induced cardioacceleration and myocardial blood flow in subjects with and without coronary artery disease. *Am. J. Cardiol.* 1974;33:327-332.
[88] Sheinman MM, Hornburn DT, Abott JA. Use of atropine in patients with acute myocardial infarction and sinus bradycardia. *Circulation* 1975;52:627-633.
[89] Massumi RA, Mason DT, Amsterdam EA, et al. Ventricular fibrillation and tachycardia after intravenous atropine for treatment of bradycardia. *N. Engl. J. Med.* 1972;287:336-338.
[90] Cooper MJ, Abinder EG. Atropine induced ventricular fibrillation: Case report and review of the literature. *Am. Heart J.* 1979;97:225-228.
[91] Cooper JA, Frieden J. Atropine in the treatment of cardiac disease. *Am. Heart J.* 1969;78: 124-127
[92] Mc Guigan H. Effect of small doses of atropine on heart rate. *JAMA* 1921;76:1338-1341
[93] Averill KH, Lamb LE. Less commonly recognized actions of atropine on cardiac rhythm. *Am. J. Med. Sci.* 1959;237:304-318.
[94] Katona PG, Lipson D, Dauchot PJ. Opposing central and peripheral effects of atropine on parasympathetic cardiac control. *Am. J. Physiol.* 1977;232:H146-H151.
[95] Schweitzer P, Mark H. The effect of atropine on cardiac arrhythmias and conduction. Part 1. *Am. Heart J.* 1980;100:119-127.
[96] Ohuchi H, Hamamichi Y, Hayashi T. Negative chronotropic response to low-dose atropine is associated with parasympathetic nerve-mediated cardiovascular response in postoperative patients with congenital heart disease. *Int. J. Cardiol.* 2005;99:455-462.
[97] Chamberlain DA, Turner P, Sneddon JM. Effects of atropine on heart rate in healthy man. *Lancet* 1967;2:12-15.
[98] Severinghaus JW, Stupfel N. Respiratory dead space increase following atropine in man, and atropine vagal or ganglionic blockade and hypothermia in dogs. *J. Appl. Physiol.* 1955;8:81-87.

[99] De Troyer AJ, Yernault JC, Rodenstein D. Effects of vagal blockade on lung mechanics in normal man. *J. Appl. Physiol.* 1979;46:217-226.

[100] Chang KC, Hahn KH. Is a-adrenoceptor blockade responsible for atropine flush? *Eur. J. Pharmacol.* 1995;284:331-334.

[101] Robenshtok E, Luria S, Tashma Z, Hourvitz A. Adverse reaction to atropine and the treatment of organophosphate intoxication. *Isr. Med. Assoc. J.* 2002;4:535-539.

[102] Khavari KA, Maickel RP. Atropine and atropine methyl bromide effects on behavior of rats. *Int. J. Neuropharmacol.* 1967;6:301-306.

[103] Albanus L. Central and peripheral effects of anticholinergic compounds. *Acta Pharmacol. Toxicol.* 1970;28:305-326.

[104] Eisenberg MS, Mengert TJ. Cardiac resuscitation. *N. Engl. J. Med.* 2001;344: 1304-1313.

[105] Engdahl J, Bang A, Lindqvist J, Herlitz J. Can we define patients with no and those with some chance of survival when found in asystole out of hospital? *Am. J. Cardiol.* 2000;86:610-614.

[106] Tortolani AJ, Risucci DA, Powell SR, Dixon R. In-hospital cardiopulmonary resuscitation during asystole. Therapeutic factors associated with 24-hour survival. *Chest* 1989;96:622-626.

[107] Greenberg HM. Bradycardia at onset of sudden death: potential mechanisms. *Ann. NY Acad. Sci.* 1984;427:241-252.

[108] Iseri LT, Humphrey SB, Siner EJ. Prehospital brady-asystolic cardiac arrest. *Ann. Intern. Med.* 1978;88:741-745.

[109] Ornato J, Perberdy M. The mystery of bradyasystole during cardiac arrest. *Ann. Emerg. Med.* 1996;27:576-587.

[110] Bunch TJ, White RD. A simplified approach to the challenging problem of resuscitation of patients who present in pulseless electrical activity. *Crit. Care Med.* 2008;36:619-620.

[111] Nadkarni VM, Larkin GL, Peberdy MA, Carey SM, Kaye W, Mancini ME. First documented rhythm and clinical outcome from in-hospital cardiac arrest among children and adults. *JAMA* 2006;295:50-57.

[112] Gueugniaud PY, Mols P, Goldstein P, et al. A comparison of repeated high doses and repeated standard doses of epinephrine for cardiac arrest outside the hospital. *N. Engl. J. Med.* 1998;339:1595-1601.

[113] Steil IG, Herbert PC, Weitzman BN, et al. High-dose epinephrine in adult cardiac arrest. *N. Engl. J. Med.* 1992;327:1045-1050.

[114] Paradis NA, Martin GB, Goetting MG, et al. Aortic pressure during human cardiac arrest. Identification of pseudo-electromechanical dissociation. *Chest* 1992;101:123-128.

[115] Brown DC, Lewis AJ, Criley MJ. Asystole and its treatment:The possible role of the parasympathetic nervous system in cardiac arrest. *JACEP* 1979;8:448-452.

[116] Gupta PK, Lichstein E, Chadda KD. Transient atrioventricular standstill. *JAMA* 1975;234:1038-1042.

[117] Coon GA, Clinton JE, Ruiz E. Use of atropine for brady-asystolic prehospital cardiac arrest. *Ann. Emerg. Med.* 1981;10:462-467.

[118] Stueven HA, Tonsfeldt DJ, Thompson BM, Whitcomb J, Kastenson E, Aprahamian C. Atropine in asystole: Human studies. *Ann. Emerg. Med.* 1984;13:815-817.

[119] Rials SJ, Tse NW. Effects of atropine on the cardiac arrest induced by propanolol and digitoxin in dogs. *J. Electrocardiogr.* 1982;15:277-289.
[120] Kasten GW, Martin ST. Successful cardiovascular resuscitation after massive intravenous bupicavaine overdosage in anesthetized dogs. *Anesth. Analg.* 1985; 64:491-497.
[121] Blecic S, Chaskis C, Vincent JL. Atropine administration in experimental electromechanical dissociation. *Am. J. Emerg. Med.* 1992;10:515-518.
[122] Vanags B, Thakur RK, Stueven HA, Aufderheide TP, Tresch DD. Interventions in the therapy of electromechanical dissociation. *Resuscitation* 1989;17:163-171.
[123] Redding JS, Raleigh RR, Thomas JD. Drug therapy in resuscitation from electromechanical dissociation. *Crit. Care Med.* 1983;11:681-684.
[124] Stiell IG, Wells GA, Field B, et al. Advanced cardiac life support in out-of-hospital cardiac arrest. *N. Engl. J. Med.* 2004;351:647-656.
[125] Stiell IG, Wells GA, Hebert PC, Laupacis A, Weitzman BN. Association of drug therapy with survival in cardiac arrest: limited role of advanced cardiac life support drugs. *Acad. Emerg. Med.* 1995;2:264-273.
[126] Engdahl J, Bang A, Lindqvist J, Herlitz J. Factors affecting short- and long-term prognosis among 1069 patients with out-of-hospital cardiac arrest and pulseless electrical activity. *Resuscitation* 2001;51:17-25.
[127] Dumot JA, Burval DJ, Sprung J, et al. Outcome of adult cardiopulmonary resuscitations at a tertiary referral center including results of "limited" resuscitations. *Arch. Intern. Med.* 2001;161:1751-1758.
[128] Chadda KD, Lichstein E, Gupta PK, et al. Bradycardia-hypotension syndrome in acute myocardial infarction. *Am. J. Med.* 1975;59:158-164.
[129] Klein MD, Barret J, Ryan TJ, et al. Atropine dose in acute myocardial infarction in man. *Cardiol.* 1975;60:193-205.
[130] Sheiinman MM, Thorburn D, Abbot JA. Use of atropine in patients with acute myocardial infarction and sinus bradycardia. *Circulation* 1975;52:627-633.
[131] Chadda KD, Lichstein E, Gupta PK, et al. Effects of atropine in patients with bradyarrhythmia complicating myocardial infarction. Usefulness of an optimum dose for overdrive. *Am. J. Med.* 1977:63:503-510.
[132] Carp C, Campeanu A, Plesea O, et al. Beneficial and adverse effects of atropine in patients with acute myocardial infarction. *Med. Intern.* 1979;17:9-22.
[133] Fiegl D, Ashkenazy J, kishon Y. Early and late atrioventricular block in acute inferior myocardial infarction. *J. Am. Col. Cardiol.* 1984;4:35-38.
[134] Stuckey JG. Arrhythmias in the prehospital phase of acute myocardial infarction. *Med. J. Austr.* 1973;2:29-32.
[135] Warren JV, Lewis RP. Beneficial effects of atropine in the prehospital phase of coronary care. *Am. J. Cardiol.* 1976;37:68-72.
[136] Antman EM, Anbe DT, Armstrong PW, et al. ACC/AHA Guidelines for the management of patients with ST-elevation myocardial infarction. *Circulation* 2004;110:588-636

[137] Emergency Cardiac Care Committee and Subcommittees, American Heart Association. Guidelines for cardiopulmonary resuscitation and emergency cardiac care. *J. Am. Med. Assoc.* 1992;268:2171-2302.

[138] Richman S. Adverse effect of atropine during myocardial infarction. *JAMA* 1974;228:1414-1416.

In: Drugs in Cardiopulmonary Resuscitation
Editor: Theodoros Xanthos

ISBN: 978-1-61122-512-9

Chapter 4

Amiodarone, Magnesium and Calcium in Cardiac Arrest

Konstantinos Stroumpoulis
University of Athens, Medical School, Greece

Abstract

Despite the use of vasopressors in cardiopulmonary resuscitation (CPR), hospital discharge rates for both in-hospital and out-of hospital cardiac arrest (CA) remain dismal. Therefore, the use of antiarrhythmic agents with potential beneficial effects in CA such as amiodarone and magnesium, and ions with substantial effects in cardiac mechanics, such as calcium, is investigated in the international literature.

Amiodarone has been found to increase survival to hospital admission in shock-refractory ventricular fibrillation (VF). Current guidelines recommend it as the antiarrhythmic of choice in refractory VF/pulseless ventricular tachycardia (VT).

On the other hand, the routine administration of magnesium and calcium during CA failed to show any benefit and therefore it is not advocated by current guidelines. Magnesium is only recommended for the treatment of shock-refractory VF in the presence of possible hypomagnesemia or torsades de pointes.

The recommendations for calcium administration in CA are limited only to pulseless electrical activity (PEA) when specific reversible causes (hypokalemia, hypocalcemia, calcium-channel blockers overdose) need to be treated. However, these treatment recommendations are based on evidence provided by trials performed following resuscitation strategies according to previous guidelines. Data from studies implementing the 2005 International Liaison Committee on Resuscitation (ILCOR) guidelines are necessary in order to better evaluate the efficacy of these agents in CA.

Introduction

Early CPR and early defibrillation significantly improve the likelihood of successful resuscitation from CA as advocated by the American Heart Association (AHA) and the

European Resuscitation Council (ERC) guidelines [1,2]. However, despite the use of vasopressors as adjuncts to CPR, hospital discharge rates for both in-hospital and out-of hospital CA remain dismal [3-6].

Therefore research in CPR, beside other interventions, was also oriented towards pharmacologic agents that were thought to be helpful through their antiarrhytmhic effects or their participation in key pathophysiological pathways.

Among those, amiodarone, magnesium and calcium occupy a significant amount of the international literature; amiodarone for its potent antiarrhythmic effects, magnesium for its antiarrhythmic and electrophysiological effects, and calcium for its crucial role in cardiac contractility, vascular tone and activation of pathophysiological pathways. These 3 agents and their role in CA will be the focus of this chapter.

Amiodarone

The use of antiarrhythmic agents is not new in the treatment protocols of CA [7,8]. The observation that premature ventricular complexes could frequently degenerate to VF in the coronary care unit [9] led to the widespread use of such agents (lidocaine, bretylium, magnesium, amiodarone) to suppress these "warning arrhythmias".

The next logical step was to use these agents as a treatment for arrhythmias in the CA setting. However, there is no evidence that the administration of any antiarrhythmic given routinely during CA increases survival to hospital discharge [1,10].

On the contrary, most antiarrhythmic medications increase the defibrillation threshold [11-16] and, theoretically, make successful defibrillation less possible. On the other hand, only one antiarrhythmic agent, amiodarone, has been found to improve short-term survival to hospital admission [17,18].

Amiodarone, an iodine-containing compound, having structural similarities to thyroxine, was developed in 1961 [19-21]. Amiodarone is lipid-soluble and concentrates in fat, muscle, liver, lungs and skin. Its high lipid solubility leads to a high volume of distribution and an unusually long elimination half-life, averaging 58 days (ranging from 10 to 103 days) [22,23]. Amiodarone is metabolized in the liver and its excretion is hepatic and biliary [21,24].

Mechanism of Action

Amiodarone possesses a wide spectrum of complex electrophysiological properties, which have not yet been completely understood. Amiodarone is categorized as a class III antiarrhythmic agent [25], prolonging the refractory period via the action potential [26].

However, this intriguing agent has several additional electrophysiological activities: it binds to sodium channels (Class IA action), it is a non-competitive beta-blocker (Class II action) and it is a (weak) calcium channel blocker (Class IV action) [21,25].

Through this multitude of actions, amiodarone prolongs action potential and refractoriness, slows atrioventricular contraction and impedes the occurrence of malignant arrhythmias.

Amiodarone in CA

After the evidence provided from several anecdotal cases and small uncontrolled studies [27-38] about amiodarone's efficacy (the reported success rates in these studies ranged from 50% to 75%) in the treatment of malignant ventricular arrhythmias, its effects were assessed in CPR trials. The assumption, therefore, was that amiodarone would be of benefit in patients with arrhythmias who can not be adequately suppressed during CPR.

Clinical Data

In 1988, a small randomized trial in Germany found that more patients treated with amiodarone were successfully resuscitated in comparison to those treated with lidocaine [39)]. In 1989, another small study reported that 11 of 14 patients in prolonged CA with recurrent VT or VF (in all patients resuscitative efforts were undertaken for at least 30 min) benefited from amiodarone administration in obtaining stable perfusing rhythm and 8 of them were discharged [40].

In 1995, 2 studies in 342 and 302 patients, respectively, reported a significant dose-related increase in the time to first event when intravenous amiodarone was administered in patients presenting with recurrent, life-threatening ventricular tachyarrhythmias or VF [26,41]. These 2 studies concluded that high-dose amiodarone (1000 mg/24 h) significantly decreased the recurrence rate of tachyarrhythmias.

To this conclusion concurred another trial (273 patients), in 1996, reporting a significant difference in the time to first recurrence of ventricular tachyarrhythmia when high-dose groups (1050 mg/24 h and 2100 mg/24 h) were compared with a 525 mg/24 h dose group [42].

Even though the abovementioned studies provided encouraging results, the reported data can not be uniformly interpreted because the majority of these studies were non-randomized, underpowered and they were not exclusively focused on CA; patients with a pulse (nevertheless suffering from tachyarrhythmia) were assessed with patients in CA. Therefore, the effectiveness of intravenous amiodarone for the treatment of refractory VT/VF was not established. This gap was partially filled by 2 studies [17,18]. In 1999, a randomized, double-blind, placebo-controlled trial, the ARREST trial, evaluated the administration of intravenous amiodarone or placebo in 504 patients with out-of-hospital CA, after receiving 3 or more unsuccessful shocks. The authors reported that amiodarone resulted in a statistically higher rate of survival to hospital admission (44% vs 34%, $p<0.03$), although no difference was reported regarding hospital discharge [17].

The same conclusions about amiodarone's efficacy were drown, in 2002, in another prospective, randomized, blinded trial, the ALIVE trial, comparing amiodarone and lidocaine in 347 patients with refractory out-of-hospital CA. Patients were randomized to either an initial 5 mg/kg bolus dose of amiodarone followed by a second 2.5 mg/kg if necessary or an initial 1.5 mg/kg bolus dose of lidocaine, repeated once if necessary. Compared to lidocaine, amiodarone led to significantly higher rates of survival to hospital admission (23% vs 11%, $p<0.005$) [18]. Even though this study was not powered to detect changes to hospital discharge rates, nevertheless, no difference was observed.

Experimental Data

Animal studies also advocate for a beneficial role of amiodarone in refractory VF and CA [43,44]. Evidence suggests that amiodarone can not replace a vasopressor and that it should always be administered with one, otherwise the resulting coronary perfusion pressure (CPP) is significantly lower [44].

Adverse Effects

All the aforementioned clinical trials report hypotension as a major adverse effect of amiodarone [17,18,26,41,42]. In clinical trials, this phenomenon appears in more than 20% of the cases [17,45] and usually requires medical intervention [26,41,42,46]. As mentioned before, amiodarone is highly lipid soluble; hence 2 chemicals were used to solubilize the pharmacologic substance. These chemicals (polysorbate 80 and benzyl alcohol) are known to exhibit negative inotropy, hypotension [47-51], and induce histamine release [52]. Furthermore, the development of hypotension was not dose related but related to the rate of drug administration [46]. The development of a new aqueous form of amiodarone seems to minimize these adverse effects even when administered rapidly, without altering the drug's efficacy [45,53]. The new form of amiodarone exhibited same rates (2%) of drug related hypotension with significantly better VT termination rates and 24-hour survival rates compared to lidocaine [45,53].

Amiodarone is also thought to have proarrhythmic effects. Bradycardia, asystole, and atrioventricular block have been reported after its use, however the do not seem to occur with greater frequency than in patients on other antiarrhythmics [17,18,26,41,42,46,54,55].

Another known adverse effect of intravenous amiodarone administration is thrombophlebitis, especially when peripheral veins are used for drug administration (incidence ranges from 8% to 25%) [46,56,57]. Aqueous amiodarone seems to have a lower incidence of thrombophlebitis [45].

Treatment Recommendations

Until the publication of the 2000 ILCOR, guidelines lidocaine was the antiarrhytmhic drug of choice [7,8]. Based on the abovementioned evidence, in the "Guidelines 2000 for Cardiopulmonary Resuscitation and Emergency Cardiovascular Care" amiodarone received a Class IIb evidence for treatment of recurrent VF/pulseless VT whereas the evidence of favor of lidocaine was classified as "indeterminate" [58].

In 2005, both AHA [1] and ERC [2] guidelines refer to amiodarone as the antiarrhythmic drug of choice in refractory VF/VT and the use of lidocaine is restricted to only when amiodarone is unavailable.

AHA guidelines advocate: "*When VF/pulseless VT persists after 2 to 3 shocks plus CPR and administration of a vasopressor, consider an antiarrhythmic such as amiodarone……. An initial dose of 300mg IV/IO can be followed by one dose of 150 mg IV/IO*" [1]. ERC guidelines recommend: "*Consider an initial intravenous dose of 300 mg amiodarone, diluted in 5% dextrose to a volume of 20 ml if VF/VT persists after the third shock.........a further dose of 150mg may be given...*" [2].

Future Research Directions

Amiodarone was administered in all the aforementioned studies if VF/VT persisted after at least three shocks; however these were delivered using the conventional three-stacked shocks strategy and under a different compression to ventilation ratio [17,18,45,53] than the 30:2 currently advocated [1,2]. Furthermore, there is a complete lack of data on the use of amiodarone in shock-refractory VF/VT when the sequence shock-CPR-shock-CPR is used. Therefore, there is no actual evidence as to when amiodarone should be administered under the current guidelines. In addition to the above, the strategy of administering amiodarone much later (3 CPR cycles = approximately 5-6 min) than the time it was actually administered in trials should probably be reexamined. New experimental and clinical trials are necessary in order to assess amiodarone's efficacy under the current guidelines.

Lastly, current evidence [59-63] suggests that VF response to therapies is time-dependent. A 3-phase model of VF evolution has been proposed: 1) the electrical phase (up to 4 min after CA onset), which responds better to immediate defibrillation, 2) the circulatory (or hemodynamic) phase (4-10 min post-CA), where administration of vasopressors is necessary for attaining CPP threshold levels and 3) the metabolic phase (after 10 min) where extensive cellular damage end endotoxin release limit the efficacy of pharmacologic interventions [59]. Therefore, a delayed administration of amiodarone could occur in the metabolic phase limiting thus the beneficial effects of this promising agent.

Furthermore, given the extremely long half-life of amiodarone [21], the possibility of interactions between amiodarone and post-resuscitative pharmacologic management can not be excluded. More specifically, this question should be addressed in the light of the data showing only a benefit to hospital admission rates and not to hospital discharge rates from amiodarone administration in refractory VF/VT [17,18].

Magnesium

Magnesium (Mg) is the second most abundant intracellular cation in the human organism [64-67]. About 60% of Mg is found in the skeleton, 39% in the intracellular space (20% in skeletal muscle) and only 1% of total body Mg is found as circulating extracellular Mg [64,65,68]. This circulating Mg is found in three forms: I) anion-complexed (to sulphate or to phosphate); II) protein-bound and III) ionized, which is the physiologically active form [66] and the most reflective of the intracellular Mg concentration [69-71].

Mechanism of Action

Mg is important in several basic physiological energy demanding processes, including muscle contraction, oxidative phosphorylation, neuromuscular excitability, cell membrane permeability and mitochondrial function [64,72-77]. Furthermore, concerning heart, Mg levels have an effect on both cellular and electrophysiological level, possessing both antiarrhythmic and vasodilatory actions [78].

On cellular level, Mg acts as a coenzyme for membrane-bound sodium-potassium adenosine triphosphatase (Na^+-K^+-ATPase) [64,79]. Mg may also affect calcium fluxes over the cell membrane by blocking both receptor-mediated and voltage-dependent calcium channels, inhibiting thus calcium influx into myocytes [80-82].

In addition to the above, Mg also competes with calcium for intracellular and extracellular sites of the cell membrane [79], and it is therefore regarded as "nature's physiologic calcium blocker" [81]. These effects lead to muscle relaxation and vasodilation on the coronary and peripheral arterial systems [68,83-86].

Furthermore, Mg may play a role in the maintenance of the normal resting membrane potential, either by blocking the slow calcium channels [81] or by facilitating the flow through the inward rectifying potassium channel [84,85,87]. Lastly, Mg has been shown to inhibit platelet aggregation. This effect is probably mediated through calcium influx blockade and inhibition of thromboxane synthesis [88].

On electrophysiological level, Mg exhibits several actions: it prolongs atrioventricular conduction time, action potential duration, and the effective refractory period, suppressing thus automaticity [80]. It also increases the energy required to induce premature ventricular contractions in experimental models [89].

On the other hand, Mg deficiency has been associated with dysrhythmias [67,90,91], ischemic heart disease and hypertension [92], respiratory muscle weakness [93], and other electrolytes disturbances [67,90]. Mg deficiency may inhibit Na^+-K^+-ATPase pump function and cause accumulation of intracellular sodium and a loss of intracellular potassium, decreasing, thus, the intracellular–to-extracellular potassium ratio. This leads to a decrease of the resting membrane potential and an increase of the Purkinje fiber excitability with consequent arrhythmia [64,79].

Furthermore, laboratory studies have associated Mg deficiency with a lack of endothelium-dependent coronary artery relaxation [94], increase of proinflamatory cytokines [95], free radical injury [96], and death from endotoxin challenge [97].

In addition to the above, Mg deficiency is associated with critical illness in both adults [67,90,98] and children [99,100] and has been found to participate in a multitude of cardiovascular, respiratory, neurological, and metabolic abnormalities seen in this context [67,75,90,92,98,100].

Causes of hypomagnesemia are not rare and may be encountered in many clinical settings. Patients under chronic diuretic therapy for hypertension may use thiazide or loop diuretics which have been associated with potassium and magnesium deficiencies, arrhythmias and sudden death [101,102]. Other causes include digoxin or aminoglycoside therapy, advanced age, diabetes, alcoholism and malabsorption [103,104]. Hypomagnesemia can therefore be often associated with hypokalemia and may contribute to arrhythmias and CA [2,105].

The abovementioned well-known electrophysiological effects of Mg along with the fact that normal concentrations are required to maintain normal cardiac conduction have led to the use of Mg sulphate in the treatment of cardiac arrhythmias related to hypomagnesemia or to torsades de pointes tachycardia [2,106-109]. Therefore, its use in torsades de pointes is not the focus if this chapter.

Magnesium in Acute Myocardial Infarction

Despite its aforementioned effects, the routine use of Mg in both acute myocardial infarction (AMI) and CA is contentious. Although one could anticipate that Mg administration would have beneficial effects in patients suffering from AMI, as early findings indicated [83,110], large studies have shown that intravenous Mg sulphate neither had any electrophysiological effect in patients with life-threatening arrhythmias nor did it decrease the incidence of ventricular arrhythmias [111-116].

Respectively, regarding survival, whereas the first sufficient size study, the LIMIT-2, including 2316 patients [111], in agreement with smaller previous studies [115,117], reported that patients assigned Mg had higher survival rates than those assigned placebo, a latter larger (58050 patients) study, the ISIS-4, reported that Mg administration in AMI did not affect mortality or the incidence of CA [116].

However, because of the different design settings and time of initiation of Mg therapy and dosage, the question as to whether Mg is beneficial in AMI has not yet been completely answered.

Magnesium in Cardiac Arrest

Mg Concentration

Serum Mg concentration has been correlated with the outcome of CA in clinical studies [118,119]. Normomagnesemia was associated with improved resuscitation rates, although it could not be determined whether it was causally related to improved outcome or it is a surrogate indicator for other factors. For example, hypomagnesemia may be indicative of increased diuretic use in patients with severe heart failure, who would be at higher risk of poor outcome after CA [118,119].

Since Mg acts as a calcium antagonist that inhibits calcium influx, it may prevent coronary spasm by vasodilation [120-123]. In the CA setting of global ischemia, experimental models show that Mg administration improves the contractile response of the stunned myocardium, limits infarct size [124] and reduces free radical concentration [125,126].

Furthermore, in case of successful resuscitation, the reperfusion following myocardial ischemia results in detrimental cytoplasmic calcium overload [127-129], which can probably be attenuated by Mg. These effects in combination with the Mg-mediated inhibition of platelet aggregation indicate that Mg may be a cardioprotective agent against myocardial reperfusion injury [130-132].

Mg administration in the same setting has been found to prevent cerebral hypoperfusion for a prolonged time during CA [133,134]. However, whether these actions are solely mediated by calcium channel blockage or other mechanisms remains to be fully elucidated.

Experimental Studies

The literature concerning the use of Mg in experimental models of CA is very limited. However, the few existing animal studies did not show any encouraging results regarding return of Spontaneous Circulation (ROSC) and survival.

Mg Administration before Cardiac Arrest

Mg administration before and during CA has been evaluated in animal studies. There are two experimental studies that evaluated Mg's effects before CA. In a rat model of hypoxia-induced CA [135], Mg given in the first minutes of hypoxia improved left ventricular pressures and immediate recovery after hypoxia. The author suggested that the possible Mg sulphate effect was an antiarrhythmic action and, possibly, myocardial relaxation during and after hypoxia. However, 7-day survival rates did not differ between Mg and control groups. Another experimental study of hyperkalemic CA in rats, despite a reported trend in improved respiratory function (possibly corroborating the observation that Mg relaxes smooth muscle tone), did not show any difference in survival times between groups (136). Although Mg displayed some potentially beneficial effects in these animal studies, it did not affect survival, leaving thus a large field of research to be explored concerning, first of all, the necessity and then the appropriate dosage and timing of Mg pretreatment.

Mg Administration during Cardiac Arrest

A VF swine model study [137] reported that the administration of Mg with epinephrine appeared to have a negative effect on aortic pressures and CPP during CPR indicating a vasodilating action of Mg. Another swine model study comparing a drug cocktail with Mg and standard advanced cardiac life support (ACLS) [138] failed to find any differences in ROSC and one-hour survival between Mg and standard ACLS.

Clinical Data

Case Reports

There are several cases (both in-hospital and out-of-hospital) reported in the international literature where refractory VF responded only to intravenous Mg administration (followed by defibrillation) [139-142]. Some of these cases where impressive, reporting restoration of spontaneous circulation and long-term complete neurologic recovery, occurring in CA victims who underwent more than one hour of CPR efforts [140,141]. In all these cases, Mg was used after all the ACLS medications were used. Dosages in these case reports varied greatly, ranging from 2 g [139] to 4 g [140] or even 8 g [141].

Clinical Trials

Under the light of the evidence provided by anecdotal cases, several studies were undertaken in order to elucidate the usefulness of Mg in sustained VF.

In 1995, a prospective cohort study including 62 CA victims found a trend toward increased resuscitation rates with Mg (2.5-5 g) use, accompanied by a trend toward post-ROSC hypotension, necessitating vasopressor support [143].

In 1997, a randomized, placebo controlled trial (MAGIC trial) failed to show any benefit to the rate of successful resuscitation, survival to 24h, survival to hospital discharge or Glasgow coma score, from Mg (2 g) administration in 156 patients with in-hospital CA [80]. Likewise in 1997, high dose Mg (5 g) was not associated with a significantly improved survival in an out of hospital CA study [144].

In 2001, another randomized, prospective, double blind, placebo controlled trial, enrolling 156 prehospital CA patients presenting with VF, failed to demonstrate that the administration of Mg sulphate (2 g) improved short or long-term survival [145]. Lastly, a study, in 2002, using the same study design, failed to show any benefit from early Mg (2-4 g) administration neither to ROSC nor to hospital discharge rates [146].

Mg infusion after ROSC has, also, been evaluated by two trials. In the MAGIC trial [80], patients who were treated with Mg and attained ROSC were given an 8 g infusion of Mg sulphate over 24 hours. There was not found any difference in any subgroup analysis between Mg and placebo. A randomized out-of-hospital CA trial [147], evaluating the infusion of Mg, diazepam or both, immediately after ROSC, failed to prove any significant improvement in neurologic outcome from CA, when using these agents.

Potential Adverse Effects of Magnesium Administration in Cardiac Arrest

It is well known that the single overriding determinant for successful defibrillation in VF is the CPP [148,149]. The restoration of adequate CPP threshold levels is the aim of chest compressions and vasopressor use in resuscitation efforts. The effects of epinephrine, the recommended vasopressor in CPR [1,2], are mostly mediated through alpha-2 adrenergic receptors which are calcium channels [150-153]. Therefore, Mg which inhibits the passage of calcium through voltage-gated calcium channels would attenuate epinephrine's effects and efficacy, as the abovementioned experimental [137] and clinical data indicate [143].

Treatment Recommendations for Mg Use in Cardiac Arrest

Based on the aforementioned data, both AHA and ERC latest (2005) guidelines state that Mg should not be routinely used in CA [1,2].

More specifically, AHA guidelines state: "*Magnesium can be considered for torsades de pointes (Class IIa recommendation), but it is not effective for treatment of cardiac arrest from other causes.*" Also, "*When VF/pulseless VT is associated with torsades de pointes, providers may administer magnesium sulphate at a dose of 1 to 2 g diluted in 10 ml D_5W IV/IO push, typically over 5 to 20 minutes.*" ERC proposes to "*give magnesium (8mmol=4ml 50% magnesium or 2g) for refractory VF if there is any suspicion of hypomagnesemia……ventricular tachyarrhythmias in the presence of possible hypomagnesaemia, torsades de pointes and digoxin toxicity*". The recommended dose is "*2 g of 50% magnesium sulphate given peripherally over 1-2 min; it may be repeated after 10-15 min*".

Limitations in the Interpretation of the Available Data

Previous Guidelines

All the available data come either from cases [139-142] or studies [80,143-146] who took place before the release of the ILCOR 2005 guidelines. Therefore, the effects of Mg after an increased compression/ventilation ratio CPR (30/2 vs. 15/2) [1,2,58] with fewer interruptions in CPR time have not been evaluated.

Furthermore, the difference in cardiac mechanics and biochemistry between 3 consecutive defibrillations and the new 2 min CPR-shock-2min CPR-shock sequence has not yet been assessed in view of Mg's actions.

Dosage, Timing, Arrest Rhythms

As abovementioned, both the experimental [125,135,137,138] and the clinical [80,143-145] studies were conducted using different Mg dosages.

Furthermore, the timing of drug administration ranged from 10 to more than 25 minutes and in some trials patients with different initial arrest rhythms (even non-shockable) were included [80,144].

Mg Concentration

As abovementioned, serum Mg accounts only for 1% of total Mg and its ionized form is the most reflective of the intracellular Mg concentration [67,69-71]. Serum Mg may also fluctuate whereas intracellular levels may remain stable [64].

On the other hand, critically ill adults [67,97] and children [99] have been shown to exhibit low ionized Mg concentration with or without a deficiency in total serum Mg. It is therefore difficult to identify patients with hypomagnesemia without measuring ionized Mg. In addition to all that, none of the aforementioned studies measured ionized Mg.

Since hypokalemia is a common concomitant of hypomagnesemia [2,23,105], perhaps, hypokalemic patients should also be targeted for treatment.

Calcium

Calcium is an extracellular cation and the most abundant mineral in the human body, deposited for the greater part in the bone skeleton [1,65]. Approximately 50% of the extracellular calcium is bound to albumin and the remaining 50% is in the biologically active, ionized form [2,154]. Ideally, in the CA setting, the ionized fraction should be measured, because serum calcium concentration does not correlate well with ionized concentration in critically ill patients (155,156). A multitude of processes depend on intracellular calcium such as enzymatic reactions, muscle contraction, cardiac contractility, platelet aggregation, surfactant production, neurotransmission, spermatozoid motility [65]. It should not be forgotten that calcium is also essential for neuromuscular function and bone strength [1].

Calcium's Actions in the Cardiovascular System

Although the extracellular concentration of calcium ions does not affect skeletal muscle contractility, it plays a vital role in the contraction of smooth muscle cells. Indeed, extracellular calcium uptake leads to smooth muscle contraction, whereas smooth muscle relaxation is performed through calcium excretion from the myocytes and calcium uptake towards the sarcoplasmic reticulum through calcium pumps in both cases [157-162].

When the action potential is propagated through the cell membrane of myocytes, it is also propagated to the membranes of the T-tubules causing the immediate release of calcium ions from the sarcoplasmic reticulum deposits towards the sarcoplasm of the muscle fibre. Then, the calcium ions are dispersed to the myofibrils where they are catalyzing actin and myosin movement, promoting thus muscular contraction. In cardiac myocytes contraction however, there is an extra amount of calcium, provided by the T-tubules during the action potential. The contraction force of cardiac muscle depends largely in extracellular calcium concentrations because the distal ends of the T-tubules are open towards the outside of myocardial fibres; hence the extracellular fluid penetrates the T-tubules. Therefore, the availability of calcium ions for cardiac muscle contraction depends on their extracellular concentration [10,65,163-165]. Hence, calcium plays a vital role in cardiac contractility and systemic vascular resistance.

Furthermore, calcium is an important factor in coagulation processes. Calcium is essential for the activation of factors IX and X and for the transformation of prothrombin to thrombin [65].

Rationale of Calcium Use in CPR

Evidence that calcium increases myocardial contractility and prolongs systole dates back to 1882, when Ringer reported that calcium had an inotropic effect on cardiac contractility [166]. That evidence was further supported by later data [10,65,163-165]. Clinical support was added in 1951, when the administration of calcium chloride successfully reversed asystole in 4 paediatric patients during cardiac surgery [167]. Hence, until the early 80's, calcium chloride administration was advocated by AHA for the treatment of patients with either asystole or PEA [168].

Calcium during CA

Whereas experimental studies [169-171] give contradictory results as to whether ionized hypocalcemia occurs during CPR, clinical studies have demonstrated that ionized hypocalcemia can occur in CA [155,172-174] and it is probably time-dependent [155,172]. It comes as a result of the increase in the intracellular calcium and it is associated with ischemia and reperfusion [127,175-180]. Possible mechanisms have been described [175,176,179] but the complete aetiology for this effect remains to be elucidated. Hypoxia and ischemia cause ATP depletion and suppress Na^+-K^+-ATPase pump, causing, thus, an accumulation of intracellular sodium and a loss of intracellular potassium. Intracellular sodium increase leads to intracellular calcium increase mediated by the sodium calcium exchange mechanism. The increased extracellular potassium leads to depolarization which affects the voltage-dependent calcium channels, facilitating thus a calcium influx and further enhancing the intracellular calcium increase [176]. Furthermore, catecholamine stimulation during CA can lead to an up-regulation of adrenergic receptors [181], which in turn induce an increase in calcium uptake [182,183]. Besides, the energy depletion leads to malfunction of the calcium pump in the sarcoplasmic reticulum with consequent calcium release and further increase of calcium's intracellular levels [175,176,179]. Other studies postulate that hypocalcemia in CA may be due primarily to extracellular complexing of calcium to iactate generated by anaerobic metabolism [155,184].

Intracellular calcium increase has some potential deleterious adverse effects on cardiac and cerebral resuscitation, since it is implicated in ischemic injury, cell death and post-anoxic tissue damage [175,185-187]. Calcium overload may also enhance coronary vasospasm and induce arrhythmias in patients with digitalis toxicity [188].

Even though the aforementioned studies leave some questions unanswered, they may however lead to a significant conclusion. The observed ionized hypocalcemia in CA is probably most of the times not causally related to CA, but it comes as a result of the CA and it is more pronounced as the arrest continues. Therefore, it is doubtful whether victims of CA would benefit from routine calcium administration, especially if one would take into account that intracellular calcium levels are already increased in this setting and that a calcium treatment would probably further accentuate cellular damage harming thus the ischemic myocardium and impairing cerebral recovery [1,2,189].

Experimental and Clinical Data

Animal studies have failed to show any benefit from calcium chloride administration in asystole or PEA [190,191]. Likewise, clinical trials in CA setting have shown no benefit from calcium administration [10,192,193]. The largest of these studies, a prospective cohort study [10], found, while controlling for significant patient factors and arrest factors, a significant association between unsuccessful resuscitation and the use of calcium (among other medications such as epinephrine).

Treatment Recommendations

Current (2005) guidelines do not support the routine use of calcium chloride during CA (AHA,ERC). More precisely, guidelines advocate for a very cautious use in very specific settings. AHA guidelines state: "*calcium should not be used routinely to support circulation in the setting of cardiac arrest. When hyperkalemia, ionized hypocalcemia (e.g., after multiple blood transfusions), or calcium channel blocker toxicity is present, use of calcium is probably helpful*" [1].

ERC guidelines state: "*Give calcium during resuscitation only when indicated specifically, i.e. in pulseless electrical activity caused by hyperkalaemia, hypocalcaemia, overdose of calcium channel-blocking drugs*" [2].

The recommended dose by the international organisms is 5-10 ml of a 10% calcium chloride solution.

Conclusion

Despite the encouraging results provided by early reports concerning amiodarone, magnesium and calcium in CA, only amiodarone administration seems to be of benefit in CA. The routine use of magnesium and calcium in CA is not recommended. Furthermore, the cases in which calcium has an indication for use in CA seem to be very limited and difficult to identify. However, all the available data come from studies following completely different resuscitation strategies than those advocated by current (2005) guidelines. Especially amiodarone and magnesium should be reevaluated in trials following new guidelines.

References

[1] American Heart Association Guidelines for cardiopulmonary resuscitation and emergency cardiovascular care. *Circulation* 2005;112(Suppl. IV):IV1-121.

[2] Nolan JP, Deakin CD, Soar J, Bottiger BW, Smith G. European Resuscitation Council Guidelines for Resuscitation 2005. Section 4. Adult advanced life support. *Resuscitation* 2005;67:S39-S86.

[3] Gueugniaud PY, David JS, Chanzy E, Hubert H, Dubien PY, Mauriaucourt P, Bragança C, Billères X, Clotteau-Lambert MP, Fuster P, Thiercelin D, Debaty G, Ricard-Hibon A, Roux P, Espesson C, Querellou E, Ducros L, Ecollan P, Halbout L, Savary D, Guillaumée F, Maupoint R, Capelle P, Bracq C, Dreyfus P, Nouguier P, Gache A, Meurisse C, Boulanger B, Lae C, Metzger J, Raphael V, Beruben A, Wenzel V, Guinhouya C, Vilhelm C, Marret E. Vasopressin and epinephrine vs. epinephrine alone in cardiopulmonary resuscitation. *N. Engl. J. Med.* 2008;359:21-30.

[4] Gueugniaud PY, Mols P, Goldstein P, Pham E, Dubien PY, Deweerdt C, Vergnion M, Petit P, Carli P. A comparison of repeated high doses and repeated standard doses of epinephrine for cardiac arrest outside the hospital. European Epinephrine Study Group. *N. Engl. J. Med.* 1998;339:1595-601.

[5] Bobrow BJ, Clark LL, Ewy GA, Chikani V, Sanders AB, Berg RA, Richman PB, Kern KB. Minimally interrupted cardiac resuscitation by emergency medical services for out-of-hospital cardiac arrest. *JAMA* 2008;299:1158-1165.

[6] Ong ME, Tan EH, Ng FS, Panchalingham A, Lim SH, Manning PG, Ong VY, Lim SH, Yap S, Tham LP, Ng KS, Venkataraman A; Cardiac Arrest and Resuscitation Epidemiology Study Group. Survival outcomes with the introduction of intravenous epinephrine in the management of out-of-hospital cardiac arrest. *Ann. Emerg. Med.* 2007;50:635-642.

[7] Guidelines for advanced life support: A statement by the Advanced Life Support Working Party of the European Resuscitation Council, 1992. *Resuscitation* 1992;24:111-121.

[8] Cummins RO ed, *Advanced Cardiac Life Support*. Dallas, TX: American Heart Association, 1997:1-17.

[9] Lown B, Fakhro AM, Hood WB, Thorn GW. The coronary care unit, new perspectives and directions. *JAMA* 1967;199:188-198.

[10] van Walraven C, Stiell IG, Wells GA, Hébert PC, Vandemheen K. Do advanced cardiac life support drugs increase resuscitation rates from in-hospital cardiac arrest? The OTAC Study Group. *Ann. Emerg. Med.* 1998;32:544-553.

[11] Babbs CF, Yim GKW, Whistler SJ, Tacker WA, Geddes LA. Elevation of ventricular defibrillation threshold in dogs by antiarrhythmic drugs. *Am. Heart J.* 1979;98:345-350.

[12] Yoon MS, Han J, Goel BG, Creamer P. Effect of procainamide on fibrillation threshold of normal and ischemic ventricles. *Am. J. Cardiol.* 1974;33:238-242.

[13] Echt DS, Black JN, Barbey JT, Coxe DR, Cato E. Evaluation of antiarrhythmic drugs on defibrillation energy requirements in dogs: sodium channel block and action potential prolongation. *Circulation* 1989;76:1106-1117.

[14] Kerber RE, Pandian NG, Jensen SR, et al. Effect of lidocaine and bretylium on energy requirements for transthoracic defibrillation: experimental studies. *J. Am. Coll. Cardiol.* 1986;7:397-405.

[15] Dorian P, Fain ES, Davy JM, Winkle RA. Lidocaine causes a reversible, concentration-dependent increase in defibrillation energy requirements. *J. Am. Coll. Cardiol.* 1986;8:327-332.

[16] Tacker WA, Niebauer JM, Baggs CF, et al. The effect of new antiarrhythmic drugs on defibrillation threshold. *Crit. Care Med.* 1980;8:177-180.

[17] Kudenchuk PJ, Cobb LA, Copass MK, et al. Amiodarone for resuscitation after out-of-hospital cardiac arrest due to ventricular fibrillation. *N. Engl. J. Med.* 1999;341:871-878.

[18] Dorian P, Cass D, Schwartz B, Cooper R, Gelaznikas R, Barr A. Amiodarone as compared with lidocaine for shock-resistant ventricular fibrillation. *N. Engl. J. Med.* 2002;346:884-890.

[19] Deltour G, Binon F, Tondeur R, et al. Studies in the benzofuran series. VI. Coronary-dilating activity of alkylated and aminoalkylated derivatives of 3-benzoylbenzofuran. *Arch. Int. Pharmacodyn. Ther.* 1962;139:247-254.

[20] Charlier R, Deltour G, Tondeur R, Binon F. Studies in the benzofuran series. VII. Preliminary pharmacological study of 2-butyl-3-(3,5-diiodo-4-beta-N-diethylaminoethoxybenzoyl)-benzofuran. *Arch. Int. Pharmacodyn. Ther.* 1962;139:255-264.

[21] Siddoway LA. Amiodarone: guidelines for use and monitoring. *Am. Fam. Physician.* 2003;68:2189-2196.

[22] *Physicians' desk reference*. 56th ed. Montvale, N.J.: Medical Economics, 2002.

[23] Jaffe AS. The use of antiarrhythmics in advanced cardiac life support. *Ann. Emerg. Med.* 1993;22:307-316.

[24] *Remington: The Science and Practice of Pharmacy*. 21st edition. Philadelphia, PA. USA. Lippincott Williams and Wilkins

[25] *Pharmacology*. 4th Edition. Harvey R, Champe P. editors. Philadelphia, PA. USA. Wolters Kluwer/Lippincott Williams and Wilkins

[26] Kowey PR, Levine JH, Herre JM, et al. Randomized, double-blind comparison of intravenous amiodarone and bretylium in the treatment of patients with recurrent, hemodynamically destabilizing ventricular tachycardia or fibrillation. *Circulation* 1995;92:3255-3263.

[27] Schutzenberger W, Leisch F, Kerschner K, Harringer W, Herbinger W. Clinical efficacy of intravenous amiodarone in the short term treatment of recurrent sustained ventricular tachycardia and ventricular fibrillation. *Br. Heart J.* 1989;62:367-371.

[28] Mooss AN, Mohiuddin SM, Hee TT, Esterbrooks DJ, Hilleman DE, Rovang KS, Sketch MH Sr. Efficacy and tolerance of high-dose intravenous amiodarone for recurrent, refractory ventricular tachycardia. *Am. J. Cardiol.* 1990;65:609-614.

[29] Nalos PC, Ismail Y, Pappas JM, Nyitray W, DonMichael TA. Intravenous amiodarone for short-term treatment of refractory ventricular tachycardia or fibrillation. *Am. Heart J.* 1991;122:1629-1632.

[30] Ochi RP, Goldenberg IF, Almquist A, Pritzker M, Milstein S, Pedersen W, Gobel FL, Benditt DG. Intravenous amiodarone for the rapid treatment of life-threatening ventricular arrhythmias in critically ill patients with coronary artery disease. *Am. J. Cardiol.* 1989;64:599-603.

[31] Figa FH, Gow RM, Hamilton RM, Freedom RM. Clinical efficacy and safety of intravenous amiodarone in infants and children. *Am. J. Cardiol.* 1994;74:573-577.

[32] Helmy I, Herre JM, Gee G, Sharkey H, Malone P, Sauve MJ, Griffin JC, Scheinman MM. Use of intravenous amiodarone for emergency treatment of life-threatening ventricular arrhythmias. *J. Am. Coll. Cardiol.* 1988;12:1015-1022.

[33] Klein RC, Machell C, Rushforth N, Standefur J. Efficacy of intravenous amiodarone as short-term treatment for refractory ventricular tachycardia. *Am. Heart J.* 1988;115:96-101.

[34] Leak D. Intravenous amiodarone in the treatment of refractory life-threatening cardiac arrhythmias in the critically ill patient. *Am. Heart J.* 1986;111:456-462.

[35] Somberg JC, Tepper D, Keefe DL. Incessant VT treated with IV amiodarone: rapid onset of action with a long half-life agent (abstr). *J. Clin. Pharmacol.* 1986;26:543.

[36] Morady F, Scheinman MM, Shen E, Shapiro W, Sung RJ, DiCarlo L. Intravenous amiodarone in the acute treatment of recurrent symptomatic ventricular tachycardia. *Am J. Cardiol.* 1983;51:156-159.

[37] Horowitz LN, Mattleman SJ, Spielman SR, Frye SJ, Greenspan AM, Swanson BM, Vlasses PH, Rotmensch HH. Intravenous amiodarone loading for ventricular tachycardia (abstr). *Circulation* 1982;66(suppl II):II-222.

[38] Greene HL. The efficacy of amiodarone in the treatment of ventricular tachycardia or ventricu[ar fibrillation. *Prng. Cardiavasc. Dis.* 1989;31:319-354.

[39] Kentsch M, Berkel H, Bleifeld W. Intravenose amiodarone-applikation bei therapierefraktarem kammerflimmern. *Intensivmedizin* 1988;25:70-74.

[40] Williams ML Woelfel A, Cascia WE, et.ah Intiavenous amiodarone during prolonged resuscitation from cardiac arrest. *Ann. Intern. Med.* 1989;110:839-842.

[41] Scheinman MM, Levine JH, Cannom DS, Friehling T, Kopelman HA, Chilson DA, Platia EV, Wilber DJ, Kowey PR. Dose-ranging study of intravenous amiodarone in patients with life-threatening ventricular tachyarrhythmias. The Intravenous Amiodarone Multicenter Investigators Group. *Circulation* 1995; 92:3264-3272.

[42] Levine JH, Massumi A, Scheinman MM, Winkle RA, Platia EV, Chilson DA, Gomes A, Woosley RL. Intravenous amiodarone for recurrent sustained hypotensive ventricular tachyarrhythmias. Intravenous Amiodarone Multicenter Trial Group. *J. Am. Coll. Cardiol.* 1996;27:67-75.

[43] Anastasiou-Nana MI, Nanas JN, Nanas SN, et al. Effects of amiodarone on refractory ventricular fibrillation in acute myocardial infarction: experimental study. *J. Am. Coll. Cardiol.* 1994;23:253-258.

[44] Paiva EF, Perondi MB, Kern KB, Berg RA, Timerman S, Cardoso LF, Ramirez JA. Effect of amiodarone on haemodynamics during cardiopulmonary resuscitation in a canine model of resistant ventricular fibrillation. *Resuscitation* 2003;58:203-208.

[45] Somberg JC, Timar S, Bailin SJ, et al. Lack of a hypotensive effect with rapid administration of a new aqueous formulation of intravenous amiodarone. *Am. J. Cardiol.* 2004;93:576-581.

[46] *Cordarone Intravenous drug label.* In: Physicians' Desk Reference. 57th Ed. Montvale, NJ: Thomson PDR, 2003;3387-3390.

[47] Gough WB, Zeiler RH, Barreca P, El-Sherif N. Hypotensive action of commercial intravenous amiodarone and polysorbate 80 in dogs. *J. Cardiovasc. Pharmacol.* 1982;4:375-380.

[48] Platou ES, Refsum H. Acute electrophysiologic and blood pressure effects of amiodarone and its solvent in the dog. *Acta Pharmacol. Toxicol. (Copenh)* 1986;58:163-168.

[49] Munoz A, Karila P, Galley P, Grolleau R. A randomized hemodynamic comparison of intravenous amiodarone with and without Tween 80. *Circulation* 1985;72(supp III):III-168.

[50] Munoz A, Karila P, Gallay P, Zettelmeier F, Messner P, Mery M, Grolleau R. A randomized hemodynamic comparison of intravenous amiodarone with and without Tween 80. *Eur. Heart J.* 1988;9:142-148.

[51] Sicart M, Besse P, Choussat A, Bricaud H. Hemodynamic effects of intravenous amiodarone in humans. *Arch. Mal. Cœur. Vaiss.* 1977;70:219-227.

[52] Masini E, Planchenault J, Pezziardi F, Gautier P, Gagnol JP. Histamine-releasing properties of Polysorbate 80 in vitro and in vivo: correlation with its hypotensive action in the dog. *Agents Actions* 1985;16:470-477.

[53] Somberg JC, Bailin SJ, Haffajee CI, et al. Intravenous lidocaine versus intravenous amiodarone (in a new aqueous formulation) for incessant ventricular tachycardia. *Am. J. Cardiol.* 2002;90:853-859.

[54] Remme WJ, van Hoogenhuyze DC, Kruyssen DA, Krauss XH, Storm CJ. Amiodarone. Haemodynamic profile during intravenous administration and effect on pacing-induced ischaemia in man. *Drugs* 1985;29(suppl 3):11-22.

[55] Path GJ, Dai XZ, Schwartz JS, Benditt DG, Bache RJ. Effects of amiodarone with and without polysorbate 80 on myocardial oxygen consumption and coronary blood flow during treadmill exercise in the dog. *J. Cardiovasc. Pharmacol.* 1991;18:11-16.

[56] Kreiss Y, Sidi Y, Gur H. Efficacy and safety of intravenous amiodarone in recent-onset atrial fibrillation: experience in patients admitted to a general internal medicine department. *Postgrad. Med. J.* 1999;75:278-281.

[57] Hilleman DE, Spinler SA. Conversion of recent-onset atrial fibrillation with intravenous amiodarone: a meta-analysis of randomized controlled trials. *Pharmacotherapy* 2002;22:66-74.

[58] American Heart Association Guidelines 2000 for Cardiopulmonary Resuscitation and Emergency Cardiovascular Care: an international consensus on science. *Circulation* 2000;102(Suppl I):1-384.

[59] Cobb LA, Fahrenbruch CE, Walsh TR, Copass MK, Olsufka M, Breskin M, Hallstrom AP. Influence of cardiopulmonary resuscitation prior to defibrillation in patients with out-of-hospital ventricular fibrillation. *JAMA* 1999;281:1182-1188.

[60] Weisfeldt ML, Becker LB. Resuscitation after cardiac arrest: a 3-phase time-sensitive model. *JAMA* 2002;288:3035-3038.

[61] Kern KB, Valenzuela TD, Clark LL, Berg RA, Hilwig RW, Berg MD, Otto CW, Newburn D, Ewy GA. An alternative approach to advancing resuscitation science. *Resuscitation* 2005;64:261-268.

[62] The Public Access Defibrillation Trial Investigators. Public-access defibrillation and survival after out-of-hospital cardiac arrest. *N Engl J Med* 2004;351:637-646.

[63] Berg RA, Hilwig RW, Kern KB, Sanders AB, Xavier LC, Ewy GA. Automated external defibrillation versus manual defibrillation for prolonged ventricular fibrillation: lethal delays of chest compressions before and after countershocks. *Ann. Emerg. Med.* 2003;42:458-467.

[64] Wester PO. Magnesium-effect on arrhythmias. *Int. J. Cardiol.* 1986;12:181-183.

[65] Guyton AG. *Textbook of Medical Physiology*. 8th edition. 1991. WB Saunders, Philadelphia PA. USA

[66] Altura BM. Introduction: importance of Mg in physiology and medicine and the need for ion selective electrodes. *Scand. J. Clin. Lab. Invest Suppl.* 1994;217:5-9.

[67] Salem M, Munoz R, Chernow B. Hypomagnesemia in critical illness. A common and clinically important problem. *Crit. Care Clin.* 1991;7:225-252.

[68] Reis AG, Ferreira de Paiva E, Schvartsman C, Zaritsky AL. Magnesium in cardiopulmonary resuscitation: critical review. *Resuscitation* 2008;77:21-25.

[69] Laughlin MR, Thompson D. The regulatory role for magnesium in glycolytic flux of the human erythrocyte. *J. Biol. Chem.* 1996;271:28977-28983.

[70] Resnick LM, Altura BT, Gupta RK, Laragh JH, Alderman MH, Altura BM. Intracellular and extracellular magnesium depletion in type 2 (non-insulin-dependent) diabetes mellitus. *Diabetologia* 1993;36:767-770.

[71] Resnick LM, Bardicef O, Altura BT, Alderman MH, Altura BM.Serum ionized magnesium: relation to blood pressure and racial factors. *Am. J. Hypertens.* 1997;10:1420-1424.

[72] Altura BM, Shah NC, Jiang XC, Li Z, Perez-Albela JL, Sica AC, Altura BT. Short-term magnesium deficiency results in decreased levels of serum sphingomyelin, lipid peroxidation, and apoptosis in cardiovascular tissues. *Am. J. Physiol. Heart Circ. Physiol.* 20091;297:H86-92.

[73] Sinert R, Zehtabchi S, Desai S, Peacock P, Altura BT, Altura BM. Serum ionized magnesium and calcium levels in adult patients with seizures. *Scand. J. Clin. Lab. Invest* 2007;67:317-326.

[74] Li J, Li W, Liu W, Altura BT, Altura BM. Peroxynitrite induces apoptosis and decline in intracellular free Mg with concomitant elevation in [Ca2+]I in rat aortic smooth muscle cells: possible roles of extracellular and intracellular magnesium ions in peroxynitrite-induced cell death. *Drug Metab. Lett.* 2007;1:85-89.

[75] Sinert R, Spektor M, Gorlin A, Doty C, Rubin A, Altura BT, Altura BM. Ionized magnesium levels and the ratio of ionized calcium to magnesium in asthma patients before and after treatment with magnesium. *Scand. J. Clin. Lab. Invest* 2005;65:659-670.

[76] Altura BM, Kostellow AB, Zhang A, Li W, Morrill GA, Gupta RK, Altura BT. Expression of the nuclear factor-kappaB and proto-oncogenes c-fos and c-jun are induced by low extracellular Mg2+ in aortic and cerebral vascular smooth muscle cells: possible links to hypertension, atherogenesis, and stroke. *Am. J. Hypertens.* 2003;16:701-707.
[77] Altura BM, Gebrewold A, Zhang A, Altura BT. Low extracellular magnesium ions induce lipid peroxidation and activation of nuclear factor-kappa B in canine cerebral vascular smooth muscle: possible relation to traumatic brain injury and strokes. *Neurosci. Lett.* 2003;341:189-192.
[78] Smith GA, Vandenberg JI, Freestone NS, Dixon HB. The effect of Mg2+ on cardiac muscle function: Is CaATP the substrate for priming myofibril cross-bridge formation and Ca2+ reuptake by the sarcoplasmic reticulum? *Biochem. J.* 2001;354:539-551.
[79] Skou JC. The (Na++K+) activated enzyme system and its relationship to transport of sodium and potassium. *Q Rev. Biophys.* 19741;7:401-434.
[80] Thel MC, Armstrong AL, McNulty SE, Califf RM, O'Connor CM. Randomised trial of magnesium in in-hospital cardiac arrest. Duke Internal Medicine Housestaff. *Lancet* 1997;350:1272-1276.
[81] Iseri LT, French JH. Magnesium: nature's physiologic calcium blocker. *Am. Heart J.* 1984;108:188-193.
[82] Levine BS, Coburn JW. Magnesium, the mimic/antagonist to calcium. *N. Engl. J. Med.* 1984;310:1253-1255.
[83] Woods KL. Possible pharmacological actions of magnersium in acute myocardial infarction. *Br. J. Clin. Pharmacol.* 1991;32:3-10.
[84] Vigorito C, Giordano A, Ferraro P, Acanfora D, De Caprio L, Naddeo C, Rengo F. Hemodynamic effects of magnesium sulfate on the normal human heart. *Am. J. Cardiol.* 1991;67:1435-1437.
[85] Nadler JL, Goodson S, Rude RK. Evidence that prostacyclin mediates the vascular action of magnesium in humans. *Hypertension* 1987;9:379-383.
[86] Rude R, Manoogian C, Ehrlich L, DeRusso P, Ryzen E, Nadler J. Mechanisms of blood pressure regulation by magnesium in man. *Magnesium* 1989;8:266-273.
[87] Vandenberg CA. Inward rectification of a potassium channel in cardiac ventricular cells depends on internal magnesium ions. *Proc. Natl. Acad. Sci. USA* 1987;84:2560-2564.
[88] Hwang DL, Yen CF, Nadler JL. Effect of extracellular magnesium on platelet activation and intracellular calcium mobilization. *Am. J. Hypertens* 1992;5:700-706.
[89] Ghani MF, Rabah M. Effect of magnesium chloride on electrical stability of the heart. *Am. Heart J.* 1977;94:600-602.
[90] Chernow B, Bamberger S, Stoiko M, Vadnais M, Mills S, Hoellerich V, Warshaw AL. Hypomagnesemia in patients in postoperative intensive care. *Chest* 1989;95:391-397.
[91] Spasov AA, Iezhitsa IN, Kharitonova MV, Gurova NA. Arrhythmogenic threshold of the myocardium under conditions of magnesium deficiency. *Bull. Exp. Biol. Med.* 2008;146:63-65.
[92] Altura BM, Zhang A, Altura BT. Magnesium, hypertensive vascular diseases, atherogenesis, subcellular compartmentation of Ca2+ and Mg2+ and vascular contractility. *Miner Electrolyte Metab.* 1993;19:323-336.
[93] Molloy DW, Dhingra S, Solven F, et al. Hypomagnesemia and respiratory muscle power. *Am. Rev. Respir. Dis.* 1984;129:497-498.

[94] Altura BT, Altura BM. Endothelium-dependent relaxation in coronary arteries requires magnesium ions. *Br. J. Pharmacol.* 1987;91:449-451.

[95] Weglicki WB, Phillips TM, Freedman AM, Cassidy MM, Dickens BF. Magnesium deficiency elevates circulating levels of inflammatory cytokines and endothelin. *Mol. Cell Biochem.* 1992;110:169-173.

[96] Weglicki WB, Bloom S, Cassidy MM, Freedman AM, Atrakchi AH, Dickens BF. Antioxidants and the cardiomyopathy of Mg-deficiency. *Am. J. Cardiovasc. Pathol.* 1992;4:210-215.

[97] Salem M, Kasinski N, Munoz R, Chernow B. Progressive magnesium deficiency increases mortality from endotoxin challenge: protective effects of acute magnesium replacement therapy. *Crit. Care Med.* 1995;23:108-118.

[98] Ryzen E. Magnesium homeostasis in critically ill patients. *Magnesium* 1989;8:201-202.

[99] Fiser RT, Torres A Jr, Butch AW, Valentine JL. Ionized magnesium concentrations in critically ill children. *Crit. Care Med.* 1998;26:2048-2052.

[100] Broner CW, Stidham GL, Westenkirchner DF, Tolley EA. Hypermagnesemia and hypocalcemia as predictors of high mortality in critically ill pediatric patients. *Crit. Care Med.* 1990;18:921-928.

[101] Grant HI, Yeston NS. Cardiac arrest secondary to emotional stress and torsade de pointes in a patient with associated magnesium and potassium deficiency. *Crit. Care Med.* 1991;19:292-294.

[102] Iseri LT. Role of magnesium in cardiac tachyarrhythmias. *Ann .J. Cardiol.* 1990;65:47K-50K.

[103] Hollifield JW. Thiazide treatment of systemic hypertension: effects on serum magnesium and ventricular ectopic activity. *Am. J. Cardiol.* 1989;63:22G-25G.

[104] Ryan MP. Diuretics and potassium/magnesium depletion. Directions for treatment. *Am J. Med.* 1987;82:38-47.

[105] Seelig M. Cardiovascular consequences of magnesium deficiency and loss: pathogenesis, prevalence and manifestations--magnesium and chloride loss in refractory potassium repletion. *Am. J. Cardiol.* 1989;63:4G-21G.

[106] Reinhart RA. Magnesium metabolism. A review with special reference to the relationship between intracellular content and serum levels. *Arch. Intern. Med.* 1988;148:2415-2420.

[107] Whang R, Ryder KW. Frequency of hypomagnesemia and hypermagnesemia. Requested vs routine. *JAMA* 1990;263:3063-3064.

[108] Manz M, Pfeiffer D, Jung W, Lueritz B. Intravenous treatment with magnesium in recurrent persistent ventricular tachycardia. *New Trends in Arrhythmias* 1991;7:437-442.

[109] Tzivoni D, Banai S, Schuger C, Benhorin J, Keren A, Gottlieb S, Stern S. Treatment of torsade de pointes with magnesium sulfate. *Circulation* 1988;77:392-397.

[110] Sueta CA, Clarke SW, Dunlap SH, et al. Effect of acute magnesium administration on the frequency of ventricular arrhythmia in patients with heart failure. *Circulation* 1994;89:660-666.

[111] Woods KL, Fletcher S, Roffe C, Haider Y. Intravenous magnesium sulphate in suspected acute myocardial infarction: results of the second Leicester Intravenous Magnesium Intervention Trial (LIMIT-2). *Lancet* 1992; 339:1553-1558.

[112] Horner SM. Efficacy of intravenous magnesium in acute myocardial infarction in reducing arrhythmias and mortality: meta-analysis of magnesium in acute myocardial infarction. *Circulation* 1992;86:774-779.

[113] Teo KK, Yusuf S, Collins R, Held PH, Peto R. Effects of intravenous magnesium in suspected acute myocardial infarction: overview of randomised trials. *BMJ* 1991;303:1499-1503.

[114] Hilton TC, Fredman C, Holt DJ, Bjerregaard P, Ira GH, Jr, Janosik DL. Electrophysiologic and antiarrhythmic effects of magnesium in patients with inducible ventricular tachyarrhythmia. *Clin. Cardiol.* 1992;15:176-180.

[115] Roffe C, Fletcher S, Woods KL. Investigation of the effects of intravenous magnesium sulphate on cardiac rhythm in acute myocardial infarction. *Br. Heart J.* 1994;71:141-145.

[116] ISIS-4 (Fourth International Study of Infarct Survival) Collaborative Group. ISIS-4: a randomised factorial trial assessing early oral captopril, oral mononitrate, and intravenous magnesium sulphate in 58 050 patients with suspected acute myocardial infarction. *Lancet* 1995;345:669-785.

[117] Smith LF, Heagerty AM, Bing RF, Barnett DB. Intravenous infusion of magnesium sulphate after acute myocardial infarction: effects on arrhythmias and mortality. *Int. J. Cardiol.* 1986;12:175-183.

[118] Cannon LA, Heiselman DE, Dougherty JM, Jones J. Magnesium levels in cardiac arrest victims: relationship between magnesium levels and successful resuscitation. *Ann. Emerg. Med.* 1987;16:1195-1199.

[119] Buylaert WA, Calle PA, Houbrechts HN. Serum electrolyte disturbances in the post-resuscitation period. *Resuscitation* 1987;17(Suppl.):S189-196.

[120] Atar D, Serebruany V, Poulton J, et al. Effects of magnesium supplementation in a porcine model of myocardial ischemia and reperfusion. *J. Cardiovasc. Pharmacol.* 1994;24:603-611.

[121] Cohen L, Kitzes R:.Magnesium sulfate in the treatment of variant angina. *Magnesium* 1984;3:46-49.

[122] Kimura T, Yasue H, Sakaino N, et al: Effects of magnesium on the tone of isolated human coronary arteries. *Circulation* 1989;79:1118-1124.

[123] Satake K, Lee J, Shimizer H, et al: Relation between severity of magnesium deficiency and frequency of anginal attacks in men with variant angina. *J. Am. Coll. Cardiol.* 1996;28:897-902.

[124] Matsusaka T, Hasebe N, Jin YT, Kawabe J, Kikuchi K. Magnesium reduces myocardial infarct size via enhancement of adenosine mechanism in rabbits. *Cardiovasc. Res.* 2002;54:568-575.

[125] Zhang Y, Davies LR, Martin SM, Bawaney IM, Buettner GR, Kerber RE. Magnesium reduces free radical concentration and preserves left ventricular function after direct current shocks. *Resuscitation* 2003;56:199-206.

[126] Garcia LA, Dejong SC, Martin SM, Smith RS, Buettner GR, Kerber RE. Magnesium reduces free radicals in an in vivo coronary occlusion-reperfusion model. *J. Am. Coll. Cardiol.* 1998;32:536-539.

[127] Shen A, Jennings R. Myocardial calcium and magnesium in acute ischemic injury. *Am J. Pathol.* 1972;67:417-440.

[128] Thandroyen F, Bellato D, Katayama A, et al. Subcellular electrolyte alterations during progressive hypoxia and following reoxygenation in isolated neonatal rat ventricular myocytes. *Circ. Res.* 1992;71:106-119.

[129] Hearse DJ. Reperfusion of the ischemic myocardium. *J. Mol. Cell Cardiol.* 1977;9:605-616.

[130] Ver Donck L, Bargers M, Verdonck F. Inhibition of sodium and calcium overload pathology in myocardium. A new cytoprotective principle. *Cardiovasc. Res.* I993;27:349-357.

[131] Klein H, Pick S, Bohle R, et al. Myocardial protection by Na+-H+ exchange inhibition in ischemic, reperfused porcine hearts. *Circulation* I995;92:912-917.

[132] Tosaki A, Szerdahelyi P, Engelman R, et al. Effects of extracellular magnesium manipulation on reperfusion-induced arrhythmias and myocardial ion shifts in isolated reperfused rat hearts. *J. Pharmacol. Exp. Ther.* 1993;267:1045-1053.

[133] White BC, Winegar CD, Wilson RF, Krause GS. Calcium blockers in cerebral resuscitation. *J. Trauma* 1983;23:788-794.

[134] Schwartz AC. Neurological recovery after cardiac arrest: clinical feasibility trial of calcium blockers. *Am. J. Emerg. Med.* 1985;3:1–10.

[135] Siemkowicz E. Magnesium sulfate solution dramatically improves immediate recovery of rats from hypoxia. *Resuscitation* 1997;35:53-59.

[136] Hollmann MW, Strumper D, Salmons VA, Washington JM, Durieux ME. Effects of calcium and magnesium pre-treatment on hyperkalaemic cardiac arrest in rats. *Eur. J. Anaesthesiol.* 2003;20:606-611.

[137] Brown CG, Griffith RF, Neely D, Hobson J, Miller B. The effect of intravenous magnesium administration on aortic, right atrial and coronary perfusion pressures during CPR in swine. *Resuscitation* 1993;26:3-12.

[138] Seaberg DC, Menegazzi JJ, Check B, MacLeod BA, Yealy DM. Use of a cardiocerebral-protective drug cocktail prior to countershock in a porcine model of prolonged ventricular fibrillation. *Resuscitation* 2001;51:301-308.

[139] Baraka A, Ayoub C, Kawkabani N. Magnesium therapy for refractory ventricular fibrillation. *J. Cardiothorac. Vasc. Anesth.* 2000;14:196-199.

[140] Tobey RC, Birnbaum GA, Allegra JR, Horowitz MS, Plosay III JJ. Successful resuscitation and neurologic recovery from refractory ventricular fibrillation after magnesium sulphate administration. *Ann. Emerg. Med.* 1992;21:92-96.

[141] Craddock L, Miller B, Clifton G, Krumbach B, Pluss W. Resuscitation from prolonged cardiac arrest with high-dose intravenous magnesium sulfate. *J. Emerg. Med.* 1991;9:469-476.

[142] Iseri LT, Chung P, Tobis J. Magnesium therapy for intractable ventricular tachyarrhythmias in normomagnesemic patients. *West J. Med.* 1983;138:823-828.

[143] Miller B, Craddock L, Hoffenberg S, et al. Pilot study of intravenous magnesium sulfate in refractory cardiac arrest: safety data and recommendations for future studies. *Resuscitation* 1995;30:3-14.

[144] Fatovich DM, Prentice DA, Dobb GJ. Magnesium in cardiac arrest (the magic trial). *Resuscitation* 1997;35:237-241.

[145] Allegra J, Lavery R, Cody R, et al. Magnesium sulfate in the treatment of refractory ventricular fibrillation in the prehospital setting. *Resuscitation* 2001;49:245-249.

[146] Hassan TB, Jagger C, Barnett DB. A randomized trial to investigate the efficacy of magnesium sulphate for refractory ventricular fibrillation. *Emerg. Med. J.* 2002;19:57-62.

[147] Longstreth Jr WT, Fahrenbruch CE, Olsufka M, Walsh TR, Copass MK, Cobb LA. Randomized clinical trial of magnesium, diazepam, or both after out-of-hospital cardiac arrest. *Neurology* 2002;59:506-514.

[148] Waalewijn RA, Nijpels MA, Tijssen JG, Koster RW. Prevention of deterioration of ventricular fibrillation by basic life support during out-of-hospital cardiac arrest. *Resuscitation* 2002;54:31-36.

[149] Paradis NA, Martin GB, Rivers EP, Goetting MG, Appleton TJ, Feingold M, Nowak RM. Coronary perfusion pressure and the return of spontaneous circulation in human cardiopulmonary resuscitation. *JAMA* 1990;263:1106-1113.

[150] Michael JR, Guerci AD, Koehler RC, Shi AY, Tsitlik J, Chandra N, Niedermeyer E, Rogers MC, Traystman RJ, Weisfeldt ML. Mechanisms by which epinephrine augments cerebral and myocardial perfusion during cardiopulmonary resuscitation in dogs. *Circulation* 1984;69:822-835.

[151] Pytte M, Kramer-Johansen J, Eilevstjønn J, Eriksen M, Strømme TA, Godang K, Wik L, Steen PA, Sunde K. Haemodynamic effects of adrenaline (epinephrine) depend on chest compression quality during cardiopulmonary resuscitation in pigs. *Resuscitation* 2006;71:369-378.

[152] Brown CG, Werman HA, Davis EA, Hobson J, Hamlin RL. The effects of graded doses of epinephrine on regional myocardial blood flow during cardiopulmonary resuscitation in swine. *Circulation* 1987;75:491-497.

[153] Brown CG, Werman HA. Adrenergic agonists during cardiopulmonary resuscitation. *Resuscitation* 1990;19:1-16.

[154] Moore EW: Ionized calcium in normal serum, ultrafiltrates and whole blood determined by ion-exchange electrodes. *J. Clin. Invest* 1970;49:318-334.

[155] Urban P, Scheidegger D, Buchmann B, Barth D. Cardiac arrest and blood ionized calcium levels. *Ann. Intern. Med.* 1988;109:110-113.

[156] Cardenas-Rivero N, Chernow B, Stoiko MA, Nussbaum SR, Todres ID. Hypocalcemia in critically ill children. *J. Pediatr.* 1989;114:946-951.

[157] Gollasch M, Löhn M, Furstenau M, Nelson MT, Luft FC, Haller H. Ca2+ channels, 'quantized' Ca2+ release, and differentiation of myocytes in the cardiovascular system. *J. Hypertens* 2000;18:989-998.

[158] Arnon A, Hamlyn JM, Blaustein MP. Na(+) entry via store-operated channels modulates Ca(2+) signaling in arterial myocytes. *Am. J. Physiol. Cell Physiol.* 2000;278:C163-173.

[159] Walker JS, Wingard CJ, Murphy RA. Energetics of crossbridge phosphorylation and contraction in vascular smooth muscle. *Hypertension* 1994;23:1106-1112.

[160] Jaggar JH, Wellman GC, Heppner TJ, Porter VA, Perez GJ, Gollasch M, Kleppisch T, Rubart M, Stevenson AS, Lederer WJ, Knot HJ, Bonev AD, Nelson MT. Ca2+ channels, ryanodine receptors and Ca(2+)-activated K+ channels: a functional unit for regulating arterial tone. *Acta Physiol. Scand.* 1998;164:577-587.

[161] Bohr DF, Webb RC. Vascular smooth muscle function and its changes in hypertension. *Am. J. Med.* 1984;77:3-16.

[162] Fleming WW. The electrogenic Na+, K+-pump in smooth muscle: physiologic and pharmacologic significance. *Annu. Rev. Pharmacol. Toxicol.* 1980;20:129-149.

[163] Stulz PM, Scheidegger D, Drop LJ, Lowenstein E, Laver MB. Ventricular pump performance during hypocalcemia: clinical and experimental studies. *J. Thorac. Cardiovasc. Surg.* 1979;78:185-194.

[164] Moss RL, Razumova M, Fitzsimons DP. Myosin crossbridge activation of cardiac thin filaments: implications for myocardial function in health and disease. *Circ. Res.* 2004;94:1290-1300.

[165] Pirani A, Vinogradova MV, Curmi PM, King WA, Fletterick RJ, Craig R, Tobacman LS, Xu C, Hatch V, Lehman W. An atomic model of the thin filament in the relaxed and Ca2+-activated states. *J. Mol. Biol.* 2006;357:707-717.

[166] Ringer S. A further contribution regarding the influence of the different constituents of the blood on the contraction of the heart. *J. Physiol.* 1882;4:29-42.

[167] Kay JH, Blalock A. The use of calcium chloride in the treatment of cardiac arrest in patients. *Surg. Gynecol. Obstet.* 1951;93:97-102.

[168] Standards and Guidelines for cardiopulmonary resuscitation (CPR) and emergency cardiac care (ECC). *JAMA* 1980;244(suppl):453-509.

[169] Best R, Martin GB, Carden DL, Tomlanovich MC, Foreback C, Nowak RM. Ionized calcium during CPR in the canine model. *Ann. Emerg. Med.* 1985;14:633-635.

[170] Niemann JT, Cairns CB. Hyperkalemia and ionized hypocalcemia during cardiac arrest and resuscitation: possible culprits for postcountershock arrhythmias? *Ann. Emerg. Med.* 1999;34:1-7.

[171] Salerno DM, Elsperger K J, Helseth R Murakami M, Chepuri V. Serum potassium, calcium and magnesium after resuscitation from ventricular fibrillation: a canine study. *J. Am. Coll. Cardiol.* 1987;10:178-185.

[172] Gando S, Igarashi M, Kameue T, Nanzaki S. Ionized hypocalcemia during out-of-hospital cardiac arrest and cardiopulmonary resuscitation is not due to binding by lactate. *Intensive Care Med.* 1997;23:1245-1250.

[173] Gando S, Tedo I, Kubota M. A comparison of serum ionized calcium in arterial and mixed venous blood during CPR. *Ann. Emerg. Med.* 1990;19:850-856.

[174] Gando S, Tedo I, Tujinaga H, et al. Variation in serum ionized calcium on cardiopulmonary resuscitation. *J. Anesth.* 1988;2:154-160.

[175] Nayler WG. The role of calcium in the ischemic myocardium. *Am. J. Pathol.* 1981;102:262-270.

[176] Nayler WG. Calcium and cell death. *Eur. Heart J.* 1983;4(suppl C):33-41.

[177] Lee HC, Smith N, Mohabir R, et al. Cytosolic calcium transients from the beating mammalian heart. *Proc. Natl. Acad. Sci. USA* 1987;84:7793-7797.

[178] Kitakaze M, Pike M, Chacko VP, et al. Direct measurement of cytosolic free calcium during ischemia and reperfusion in ferret hearts. *Circulation* 1987;76(suppl IV):IV-380.

[179] Shapiro HM. Post-cardiac arrest therapy: Calcium entry blockade and brain resuscitation. *Anesthesiology* 1985;62:384-387.

[180] Steen PA, Gisvold 8E, Milde JH, et al. Nimodipine improves outcome when given after complete cerebral ischemia in primates. *Anesthesiology* 1985;62:406-414.

[181] Zhong JQ, Dorian P. Epinephrine and vasopressin during cardiopulmonary resuscitation. *Resuscitation* 2005;66:263-269.

[182] Corr PB, Shayman JA, Kramer JB, et al. increased a2-adrenergic receptors in ischemic cat myocardium. *J. Clin. Invest.* 1981;67:1232-1236.
[183] Schömig A, Richardt G.The role of catecholamines in ischemia. *J. Cardiovasc. Pharmacol.* 1990;16 Suppl 5:S105-112.
[184] Cairns CB, Niemann JT, Pelikan PCD, Sharma J. Ionized hypocalcemia during prolonged cardiac arrest and closed-chest CPR in a canine model. *Ann. Emerg. Med.* 1991;20:1178-1182.
[185] White BC, Gadzinski DS, Hoehner PJ, et al. Effect of flunarizine on canine cerebral cortical blood flow and vascular resistance post cardiac arrest. *Ann. Emerg. Med.* 1982;11:119-126.
[186] Shen AC, Jennings RB. Kinetics of calcium accumulation in acute myocardial ischemic injury. *Am. J. Pathol.* 1972;67: 441-452.
[187] Katz AM, Reuter H. Cellular calcium and cardiac cell death. *Am. J. Cardiol.* 1979;44:188-190.
[188] Paraskos JA. Cardiovascular pharmacology. III: Atropine, calcium, calcium blockers, and beta-blockers. *Circulation* 1986;74:IV86-89.
[189] Carlon GC, Howland WS, Kahn RC, Schweizer O. Calcium chloride administration in normocalcemic critically ill patients. *Crit. Care Med.* 1980;8:209-212.
[190] Niemann JT, Adomian GE, Garner D, Rosborough JP. Endocardial and transcutaneous cardiac pacing, calcium chloride, and epinephrine in postcountershock asystole and bradycardias. *Crit. Care Med.* 1985;13:699-704.
[191] Blecic S, De Backer D, Huynh CH, Deleuze M, Domb M, Luypaert P, Vincent JL. Calcium chloride in experimental electromechanical dissociation: a placebo-controlled trial in dogs. *Crit. Care Med.* 1987;15:324-327.
[192] Stueven HA, Thompson B, Aprahamian C, Tonsfeldt DJ, Kastenson EH. The effectiveness of calcium chloride in refractory electromechanical dissociation. *Ann. Emerg. Med.* 1985;14:626-629.
[193] Stueven H, Thompson BM, Aprahamian C, Darin JC. Use of calcium in prehospital cardiac arrest. *Ann. Emerg. Med.* 1983;12:136-139.

In: Drugs in Cardiopulmonary Resuscitation
Editor: Theodoros Xanthos

ISBN: 978-1-61122-512-9

Chapter 5

Anti-Ischemic Therapy in Acute Coronary Syndromes

Konstantinos A. Ekmektzoglou
University of Athens, Medical School

Abstract

A primary challenge in the development of clinical practice guidelines is keeping pace with the stream of new data upon which recommendations are based.

Management of a patient with Acute Coronary Syndromes (ACS), although tailored in specific algorithms, proves everyday to be challenging so as not only to make the diagnosis as soon as possible but also to go on establishing the appropriate therapeutic protocol.

This last one is of particular importance since the pathophysiology of ACS is not the same. Anti-ischemic therapy remains a cornerstone in the treatment of all ACS patients providing pain relief and improving the prognosis of patients with unstable angina/Non-ST-segment elevation myocardial infarction (UA/NSTEMI) and ST-segment elevation myocardial infarction (STEMI).

Introduction

UA/NSTEMI and STEMI, although constituting the term ACS, do not share the same underlying pathophysiology. This difference calls for different therapeutic approaches.

In UA/NSTEMI, the therapeutic goal is to prevent further thrombosis and to allow endogenous fibrinolysis to dissolve the thrombus and reduce the degree of coronary stenosis with revascularization being used to increase blood flow and prevent reocclusion or recurrent ischemia.

On the other hand, in STEMI, a coronary artery or its branch is usually totally occluded. Therefore, immediate pharmacological or catheter-based reperfusion is the initial approach, with the goal of obtaining normal coronary blood flow.

Other therapies, such as anti-ischemic and lipid-lowering therapies, are used in both cases, since they do not target the initial pathophysiological process, but are used to provide patient comfort and stabilize plaques over the long term [1].

This chapter focuses on the pharmacology of the anti-ischemic therapy in patients with ACS.

Morphine

Morphine, the prototypical opioid agonist, has long been known to relieve severe pain with remarkable efficacy. Morphine (Figure 1) is a member of the morphinan-framed alkaloids, which are present in the poppy plant, the source of crude opium from which the pure alkaloid morphine was isolated in 1803 (with its name been given after Morpheus, the Greek god of dreams). It remains the standard against which all drugs that have strong analgesic action are compared. Opioid drugs include full agonists, partial agonists, and antagonists, with morphine, being a full agonist at the μ opioid receptor. Morphine produces analgesia through actions at regions in the brain that contain peptides which have opioid-like pharmacologic properties, with these endogenous substances being referred to as endogenous opioid peptides [1]. Three families of endogenous opioid peptides have been described in detail: the enkephalins, endorphins, and dynorphins. A novel endogenous opioid peptide was cloned in 1995 [2,3]. This peptide is called orphanin FQ (OFQ) or nociceptin (N). Each endogenous opioid peptide exhibits different activity for the opioid receptors subtypes (which will be discussed below), explaining, therefore, their diverse pharmacological effects [1].

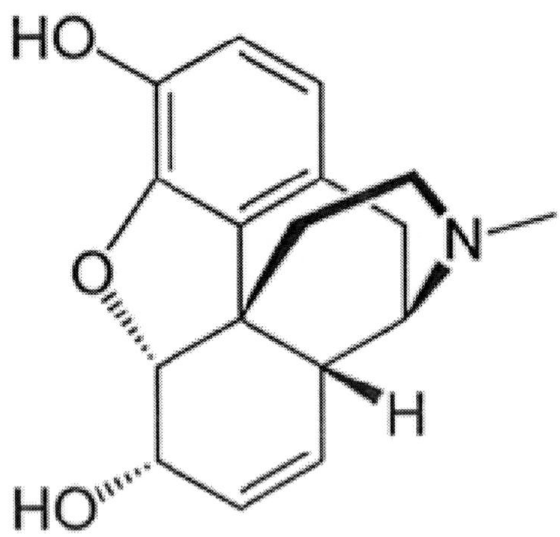

Figure 1. Structure of morphine.

Pharmacokinetics

Morphine is well absorbed when given by subcutaneous, intramuscular, and oral routes. However, the oral dose may need to be much higher than the parenteral dose to elicit a therapeutic effect (the first-pass effect, i.e., the phenomenon of drug metabolism whereby the concentration of a drug is greatly reduced before it reaches the systemic circulation, is responsible for that), making the prediction of an effective oral dose difficult.

Intranasal delivery of morphine can result in rapid therapeutic blood levels by avoiding first-pass metabolism. Other routes of opioid administration include oral mucosal and the application of transdermal patches, which can provide delivery of potent analgesics over days [4].

The uptake of morphine by various organs and tissues is a function of both physiologic and chemical factors.

Although all opioids bind to plasma proteins with varying affinity, the drugs rapidly leave the blood compartment and localize in highest concentrations in tissues that are highly perfused such as the brain, lungs, liver, kidneys, and spleen. Drug concentrations in skeletal muscle may be much lower, but this tissue serves as the main reservoir because of its greater bulk [4].

The metabolism of morphine, whose half-life is between 3 to 4 h, occurs not only in the liver, but may also take place in the brain and the kidneys. Morphine is converted in large part to polar metabolites (mostly glucuronides), mainly eliminated via bile and urine.

Morphine, which contains free hydroxyl groups, is primarily conjugated to morphine-3-glucuronide (M3G), a compound with neuroexcitatory properties. Moreover, approximately 10% of morphine is metabolized to morphine-6-glucuronide (M6G), an active metabolite with greater analgesic potency than morphine.

Glucuronides as a rule are considered as highly polar metabolites unable to cross the blood-brain barrier; however, accumulation of these metabolites may produce unexpected side effects in patients with renal failure or when exceptionally large doses of morphine are administered (seizures or enhanced and prolonged opioid action) [5,6].

Pharmacodynamics

Opioid agonists produce analgesia by binding to receptors, located primarily in brain and spinal cord regions involved in the transmission and modulation of pain.

Three major classes of opioid receptors (μ, δ, κ) that are members of the G protein-coupled family of receptors and show significant amino acid sequence homologies have been identified in various nervous system sites and in other tissues [7].

Multiple receptor subtypes have also been proposed based on pharmacologic criteria (μ_1, μ_2, δ_1, δ_2, κ_1, κ_2, κ_3,). The principle receptor for the OFQ or N system, mentioned above, is the G protein-coupled orphanin opioid-receptor-likesubtype 1 (ORL1) [4].

At the molecular level, opioid receptors form a family of proteins that physically couple to G proteins and through this interaction affect ion channel gating, modulate intracellular calcium (Ca^{2+}) disposition, inhibit adenylyl cyclase (reducing the intracellular cyclic adenosine monophosphate - cAMP - content) and alter protein phosphorylation.

The opioids have two well-established direct actions on neurons: (1) they close voltage-gated Ca^{2+} channels on presynaptic nerve terminals and, thereby, reduce transmitter release and (2) they hyperpolarize, and thus inhibit, postsynaptic neurons by opening potassium (K^+) channels, therefore, reducing neuronal excitability [4].

As noted above, morphine is a full agonist at the μ opioid receptor and therefore responsible for many effects, discussed in detail below (supraspinal and spinal analgesia;

sedation; inhibition of respiration; slowed gastrointestinal transit; modulation of hormone and neurotransmitter release).

However, morphine has been shown to act at κ and δ receptor sites as well; it is unclear to what extent this contributes to its analgesic action.

Opioid receptor binding sites have been identified using high-affinity radioligand binding with antibodies to unique peptide sequences in each receptor subtype. M, κ and δ receptors are present in high concentrations in the dorsal horn of the spinal cord, both on spinal cord pain transmission neurons and on the primary afferents that relay the pain message to them [4,8].

Morphine inhibits the release of excitatory transmitters from these primary afferents and, directly, inhibits the dorsal horn pain transmission neuron. Thus, opioids exert a powerful analgesic effect directly upon the spinal cord (spinal action). Systemically administered morphine is responsible for supraspinal actions (respiratory depression, nausea, vomiting, sedation).

Different combinations of opioid receptors are found in the supraspinal regions implicated in pain transmission and modulation (rostral ventral medulla, locus ceruleus, midbrain periaqueductal gray area) where morphine directly inhibits neurons.

Animal and human clinical studies demonstrate that both endogenous and exogenous opioids can also produce opioid-mediated analgesia at sites outside the central nervous system (CNS), where, activation of peripheral receptors results in a decrease in sensory neuron activity and transmitter release [4].

The development of tolerance and dependence with repeated use is a characteristic feature of all the opioid drugs. In tolerance, which can be detected within 12-24 hours of morphine administration, the drug loses its effectiveness and an increased dose is required to produce the same physiological response.

Dependence refers to a disturbance of the homeostatic set point of the organism if the drug is stopped, resulting in withdrawal.

Tolerance and dependence are physiological responses seen in all patients and are not predictors of addiction and are believed to be the cause of receptor desensitization (or lack of desensitization) and uncoupling, internalization, and sequestration after chronic exposure to opioids and persistent activation of μ receptors. All these hypotheses are under ongoing investigation [1,4,9,10].

In addition to the development of tolerance, persistent administration of opioid analgesics has been observed to increase the sensation of pain.

Effects, Toxicity and Clinical Use

The effects of morphine (along with its related toxicity) are depicted in Table 1. Regarding its clinical use, morphine is prescribed for analgesia (acute - myocardial infarction, multiple injuries -, chronic - cancer -, and post-operative) and as an adjunct in general anesthesia. Its role in the treatment of pulmonary edema associated with left ventricular failure (reduced cardiac preload and afterload) remains under intense scrutiny, with newer trends regarding its use advocating against its place in the clinical setting [4,11].

Table 1. Effects of morphine

Central Nervous System	Peripheral
Analgesia	**Cardiovascular system**
Euphoria	None
Sedation	Hypotension
Respiratory depression	Cerebral vasodilation, CVR decrease, CBF and ICP increase
Body temperature reduction	**Gastrointestinal system**
GnRH, CRH, LH, FSH, ACTH, b-endorphin, testosterone and cortisol reduction	Biliary, pancreatic, and intestinal secretions reduction
Prolactin increase	Gastric motility decrease
Antidiuresis	Small intestine: resting tone increased
Cough suppression	Large intestine: diminished propulsive peristaltic waves and increased tone
Convulsions	Sphincter of Oddi constriction
Miosis	Biliary colic
Truncal rigidity	Constipation
Nausea and vomiting	**Smooth muscle**
	Decrease uterine tone, frequency, and amplitude of contractions
	Tone and amplitude of ureter contractions increase
	Urinary voiding reflex inhibition, external sphincter tone and bladder volume increase
	Renal system
	GFR decrease
	Integumentary system
	Cutaneous blood vessel dilation
	Pruritus
	Urticaria
	Immune system
	Immunosuppression and increased susceptibility to infection and tumor spread (NK cell cytolytic activity and lymphocyte proliferative response inhibition)

GnRH: gonadotropin-releasing hormone; CRH: corticotropin-releasing hormone; LH: luteinizing hormone; FSH: follicle-stimulating hormone; ACTH: Adrenocorticotropic hormone; CVR: cerebral vascular resistance; CBF: cerebral blood flow; ICP: intracranial pressure; GFR: glomerular filtration rate; NK: Natural killer

Morphine in Acute Coronary Syndromes

Since retrospective data have put the use of morphine in patients with UA/NSTEMI under intense scrutiny, taking into consideration its potentially adverse effects which will be analyzed below, the recommendation for morphine for analgesia is Class I only for patients with STEMI, since continuing pain requires relief whether these patients have received or are not candidates for reperfusion [12]. Even though no randomized trials have defined the unique contribution of morphine to the therapeutic scheme or its optimal administration schedule, morphine sulfate (2 to 4 mg intravenously - IV - with increments of 2 to 8 mg repeated at 5- to 15-minute intervals) is the analgesic of choice for management of pain associated with STEMI. Morphine should be given to patients whose symptoms are not relieved despite nitroglycerin (NTG) (e.g., after 3 serial sublingual NTG tablets) or whose symptoms recur despite adequate anti-ischemic therapy. Since the pain of STEMI has a clear relationship to the underlying ischemia, interventions that affect the oxygen supply-demand relationship (i.e., by either increasing supply or decreasing demand – as done through morphine) may lessen the pain of STEMI [13].

Morphine has also hemodynamic effects, which could prove potentially beneficial in UA/NSTEMI. However, the recommendation for morphine pain relief has been reduced to a Class IIa recommendation for that patient population, due to the CRUSADE Initiative, a non-randomized, retrospective, observational registry, that suggested that its use, either alone or in combination with nitroglycerin for NSTEMI patients, was associated with higher mortality [14]. Morphine causes venodilation and can produce modest reductions in heart rate (through increased vagal tone) and systolic blood pressure (BP) to further reduce myocardial oxygen demand. The major adverse reaction to morphine is an exaggeration of its therapeutic effect, causing hypotension, especially in the presence of volume depletion and/or vasodilator therapy. The concomitant use of atropine in 0.5- to 1.5-mg doses IV may be helpful in reducing the excessive vagomimetic effects of morphine if significant bradycardia or hypotension occurs. Although rare, respiratory depression is the most serious complication of morphine; the narcotic reversing agent naloxone, 0.1 to 0.2 mg IV, can be given initially if indicated and repeated after 15 minutes if necessary [9,15].

Ca^{2+} Channel Blockers

Since it was known, almost 200 years ago, that Ca^2 influx in the cell was necessary for the contraction of smooth and cardiac muscle, the use of drugs that could block this influx (by binding to specific receptors that mediate the entry of extracellular Ca^{2+} into these cells in response to electrical depolarization) and, therefore, inhibit muscle contraction, came into play in the clinical setting. It was almost 50 years ago, that it was shown that the effect of the diphenylpiperazine analogs in preventing agonist-induced vascular smooth muscle contraction could be overcome by raising the concentration of Ca^{2+} in the extracellular medium. Although many hormones increase Ca^{2+} influx through so-called receptor-operated channels, high external concentrations of K^+ and depolarizing electrical stimuli increase Ca^{2+} influx through voltage-sensitive or "potential operated" channels. The Ca^{2+} channel antagonists produce their effects by binding to the α_1 subunit of these voltage-sensitive (L-type) Ca^{2+} channels which will be discussed below [16].

Ca^{2+} channel blockers that are part of the therapeutic protocol in patients with ACS include nifedipine (Figure 2), the prototype of the dihydropyridine family of Ca^{2+} channel blockers, verapamil (Figure 3), a phenylalkylamine and the first clinically useful member of this group that was the result of attempts to synthesize more active analogs of papaverine (a vasodilator alkaloid found in the opium poppy) and diltiazem (Figure 4), a benzothiazepine.

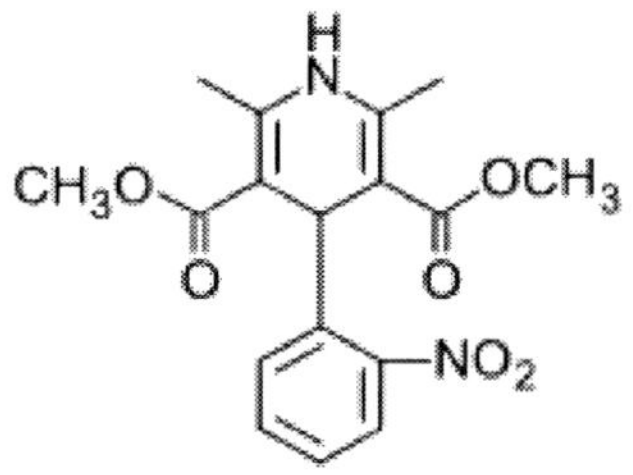

Figure 2. Structure of nifedipine.

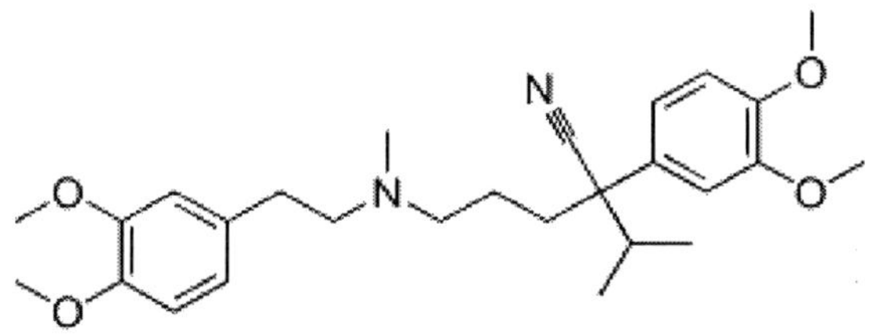

Figure 3. Structure of verapamil.

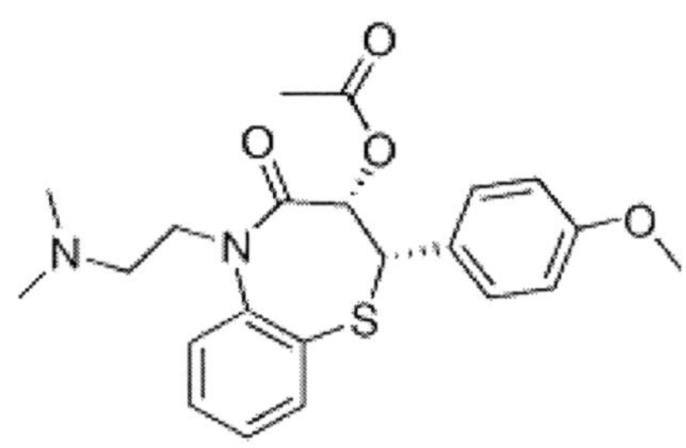

Figure 4. Structure of diltiazem.

Pharmacokinetics

The Ca^{2+} channel blockers are orally active agents and are characterized by high first-pass effect, high plasma protein binding (their elimination half-lives vary widely) and extensive metabolism. Verapamil and diltiazem are also used by the IV route. The effects of these drugs are evident within 30 to 60 minutes of an oral dose. For comparison, peak effects of verapamil (whose half-life is 6 h) occur within 15 minutes of its IV administration. For diltiazem and nifedipine the half-life is less (4 h). During repeated oral administration, bioavailability and half-life may increase because of saturation of hepatic metabolism. Diltiazem is metabolized in desacetyldiltiazem, which has about one-half of diltiazem's potency as a vasodilator. Norverapamil, the metabolic product of verapamil, is biologically active but much less potent than the parent compound. The metabolites of the nifedipine are inactive or weakly active. In patients with liver failure, the bioavailability of any Ca^{2+} channel blocker may be increased, so the physician should be careful in decreasing the dosage accordingly [16-18].

Pharmacodynamics

Voltage-sensitive channels contain domains of homologous sequence that are arranged in tandem within a single large subunit. In addition to the major channel-forming subunit (termed α_1), Ca^{2+} channels contain several other associated subunits (termed α_2, β, γ, and δ). Voltage-sensitive Ca^{2+} channels have been divided into at least three subtypes (L, N, and T) based on their conductances and sensitivities to voltage [19,20]. P/Q and R channels also have been identified. Only the L-type channel (the most prominent receptor type in cardiac and smooth muscle) is sensitive to the dihydropyridine Ca^{2+} channel blockers like nifedipine, while verapamil and diltiazem appear to bind to closely related but not identical receptors in another region [21]. After closure of Ca^{2+} channels, a finite period of time is required before the channels can open again in response to a stimulus. In the vascular tissue, at least three distinct mechanisms may be responsible for contraction of vascular smooth muscle cells. First, the voltage-sensitive Ca^{2+} channels discussed above. Second, agonist-induced contractions that occur without depolarization of the membrane result in the release of intracellular Ca^{2+} from the sarcoplasmic reticulum, which in turn mediates further influx of extracellular Ca^{2+} [22]. Third, receptor-operated Ca^{2+} channels allow the entry of extracellular Ca^{2+} in response to receptor occupancy. An increase in cytosolic Ca^{2+} results in enhanced binding of Ca^{2+} to calmodulin which, in turn, activates myosin light-chain kinase, with resulting phosphorylation of the myosin light chain. This promotes interaction between actin and myosin and, hence, contraction of smooth muscle. Ca^{2+} channel antagonists inhibit the voltage-dependent Ca^{2+} channels in vascular smooth muscle at significantly lower concentrations than are required to interfere with the release of intracellular Ca^{2+} or to block receptor-operated Ca^{2+} channels [16]. In the cardiac muscle, Ca^{2+} binds to troponin, relieving the inhibitory effect of troponin on the contractile apparatus and permitting a productive interaction of actin and myosin leading to contraction. Since depolarization largely depends on the movement of Ca^{2+}, Ca^{2+} channel blockers reduce the impulse generation (slow response, or Ca^{2+}-dependent, action potentials) in the sinoatrial (SA) node and the conduction in the atrioventricular (AV) node [17]. Skeletal muscle is not depressed by the Ca^{2+} channel blockers because it uses intracellular pools of Ca^{2+} to support excitation-contraction coupling and does not require as much transmembrane Ca^{2+} influx [17].

Effects, Toxicity and Clinical Use

Nifedipe has a greater ratio of vascular smooth muscle effects relative to cardiac effects than do diltiazem and verapamil. It does not decrease AV conduction and therefore can be used more safely than verapamil or diltiazem in the presence of AV conduction abnormalities. Although nifedipine has a direct negative inotropic effect *in vitro*, the decrease in arterial BP, due to selective dilation of arterial resistance vessels, elicits sympathetic reflexes with resulting tachycardia and positive inotropy. Contractility and segmental ventricular function are improved, and heart rate and cardiac output are increased modestly [16,17,23]. Verapamil is a less potent vasodilator *in vivo* than nifedipine and with direct negative chronotropic, dromotropic, and inotropic effect in the heart. IV verapamil causes a decrease in arterial BP owing to a decrease in vascular resistance. However its' direct negative chronotropic effect abolishes any reflex tachycardia. This intrinsic negative inotropic effect is partially offset by both a decrease in afterload and the reflex increase in adrenergic tone. Thus, in patients without congestive heart failure (CHF), ventricular performance is not impaired and actually may improve, especially if ischemia limits performance. In contrast, in patients with CHF, IV verapamil can cause a marked decrease in contractility and left ventricular function. Oral administration of verapamil reduces peripheral vascular resistance and blood pressure, often with minimal changes in heart rate [16,17]. IV administration of diltiazem can result initially in a marked decrease in peripheral vascular resistance and arterial blood pressure, which elicits a reflex increase in heart rate and cardiac output. Heart rate then falls below initial levels because of the direct negative chronotropic effect of the agent. Oral administration of diltiazem decreases both heart rate and mean arterial BP. While diltiazem and verapamil produce similar effects on the SA and AV nodes, the negative inotropic effect of diltiazem is more modest [16,17]. Verapamil and diltiazem also possess a nonspecific antiadrenergic effect, which may contribute to peripheral vasodilation. SA and AV nodal tissues are affected markedly by verapamil and moderately by diltiazem. Thus, verapamil and diltiazem decrease AV nodal conduction and are effective in the management of supraventricular reentry tachycardia and in decreasing ventricular responses in atrial fibrillation (AF) or flutter. The effects of Ca^{2+} channel blockers on diastolic ventricular relaxation (the lusitropic state of the ventricle) are complex. The sum total of these effects in any given patient cannot be determined *a priori* [16,17]. In addition to ACS patients (discussed in detail below), Ca^{2+} channel blockers have well-documented efficacy in hypertension. They also show promise in a variety of other conditions, including hypertrophic cardiomyopathy, migraine, Raynaud's phenomenon and preterm labor (stop preterm uterine contractions *in vitro)* [17]. The most important effects of Ca^{2+} channel blockers in smooth and cardiac muscle are summarized in Table 2. The most important toxic effects reported for the Ca^{2+} channel blockers are direct extensions of their therapeutic action. Cardiac depression, including cardiac arrest, bradycardia, AV block, and heart failure, especially in patients with SA node disease, in patients who exhibit AV nodal conduction disturbances or in the presence of β-adrenergic receptor blockade are such. Minor toxicity includes flushing, dizziness, nausea, constipation, coughing, wheezing, headache, digital dysesthesia, hypotension, peripheral and pulmonary edema.

Less common side effects include rash, somnolence, and occasional minor elevations of liver function tests. Some Ca^{2+} channel antagonists (especially verapamil) can cause an increase in the concentration of digoxin in plasma.

Table 2. Most important effects of Ca^{2+} channel blockers in smooth and cardiac muscle

Smooth muscle relaxation
Vascular – mostly arteries (BP lowering, PVR reduction, coronary arterial tone reduction, coronary blood flow increase)
Bronchiolar
Gastrointestinal
Uterine
Cardiac muscle
SA node impulse generation and AV node conduction reduced or blocked
Cardiac contractility reduction (excitation-contraction coupling lowering)
Cardiac output and rate reduction

BP: blood pressure; PVR: peripheral vascular resistance; SA: sinoatrial; AV: atrioventricular

Caution must be exerted by the physician when combining verapamil or diltiazem with β-blockers. Complete AV block and depression of ventricular function may ensue. In the presence of overt heart failure, all Ca^{2+} channel blockers can cause further worsening of heart failure as a result of their negative inotropic effect [16].

Ca^{2+} Channel Blockers in ACS

Verapamil and diltiazem are a reasonable therapeutic approach, according to the American College of Cardiology/American Heart Association (ACC/AHA) guidelines, for those patients in whom beta-blockers are ineffective or contraindicated for relief of ongoing ischemia or control of a rapid ventricular response with AF or atrial flutter after STEMI in the absence of CHF, left ventricular dysfunction, or AV block [15]. Long-term treatment with verapamil in patients after an acute myocardial infarction (AMI) revealed a significant reduction in major events (death or reinfarction) [24]. Verapamil's positive effect was found in patients that did not exhibit heart failure, making the former detrimental to patients with heart failure or bradyarrhythmias during the first 24 to 48 hours after a STEMI [25-27]. Alternatively, studies regarding the effect of diltiazem on mortality and reinfarction after myocardial infarction revealed a reduction in cardiac events (including the frequency of refractory postinfarction angina) only in those patients without pulmonary congestion, rendering of particular clinical importance the detrimental mortality effect of diltiazem in patients with left ventricular dysfunction [28,29]. The INTERCEPT trial showed that although diltiazem did not reduce the cumulative occurrence of cardiac death, non-fatal reinfarction, or refractory ischaemia during a 6-month follow-up of patients with AMI, but without CHF, who first received thrombolytic agents, it did reduce all composite endpoints of non-fatal cardiac events, and, especially, the need for myocardial revascularization [30]. Nifedipine not only does not reduce the incidence of reinfarction or mortality when given in patients with STEMI, but it has also been shown not to reduce infarct size, as determined by enzyme level, in patients with AMI [31-35]. On the contrary, nifedipine has been shown to cause an increase in total mortality in patients with coronary artery disease (CAD) [36]. Nifedipine could prove to be catastrophic in patients with hypotension or tachycardia, since, according to a proposed theory in these patients, it may induce a reduction in coronary perfusion pressure (CPP), disproportionate dilatation of the coronary arteries adjacent to the ischemic area, and a reflex activation of the sympathetic nervous system, with an increase in myocardial oxygen demands [15,37].

Inhibitors of the Renin-Angiotensin-Aldosterone System

The renin-angiotensin system participates significantly in the pathophysiology of hypertension, congestive heart failure, myocardial infarction, and diabetic nephropathy. The kidneys release renin (a pressor substance) when the renal arterial pressure is reduced, when the sympathetic system is stimulated and when the sodium (Na^{2+}) concentration is increased at the distal renal tubule or when its delivery is reduced.

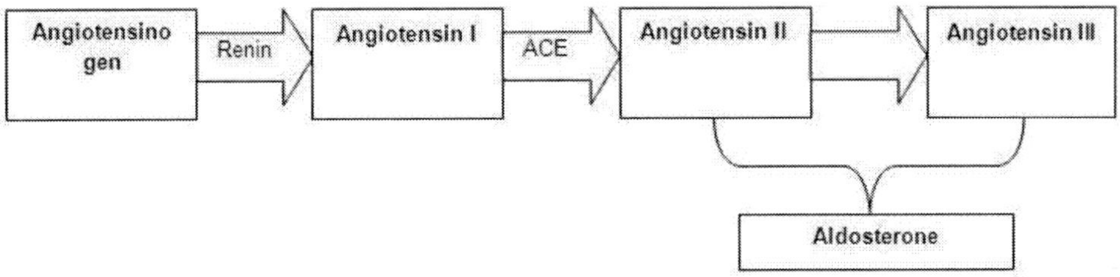

ACE: angiotensin-converting enzyme

Figure 5. The renin-angiotensin-aldosterone system.

Then, angiotensinogen (an inactive precursor globular glycoprotein) is converted to angiotensin I (through the action of renin), which in turn is converted to angiotensin II (a vasoconstrictor agent), through the angiotensin-converting enzyme (ACE), an ectoenzyme and glycoprotein. Finally, angiotensin II is converted in the adrenal gland to angiotensin III. Angiotensin II and III both stimulate aldosterone release (Figure 5). ACE is identical to kininase II, the enzyme that inactivates bradykinin, which works at least in part by stimulating release of nitric oxide and prostacyclin (leading to vasodilation) [38,39]. The functions of angiotensin II are depicted in Table 3 [38]. The renin-angiotensin-aldosterone system can be inhibited at i) the renin release (through β-adrenoceptor antagonists, ii) the renin activity (through renin inhibitors), iii) the ACE (through ACE inhibitors), iv) the angiotensin II type 1 (AT_1) receptors (through AT_1-receptor antagonists) and v) the aldosterone receptors (through aldosterone receptor antagonists) [40]. For our purposes, we will examine the last 3 categories, as the first 2 have no place in the ACS therapeutic protocol.

Table 3. Angiotensin II functions

Total peripheral resistance increase
Direct vasoconstriction
Enhancement of peripheral noradrenergic neurotransmission
Effects on the CNS (sympathetic tone increase, dipsogenic effect, vasopressin and ACTH release)
Release of catecholamines from the adrenal medulla
Renal function altering
Sodium reabsorption in the renal tubules
Release of aldosterone from the adrenal cortex
Altered renal hemodynamics (constriction the renal vascular smooth muscle, by renal sympathetic tone enhancement and renal adrenergic transmission facilitation)
Cardiovascular structure altering
Nonhemodynamically mediated effects (migration, proliferation, hypertrophy, and/or synthetic capacity of vascular smooth muscle cells, cardiac myocytes, and fibroblasts stimulation)
Hemodynamically mediated effectse (cardiac preload and afterload increase)

CNS: central nervous system; ACTH: adrenocorticotropic hormone

ACE Inhibitors

ACE inhibitors can be classified into three broad groups based on chemical structure: (1) sulfhydryl-containing ACE inhibitors, structurally related to captopril (Figure 6) (e.g., zofenopril); (2) dicarboxyl-containing ACE inhibitors, structurally related to enalapril (Figure 7) (e.g., lisinopril, ramipril, trandolapril); and (3) phosphorus-containing ACE inhibitors, structurally related to fosinopril (Figure 8).[38]

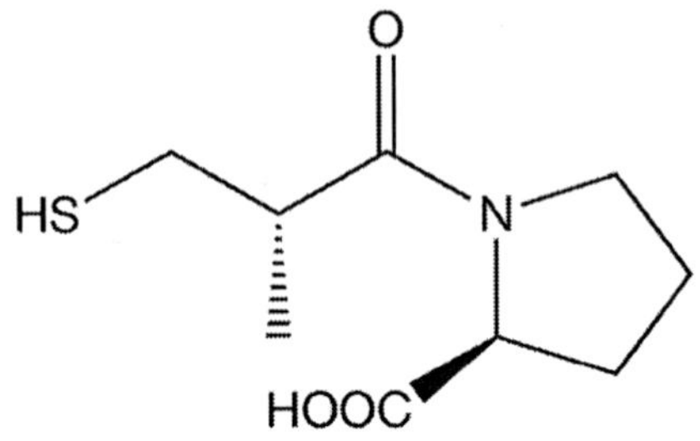

Figure 6. Structure of captopril.

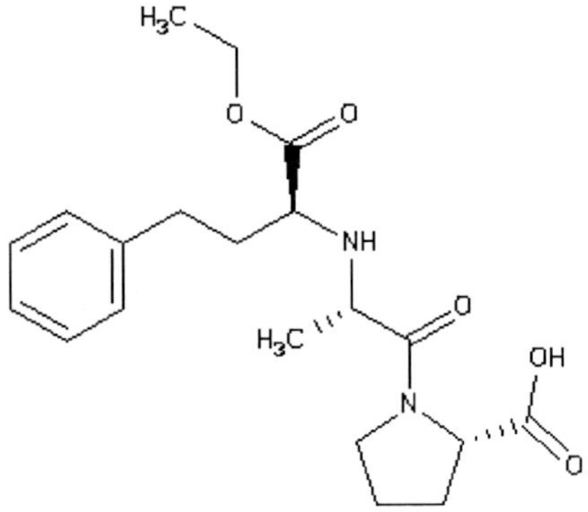

Figure 7. Structure of enalapril.

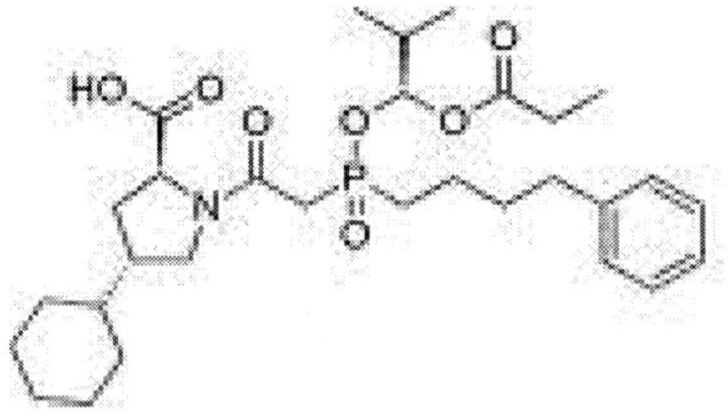

Figure 8. Structure of fosinopril.

Pharmacokinetics

Many ACE inhibitors are ester-containing prodrugs that are much less potent but have a much better oral bioavailability than the active molecules. Since ACE inhibitors are cleared predominantly by the kidneys, dosages of these drugs should be reduced in patients with renal failure.

Captopril, when administered orally, is absorbed rapidly and has a bioavailability of about 75%. Peak concentrations in plasma occur within an hour, with the drug being cleared rapidly with a half-life of approximately 2 hours. Most of the drug is eliminated in urine, almost half as captopril and the rest as captopril disulfide dimers and captopril-cysteine disulfide. Captopril should not be administered with meals but at least 1 hour after, since food reduces the oral bioavailability of captopril by 25% to 30% [38-40]. Enalapril maleate, is hydrolyzed by esterases in the liver to produce the active dicarboxylic acid, enalaprilat, which is a highly potent ACE inhibitor. Enalapril is absorbed rapidly when given orally and has an oral bioavailability of about 60%. Although peak concentrations of enalapril in plasma occur within an hour, enalaprilat concentrations peak only after 3 to 4 hours. Enalaprilat has a plasma half-life of about 11 hours. Nearly all the drug is eliminated by the kidneys as either intact enalapril or enalaprilat [38-40]. Lisinopril, although the lysine analogue of enalaprilat, in contrast to enalapril (which is inactive), is active. Lisinopril is absorbed slowly and incompletely (about 30%) after oral administration; peak concentrations in plasma are achieved in about 7 hours. It is cleared as the intact compound by the kidney, and its half-life in plasma is about 11 hours. Lisinopril does not accumulate in tissues [38-40]. Approximately 10% and 70% of an oral dose of trandolapril is bioavailable as trandolapril and trandolaprilat (its metabolic byproduct), respectively. Trandolaprilat is about eight times more potent than trandolapril. Trandolapril is also converted to inactive metabolites. The metabolic byproducts are recovered in the urine and feces. Peak concentrations of trandolaprilat in plasma are achieved in 4 to 10 hours. Trandolaprilat displays biphasic elimination kinetics with an initial half-life of about 10 hours (the major component of elimination), followed by a more prolonged half-life owing to slow dissociation of trandolaprilat from tissue ACE [38-40]. Ramipril is metabolized into ramiprilat (the active ACE inhibitor) by hepatic esterases. Ramipril is also metabolized to inactive metabolites. The products of metabolism are excreted predominantly by the kidneys. Ramipril is absorbed rapidly (peak concentrations of ramipril are achieved in 1 hour, while peak concentrations of ramiprilat in plasma are achieved in about 3 hours). Ramiprilat displays triphasic elimination kinetics with half-lives of 2 to 4 hours, 9 to 18 hours, and greater than 50 hours. This triphasic elimination is due to extensive distribution to all tissues (initial half-life), clearance of free ramiprilat from plasma (intermediate half-life), and dissociation of ramiprilat from tissue ACE (terminal half-life) [38-40]. The absorption rate of the medications above (except for enalapril and lisinopril) is reduced by food, so care must be taken so as to avoid co-administration with meals.

Effects, Toxicity and Clinical Use

ACE inhibitors affect capacitance and resistance vessels reducing cardiac load as well as arterial pressure. They do not affect cardiac contractility, so cardiac output normally increases. They act preferentially on angiotensin-sensitive vascular beds, which include those of the kidney, heart and brain. This selectivity may be important in sustaining adequate perfusion of these vital organs in the face of reduced perfusion pressure. Elevated plasma renin activity (PRA) renders patients hyperresponsive to ACE inhibitor-induced hypotension, and initial dosages of all ACE inhibitors should be reduced in patients with high plasma levels of renin (e.g., patients with heart failure and salt-depleted patients). Unlike direct vasodilators, these agents do not result in reflex sympathetic activation and can be used safely in persons with ischemic heart disease. Baroreceptor function and cardiovascular reflexes are not compromised, and responses to postural changes and exercise are little impaired [38-40].

ACE inhibitors should be given to all patients with impaired left ventricular systolic function. Inhibition of ACE in patients with systolic dysfunction prevents or delays the progression of heart failure, decreases the incidence of sudden death and myocardial infarction, decreases hospitalization, and improves quality of life. The mechanisms by which ACE inhibitors improve outcome in patients with systolic dysfunction are not completely understood. ACE inhibitors reduce plasma levels of plasminogen activator inhibitor-1 and improve endothelial vasomotor dysfunction in patients with CAD [38,39,41,42]. In patients with type 1 diabetes mellitus (DM) and diabetic nephropathy, captopril prevents or delays the progression of renal disease [38,39]. Specific renoprotection by ACE inhibitors is more difficult to demonstrate in type 2 diabetics, with some studies providing positive results [43-45], whereas others do not demonstrate blood pressure-independent renoprotection [46]. Several mechanisms participate in the renal protection afforded by ACE inhibitors (reduction of glomerular capillary pressure, increase of the permeability selectivity of the filtering membrane). As far as toxicity is concerned, severe hypotension can occur after initial doses of any ACE inhibitor in patients who are hypovolemic due to diuretics, salt restriction, or gastrointestinal fluid loss. Other adverse effects common to all ACE inhibitors include acute renal failure (particularly in patients with bilateral renal artery stenosis or stenosis of the renal artery of a solitary kidney) [38,39]. ACE inhibitors may cause hyperkalemia in patients with renal insufficiency (e.g., due to DM) or in patients taking K^+-sparing diuretics, K^+ supplements, β-adrenergic receptor blockers, or non-steroidal anti-inflammatory drugs (NSAIDs) [38]. Dry cough may appear, sometimes accompanied by wheezing, and angioedema. Bradykinin and substance P seem to be responsible for the cough and angioedema seen with ACE inhibition. This adverse effect may be mediated by the accumulation in the lungs of bradykinin, substance P, and/or prostaglandins, induction of tissue-specific autoantibodies, or inhibition of complement 1-esterase inhibitor [38,39]. However, ACE inhibitors induced cough can be reduced by other pharmaceutical pathways (thromboxane antagonism, aspirin, iron supplementation) [47-49]. Once ACE inhibitors are stopped, the cough disappears [50].

Although it is rare, angioedema of the intestine (visceral angioedema) also has been reported in association with ACE inhibitors. Visceral angioedema is characterized by emesis, watery diarrhea, and abdominal pain [38,39].The use of ACE inhibitors is contraindicated during the second and third trimesters of pregnancy because of the risk of fetal hypotension, anuria, and renal failure, sometimes associated with fetal malformations (oligohydramnios, fetal calvarial hypoplasia, fetal pulmonary hypoplasia, fetal growth retardation) [51]. ACE inhibitors may cause neutropenia or proteinuria. However, proteinuria is not a contraindication for ACE inhibitors because ACE inhibitors are renoprotective in certain renal diseases associated with proteinuria, *e.g.,* diabetic nephropathy [38,39]. Minor toxic effects seen more typically include altered sense of taste (dysgeusia), allergic skin rashes (a maculopapular rash that may or may not itch), and drug fever, which may occur in as many as 10% of patients. Glycosuria, hepatotoxicity and acute renal failure may also develop [38,39,52-54].

Important drug interactions include those with K^+ supplements or K^+-sparing diuretics, which can result in hyperkalemia. Nonsteroidal anti-inflammatory drugs may impair the hypotensive effects of ACE inhibitors Antacids may reduce the bioavailability of ACE inhibitors [38,39]. The clinical uses of ACE inhibitors are summarized in Table 4 [40].

Table 4. Clinical uses of ACE inhibitors

Hypertension
Diabetic nephropathy
Progressive renal insufficiency
Scleroderma renal crisis
Following AMI (especially with ventricular dysfunction)
Cardiac failure
At high risk of myocardial ischemia

AMI: Acute myocardial infarction

AT_1-Receptor Antagonists

AT_1-receptor antagonists potently and selectively inhibit most of the biological effects of angiotensin II (described above).

Although both classes of drugs block the renin-angiotensin system, AT_1-receptor antagonists differ from ACE inhibitors in several important aspects:

(1) AT_1-receptor antagonists reduce activation of AT_1 receptors more effectively than do ACE inhibitors.
(2) AT_1-receptor antagonists permit activation of AT_2 receptors,
(3) ACE inhibitors may increase angiotensin levels more than AT_1-receptor antagonists [38,39].

Pharmacokinetics

The nonpeptide AT_1-receptor antagonists valsartan candesartan, losartan, eprosartan, irbesartan and telmesartan are orally active, with a low oral bioavailability and high protein binding (>90%). Candesartan (the active form, Figure 9) is the product of the complete hydrolyzation of candesartan cilexetil (an inactive ester prodrug), during absorption from the gastrointestinal tract. Peak plasma levels are obtained 3 to 4 hours after oral administration, and the plasma half-life is about 9 hours. Plasma clearance of candesartan is due to renal elimination (33%) and biliary excretion (67%). The plasma clearance of candesartan is affected in patients with renal failure [38,39].

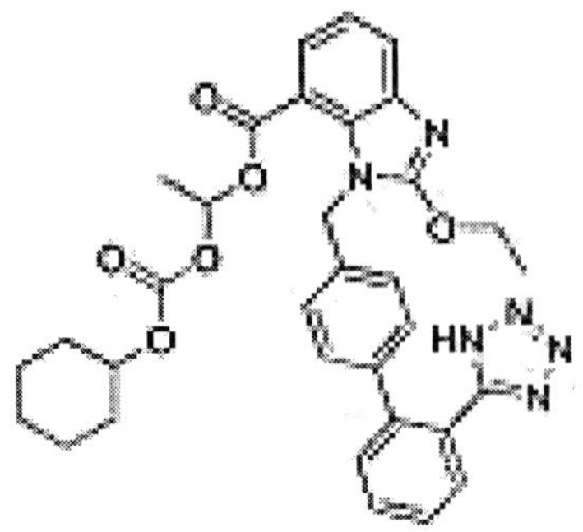

Figure 9. Structure of candesartan.

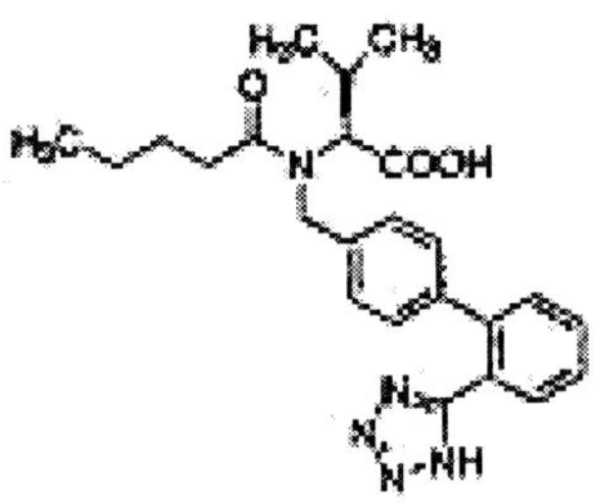

Figure 10. Structure of valsartan.

The peak plasma levels and the plasma half of valsartan (Figure 10) are identical to those of candersartan. Food markedly decreases absorption. Valsartan is cleared from the circulation by the liver (about 70% of total clearance). The plasma clearance of valsartan is affected by hepatic but not renal insufficiency [38,39].

Pharmacodynamics

The effects of angiotensins are exerted through specific heptahelical G protein-coupled receptors [55]. The two subtypes of angiotensin receptors are designated as AT_1 and AT_2 [56-58]. Most of the known actions of angiotensin II are mediated by the AT_1 receptor subtype. AT_1 receptors activate a large array of signal-transduction systems to produce effects that vary with cell type and that are a combination of primary and secondary responses. Less is known about AT_2 receptor-effector coupling, where the signal transduction pathways are still being investigated [59-63]. Most of the known actions of angiotensin II are mediated by the AT_1 receptor. Binding of angiotensin II to AT_1 receptors in vascular smooth muscle results in activation of phospholipase C and generation of inositol trisphosphate and diacylglycerol. These events, which occur within seconds, result in smooth muscle contraction. In other tissues, different signal transduction mechanisms are used (e.g., inhibition of adenylyl cyclase) [39].

Effects, Toxicity and Clinical Use

AT_1-receptor antagonists have a renoprotective function in patients with type 2 DM [64-66]. Also, AT_1-receptor antagonists (like irbesartan) may also prevent the recurrence of AF [67]. Losartan is reported to be safe and highly effective in the treatment of portal hypertension in patients with cirrhosis and portal hypertension [68]. Unlike ACE inhibitors, the angiotensin-II receptor antagonists are not significantly associated with cough or angioedema. Dizziness is a drug-related side effect that occurs in a small percentage of patients. Infrequent adverse effects with a possible causal association include nausea, headache, upper respiratory tract infection, back pain, fatigue, diarrhea, dyspepsia, nasal congestion, sinusitis and pharyngitis. Rarely, liver function tests and serum bilirubin concentrations may become elevated. AT_1-receptor antagonists have teratogenic potential and should be discontinued before the second trimester of pregnancy. AT_1-receptor antagonists should be used cautiously in patients whose arterial BP or renal function is highly dependent on the renin-angiotensin system (*e.g.*, renal artery stenosis). In such patients, they can cause hypotension, oliguria, progressive azotemia, or acute renal failure. AT_1-receptor antagonists may cause hyperkalemia in patients with renal disease or in patients taking K^+ supplements or K^+-sparing diuretics [38-40]. All AT_1-receptor antagonists are approved for the treatment of hypertension. In addition, AT_1-receptor antagonists are approved for diabetic nephropathy, for stroke prophylaxis, and, finally, for heart failure in patients who cannot tolerate or have an unsatisfactory response to ACE inhibitors [38,39]. Valsartan is indicated for use in patients with heart failure and in post-myocardial infarction (as discussed below). It has, also shown to reduce the risk of developing new-onset DM in hypertensive patients at high risk of cardiac events compared with Ca^{2+} antagonist treatment. In diabetic patients with microalbuminuria, valsartan has been shown to have benefits beyond those attributable to BP lowering alone [38,39].

Aldosterone Antagonists

Spironolactone (a synthetic steroid, Figure 11) and its analogue eplerenone (Figure 12), which differs from the former by replacement of a 17-α-thioacetyl group with a carbomethoxy group and by the fact that it has greater selectivity for the aldosterone receptor than spironolactone, act as competitive antagonists to aldosterone. These diuretic compounds antagonize the effects of aldosterone at the late distal tubule and cortical collecting tubule of the kidney. This inhibition may occur by direct pharmacologic antagonism of mineralocorticoid receptors [38-40].

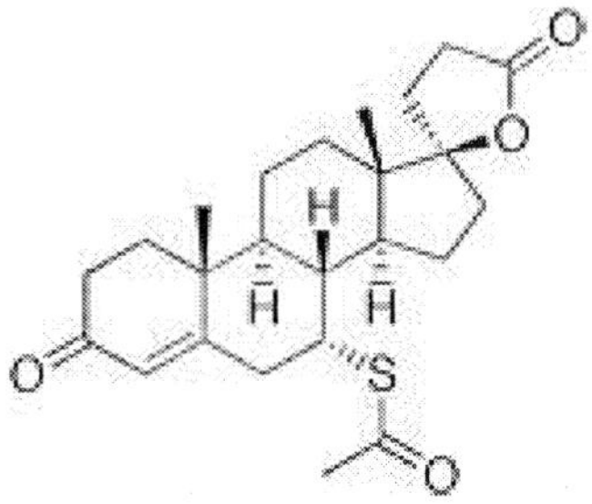

Figure 11. Structure of spironolactone.

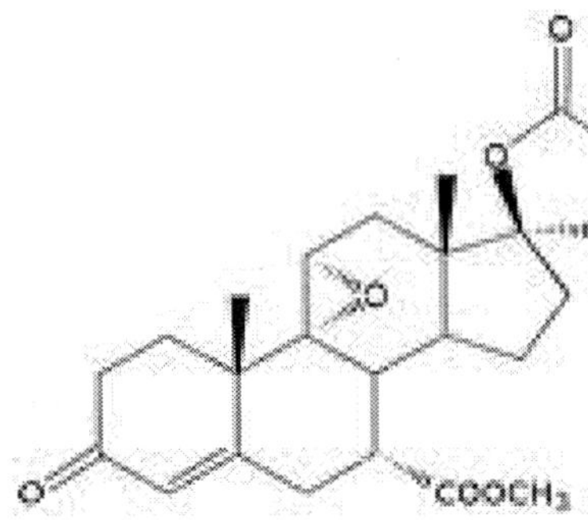

Figure 12. Structure of eplerenone.

Pharmacokinetics

Spironolactone is well absorbed from the gut. Its plasma half-life is only 10 minutes, but its active metabolite, canrenone, has a plasma half-life of 16 hours. Spironolactone has a rather slow onset of action, requiring several days before full therapeutic effect is achieved.

Eplerenone has a shorter elimination half-life than canrenone and has no active metabolites. Its onset and duration of action are determined by the kinetics of the aldosterone response in the target tissue [38-40].

Pharmacodynamics

Spironolactone and eplerenone reduce Na^+ absorption and K^+ secretion in the collecting tubules and ducts, since aldosterone, which regulates this process, is inhibited. They have very limited diuretic action when used singly, because distal Na^+/K^+ exchange accounts for reabsorption of only 2% of filtered Na^+. These aldosterone antagonists act also in the intercalated cells of the collecting tubule of the kidney by inhibiting hydrogen cation (H^+) secretion [38-40].

Effects, Toxicity and Clinical Use

These agents can cause mild, moderate, or even life-threatening hyperkalemia. The risk of this complication is greatly increased in the presence of renal disease or of other drugs that reduce renin (like NSAIDs) or angiotensin II activity (ACE inhibitors, AT_1-receptor antagonists) and, especially, when they are used as the sole diuretic agent. Also, by inhibiting H^+ secretion in parallel with K^+ secretion (as described above), these K^+-sparing diuretics can cause acidosis similar to that seen with type IV renal tubular acidosis [38]. These synthetic steroids may cause endocrine abnormalities by effects on other steroid receptors. Gynecomastia, menstrual disorder, testicular atrophy, impotence and benign prostatic hyperplasia have all been reported with spironolactone but not with eplerenone, which has lower affinity for these receptors [38]. Gastrointestinal upset is quite common. The physician should be very cautious when administering aldosterone antagonists in patients with liver failure. Dosing must be carefully adjusted for spironolactone due to its impaired metabolism.

Strong CYP3A4 inhibitors (eg, ketoconazole, itraconazole) can markedly increase blood levels of eplerenone, with potential deleterious results regarding its toxicity profile [38,39].

The clinical uses of aldosterone antagonists are summarized on Table 5 [38,39].

Table 5. Clinical uses of aldosterone antagonists

Hypertension
Heart failure
ACS
Prevents hypokalaemia when combined with K^+-losing (i.e. loop or thiazide) diuretics
Primary hyperaldosteronism (Conn's syndrome)
Resistant essential hypertension (especially low-renin hypertension)
Secondary hyperaldosteronism (hepatic cirrhosis, heart failure, nephrotic syndrome)

ACS: acute coronary syndromes

Inhibitors of the Renin-Angiotensin-Aldosterone System in ACS

The recommendation given by the ACC/AHA that ACE inhibitors should be administered orally within the first 24 hours of STEMI to patients with anterior infarction, pulmonary congestion, or left ventricular ejection fraction (LVEF) less than 0.40, in the absence of hypotension (systolic BP less than 100 mm Hg or less than 30 mm Hg below baseline) or known contraindications to that class of medications was based on several large trials that revealed reduced mortality rates when ACE inhibitors were given. ACE inhibitors should also be considered for administration to patients without these features (class IIa recommendation) [69]. An IV ACE inhibitor should not be given to patients within the first 24 hours of STEMI because of the risk of hypotension [15].

More specifically, the ISIS-4 Collaborative Group showed that the benefits of captopril when administered in patients with suspected AMI not only significantly reduced 5-week mortality but also appeared to be larger in certain higher-risk groups, such as those presenting with a history of previous myocardial infarction or with heart failure [70]. The CCS-1 Collaborative Group verified the aforementioned results [71]. The SAVE investigators revealed that in post-myocardial infarction patients with asymptomatic left ventricular dysfunction, long-term administration of captopril reduced recurrence of myocardial infarction and the need for cardiac revascularization but had no influence on the rate of hospitalization with a discharge diagnosis of UA [72].

Long-term use of ACE inhibitors has been also shown to be beneficial for many patients with high-risk chronic CAD. The Trace Study Group showed that ACE inhibition with trandolapril after myocardial infarction, complicated by left ventricular dysfunction, appeared to be of considerable importance in patients with DM by saving lives and substantially reducing the risk of progression to severe heart failure [73]. Taking the study one step further, the beneficial effect on mortality and hospitalization rates was maintained for at least 10-12 years [74]. Ramipril significantly reduced the rates of death, MI, and stroke in a broad range of high-risk patients not known to have a low LVEF or heart failure [75]. Enalapril reduced mortality rates in patients with myocardial infarction or in those who recently had a myocardial infarction and left ventricular systolic dysfunction [76]. The only trial that did not show a benefit with enalapril was the CONSENSUS II study, in which patients that were randomly assigned within the first day to receive either IV enalapril or placebo, exhibited no difference regarding mortality [77]. Lisinopril, started within 24 h from AMI symptoms, produced significant reductions in overall mortality [78]. The SMILE study showed the same results for zofenopril [79].

AT_1-receptor antagonists can also substitute ACE inhibitors for patients who cannot tolerate the later [69]. Valsartan was found to be as effective as captopril in patients at high risk for cardiovascular events after myocardial infarction; however, the same does not hold when combining valsartan with captopril, as their co-administration increased the rate of adverse events without improving survival [80]. Although not in the acute care setting, treatment of patients with chronic heart failure with candesartan (at least half of whom had an myocardial infarction) in the CHARM-Overall program showed a reduction in cardiovascular deaths and hospital admissions for heart failure, independent of ejection fraction or baseline treatment [81].

Long-term aldosterone receptor blockade should be prescribed for UA/NSTEMI patients without significant renal dysfunction or hyperkalemia who are already receiving therapeutic doses of an ACE inhibitor, have an LVEF less than or equal to 0.40, and have either symptomatic heart failure or DM [69]. A double-blind, placebo-controlled study evaluating the effect of eplerenone, a selective aldosterone blocker, on morbidity and mortality among patients with AMI complicated by left venntricular dysfunction and heart failure reduced morbidity and mortality rates [82]. This finding was validated by the Randomized Aldactone Evaluation Study Investigators, where blockade of aldosterone receptors by spironolactone, in addition to standard therapy, substantially reduced the risk of both morbidity and death among patients with severe heart failure [83].

Others

Ranolazine was approved only a few years ago for administration (alone or in combination with nitrates, beta-blockers or amlodipine) in patients with chronic refractory angina who do not respond to standard antianginal therapy [84]. Although the mechanism of its action is not fully understood, the recommended initial dose is 500 mg orally twice daily, with a maximum dose of 1000 mg twice daily [69,85]. The MERLIN-TIMI 36 randomized trial showed that the addition of ranolazine to standard treatment for ACS, while not effective in reducing major cardiovascular events, did not adversely affect the risk of all-cause death or symptomatic documented arrhythmia, rendering ranolazine a safe option for symptom relief after UA/NSTEMI, but with no significant improval in cardiovascular deaths, myocardial infarction, or recurrent ischemia [86].

Nicorandil, an ATP sensitive K^+ channel opener, with 'cardioprotective' effects, when added to aggressive anti-anginal treatment for UA, reduced transient myocardial ischaemia as well as non-sustained ventricular, and supraventricular arrhythmia compared to placebo. Its anti-arrhythmic activity is thought to be based to its anti-ischaemic action [87]. However, nicorandil has not been approved in the United States of America [69].

Magnesium, although thought to reduce mortality rates in STEMI patients, as evidenced by studies such as the LIMIT-2 trial, was later shown to have no benefit [70,88-90]. ACC/AHA guidelines suggest that it is reasonable that documented magnesium deficits be corrected, especially in patients receiving diuretics before the onset of STEMI and that episodes of torsade de pointes-type ventricular tachycardia (VT) associated with a prolonged QT interval be treated with 1 to 2 gr of magnesium administered as an IV bolus over 5 minutes. In the absence of documented electrolyte deficits or torsade de pointes-type VT, routine IV magnesium should not be administered to STEMI patients at any level of risk [15].

An insulin infusion to normalize blood glucose is recommended for patients with STEMI and complicated courses. During the acute phase (first 24 to 48 hours) of the management of STEMI in patients with hyperglycemia, it is reasonable to administer an insulin infusion to normalize blood glucose even in patients with an uncomplicated course. It is during that time that, not only the decreased insulin sensitivity contributes to impaired glucose utilization but, also, that free fatty acid levels and the concentration of their metabolites increase, potentiating ischemic injury through several mechanisms: direct myocardial toxicity, increased oxygen demand, and direct inhibition of glucose oxidation. It has been suggested that agents that support glucose oxidation, like insulin, could reduce postischemic contractile dysfunction. It has also been stipulated that insulin may improve the fibrinolytic profile of patients with STEMI. After the acute phase, it is reasonable to individualize treatment of diabetics [15,91,92].

Conclusion

During the last decades, huge advances have been made in our understanding of the pathophysiology of ACS; these have been accompanied by important breakthroughs in the management of this condition. Accurate diagnosis of ACS has life-saving implications and requires a careful assessment of both the patient's history and the findings on physical examination, 12-lead electrocardiogram (ECG), and cardiac biomarker assays. Anti-ischemic therapy remains a cornerstone in the treatment of patients with STEMI, NSTEMI or UA, and it is the treating physician and medical staff responsibility to tailor it as soon as possible so as to relief the patient from pain and improve ACS prognosis.

References

[1] Gutstein HB, Akil H. Opioid analgesics. In: *Goodman and Gilman's The Pharmacological Basis of Therapeutics*, Brunton LL, Lazo JS, Parker KL, eds. *11th edition*, New York: McGraw-Hill, *2006, 547-590.*

[2] Meunier JC, Mollereau C, Toll L, Suaudeau C, Moisand C, Alvinerie P, Butour JL, Guillemot JC, Ferrara P, Monsarrat B, et al. Isolation and structure of the endogenous agonist of opioid receptor-like ORL1 receptor. *Nature* 1995;377:532-535.

[3] Reinscheid RK, Nothacker HP, Bourson A, Ardati A, Henningsen RA, Bunzow JR, Grandy DK, Langen H, Monsma FJ Jr, Civelli O. Orphanin FQ: a neuropeptide that activates an opioidlike G protein-coupled receptor. *Science* 1995;270:792-794 .

[4] Schumacher MA, Basbaum AI, Way WL. Opioid analgesics and antagonists. In: *Basic and clinical pharmacology*, Katzung BG ed. 10th edition, Boston: 2006, 489-510.

[5] Analgesic drugs. In: *Rang and Dale's pharmacology*, Rang HP, Dale MM, Ritter JM, Flower RJ, eds. 6th edition, Philadelphia, Churchill Livingstone: 2007, 562-584.

[6] Christrup LL. Morphine metabolites. *Acta Anaesthesiol. Scand.* 1997;41:116-122.

[7] Waldhoer M, Bartlett SE, Whistler JL. Opioid receptors. *Annu. Rev. Biochem.* 2004;73:953-990.

[8] Mansour A, Fox CA, Akil H, Watson SJ. Opioid-receptor mRNA expression in the rat CNS: anatomical and functional implications. *Trends Neurosci.* 1995;18:22-29.

[9] Stefano GB, Kream RM, Esch T. Revisiting tolerance from the endogenous morphine perspective. *Med. Sci. Monit.* 2009;15:RA189-198.

[10] Ueda H, Ueda M. Mechanisms underlying morphine analgesic tolerance and dependence. *Front Biosci.* 2009;14:5260-5272.

[11] Sosnowski MA. Review article: lack of effect of opiates in the treatment of acute cardiogenic pulmonary oedema. *Emerg. Med. Australas.* 2008;20:384-390.

[12] Antman EM, Hand M, Armstrong PW, Bates ER, Green LA, Halasyamani LK, Hochman JS, Krumholz HM, Lamas GA, Mullany CJ, Pearle DL, Sloan MA, Smith SC Jr; 2004 Writing Committee Members, Anbe DT, Kushner FG, Ornato JP, Jacobs AK, Adams CD, Anderson JL, Buller CE, Creager MA, Ettinger SM, Halperin JL, Hunt SA, Lytle BW, Nishimura R, Page RL, Riegel B, Tarkington LG, Yancy CW. 2007 Focused Update of the ACC/AHA 2004 Guidelines for the Management of Patients With ST-Elevation Myocardial Infarction: a report of the American College of Cardiology/American Heart Association Task Force on Practice Guidelines: developed in collaboration With the Canadian Cardiovascular Society endorsed by the American Academy of Family Physicians: 2007 Writing Group to Review New Evidence and Update the ACC/AHA 2004 Guidelines for the Management of Patients With ST-Elevation Myocardial Infarction, Writing on Behalf of the 2004 Writing Committee. *Circulation* 2008;117:296-329.

[13] Hochman JS, Califf RM. Acute myocardial infarction. In: Smith TW. *Cardiovascular therapeutics: a companion to Braunwald's heart disease*, 2nd ed. Philadelphia, PA: WB Saunders Co Ltd; 2001:235-291.

[14] Meine TJ, Roe MT, Chen AY, Patel MR, Washam JB, Ohman EM, Peacock WF, Pollack CV Jr, Gibler WB, Peterson ED; CRUSADE Investigators. Association of intravenous morphine use and outcomes in acute coronary syndromes: results from the CRUSADE Quality Improvement Initiative. *Am. Heart J.* 2005;149:1043-1049.

[15] Antman EM, Anbe DT, Armstrong PW, Bates ER, Green LA, Hand M, Hochman JS, Krumholz HM, Kushner FG, Lamas GA, Mullany CJ, Ornato JP, Pearle DL, Sloan MA, Smith SC Jr; American College of Cardiology; American Heart Association; Canadian Cardiovascular Society. ACC/AHA guidelines for the management of patients with ST-elevation myocardial infarction--executive summary. A report of the American College of Cardiology/American Heart Association Task Force on Practice Guidelines (Writing Committee to revise the 1999 guidelines for the management of patients with acute myocardial infarction). *J. Am. Coll. Cardiol.* 2004;44:671-719.

[16] Katzung BG, Chatterjee K. Vasodilators and the treatment of angina pectoris. In: *Basic and clinical pharmacology*, Katzung BG ed. 10th edition, Boston: 2006, 183-97

[17] Michel T. Treatment of myocardial ischemia. In: *Goodman and Gilman's The Pharmacological Basis of Therapeutics*, Brunton LL, Lazo JS, Parker KL, eds. *11th edition*, New York: McGraw-Hill, *2006, 823-44*

[18] Abernethy DR, Schwartz JB. Calcium-antagonist drugs. *N. Engl. J. Med.* 1999;341:1447-1457.

[19] Schwartz A. Molecular and cellular aspects of calcium channel antagonism. *Am J Cardiol* 1992;70:6F-8F.

[20] Tsien RW, Lipscombe D, Madison DV, Bley KR, Fox A. Multiple types of neuronal calcium channels and their selective modulation. *Trends Neurosci.* 1988;11:431-438.

[21] Hockerman GH, Peterson BZ, Johnson BD, Catterall WA. Molecular determinants of drug binding and action on L-type calcium channels. *Annu. Rev. Pharmacol. Toxicol.* 1997;37:361-396.

[22] Berridge MJ. Inositol trisphosphate and calcium signalling. *Nature* 1993;361:315-325.

[23] Serruys PW, Hooghoudt TE, Reiber JH, Slager C, Brower RW, Hugenholtz PG. Influence of intracoronary nifedipine on left ventricular function, coronary vasomotility, and myocardial oxygen consumption. *Br. Heart J.* 1983;49:427-441.

[24] Effect of verapamil on mortality and major events after acute myocardial infarction (the Danish Verapamil Infarction Trial II--DAVIT II). *Am. J. Cardiol.* 1990;66:779-785.

[25] Held PH, Yusuf S. Effects of beta-blockers and calcium channel blockers in acute myocardial infarction. *Eur. Heart J.* 1993;14 Suppl F:18-25.

[26] Gheorghiade M. Calcium channel blockers in the management of myocardial infarction patients. *Henry Ford Hosp. Med. J.* 1991;39:210-216.

[27] Hilton TC, Miller DD, Kern MJ. Rational therapy to reduce mortality and reinfarction following myocardial infarction. *Am. Heart J.* 1991;122:1740-1750.

[28] The effect of diltiazem on mortality and reinfarction after myocardial infarction. The Multicenter Diltiazem Postinfarction Trial Research Group. *N. Engl. J. Med.* 1988;319:385-392.

[29] Gibson RS, Boden WE, Theroux P, Strauss HD, Pratt CM, Gheorghiade M, Capone RJ, Crawford MH, Schlant RC, Kleiger RE, et al. Diltiazem and reinfarction in patients with non-Q-wave myocardial infarction. Results of a double-blind, randomized, multicenter trial. *N. Engl. J. Med.* 1986;315:423-429.

[30] Boden WE, van Gilst WH, Scheldewaert RG, Starkey IR, Carlier MF, Julian DG, Whitehead A, Bertrand ME, Col JJ, Pedersen OL, Lie KI, Santoni JP, Fox KM. Diltiazem in acute myocardial infarction treated with thrombolytic agents: a randomised placebo-controlled trial. Incomplete Infarction Trial of European Research Collaborators Evaluating Prognosis post-Thrombolysis (INTERCEPT). *Lancet* 2000;355:1751-1756.

[31] Muller JE, Morrison J, Stone PH, Rude RE, Rosner B, Roberts R, Pearle DL, Turi ZG, Schneider JF, Serfas DH, et al. Nifedipine therapy for patients with threatened and acute myocardial infarction: a randomized, double-blind, placebo-controlled comparison. *Circulation* 1984;69:740-747.

[32] Wilcox RG, Hampton JR, Banks DC, Birkhead JS, Brooksby IA, Burns-Cox CJ, Hayes MJ, Joy MD, Malcolm AD, Mather HG, et al. Trial of early nifedipine in acute myocardial infarction: the Trent study. *Br. Med. J. (Clin Res Ed)* 1986;293:1204-1208.

[33] Secondary prevention reinfarction Israeli nifedipine trial (SPRINT). A randomized intervention trial of nifedipine in patients with acute myocardial infarction. The Israeli Sprint Study Group. *Eur. Heart J.* 1988;9:354-364.

[34] Goldbourt U, Behar S, Reicher-Reiss H, Zion M, Mandelzweig L, Kaplinsky E. Early administration of nifedipine in suspected acute myocardial infarction. The Secondary

Prevention Reinfarction Israel Nifedipine Trial 2 Study. *Arch. Intern. Med.* 1993;153:345-353.

[35] Sirnes PA, Overskeid K, Pedersen TR, Bathen J, Drivenes A, Frøland GS, Kjekshus JK, Landmark K, Rokseth R, Sirnes KE, et al. Evolution of infarct size during the early use of nifedipine in patients with acute myocardial infarction: the Norwegian Nifedipine Multicenter Trial. *Circulation* 1984;70:638-644.

[36] Furberg CD, Psaty BM, Meyer JV. Nifedipine. Dose-related increase in mortality in patients with coronary heart disease. *Circulation* 1995;92:1326-1331.

[37] Buring JE, Glynn RJ, Hennekens CH. Calcium channel blockers and myocardial infarction. A hypothesis formulated but not yet tested. *JAMA* 1995;274:654-655.

[38] Jackson EK. Renin and angiotensin. In: *Goodman and Gilman's The Pharmacological Basis of Therapeutics*, Brunton LL, Lazo JS, Parker KL, eds. *11th edition*, New York: McGraw-Hill, *2006, 789-822*

[39] Reid IA. Vasoactive peptides. In: *Basic and clinical pharmacology*, Katzung BG ed. 10th edition, Boston: 2006, 277-92

[40] The vascular system. In: *Rang and Dale's pharmacology*, Rang HP, Dale MM, Ritter JM, Flower RJ, eds. 6th edition, Philadelphia, Churchill Livingstone: 2007, 285-306

[41] Vaughan DE, Rouleau JL, Ridker PM, Arnold JM, Menapace FJ, Pfeffer MA. Effects of ramipril on plasma fibrinolytic balance in patients with acute anterior myocardial infarction. HEART Study Investigators. *Circulation* 1997;96:442-447.

[42] Brown NJ, Agirbasli M, Vaughan DE. Comparative effect of angiotensin-converting enzyme inhibition and angiotensin II type 1 receptor antagonism on plasma fibrinolytic balance in humans. *Hypertension* 1999;34:285-290.

[43] Ravid M, Brosh D, Levi Z, Bar-Dayan Y, Ravid D, Rachmani R. Use of enalapril to attenuate decline in renal function in normotensive, normoalbuminuric patients with type 2 diabetes mellitus. A randomized, controlled trial. *Ann. Intern. Med.* 1998;128:982-988.

[44] Ravid M, Lang R, Rachmani R, Lishner M. Long-term renoprotective effect of angiotensin-converting enzyme inhibition in non-insulin-dependent diabetes mellitus. A 7-year follow-up study. *Arch. Intern. Med.* 1996;156:286-289.

[45] Ravid M, Savin H, Jutrin I, Bental T, Katz B, Lishner M. Long-term stabilizing effect of angiotensin-converting enzyme inhibition on plasma creatinine and on proteinuria in normotensive type II diabetic patients. *Ann. Intern. Med.* 1993;118:577-581.

[46] Brenner BM, Cooper ME, de Zeeuw D, Keane WF, Mitch WE, Parving HH, Remuzzi G, Snapinn SM, Zhang Z, Shahinfar S; RENAAL Study Investigators. Effects of losartan on renal and cardiovascular outcomes in patients with type 2 diabetes and nephropathy. *N. Engl. J. Med.* 2001;345:861-869.

[47] Moline PL, Strocchi E, Zanardi M, Milani M, Ambrosioni E. Thromboxane antagonism and cough induced by angiotensin-converting-enzyme inhibitor. *Lancet* 1997;350:15-18.

[48] Tenenbaum A, Grossman E, Shemesh J, Fisman EZ, Nosrati I, Motro M. Intermediate but not low doses of aspirin can suppress angiotensin-converting enzyme inhibitor-induced cough. *Am. J. Hypertens.* 2000;13:776-782.

[49] Lee SC, Park SW, Kim DK, Lee SH, Hong KP. Iron supplementation inhibits cough associated with ACE inhibitors. *Hypertension* 2001;38:166-170.

[50] Israili ZH, Hall WD. Cough and angioneurotic edema associated with angiotensin-converting enzyme inhibitor therapy. A review of the literature and pathophysiology. *Ann. Intern. Med.* 1992;117:234-242.
[51] Brent RL, Beckman DA. Angiotensin-converting enzyme inhibitors, an embryopathic class of drugs with unique properties: information for clinical teratology counselors. *Teratology* 1991;43:543-546.
[52] Cressman MD, Vidt DG, Acker C. Renal glycosuria and azotemia after enalapril maleate (MK-421). *Lancet* 1982;2:440.
[53] Hagley MT, Hulisz DT, Burns CM. Hepatotoxicity associated with angiotensin-converting enzyme inhibitors. *Ann. Pharmacother.* 1993;27:228-231.
[54] Wynckel A, Ebikili B, Melin JP, Randoux C, Lavaud S, Chanard J. Long-term follow-up of acute renal failure caused by angiotensin converting enzyme inhibitors. *Am. J. Hypertens.* 1998;11:1080-1086.
[55] de Gasparo M, Catt KJ, Inagami T, Wright JW, Unger T. International union of pharmacology. XXIII. The angiotensin II receptors. *Pharmacol. Rev.* 2000;52:415-472.
[56] Whitebread S, Mele M, Kamber B, de Gasparo M. Preliminary biochemical characterization of two angiotensin II receptor subtypes. *Biochem. Biophys. Res. Commun.* 1989;163:284-291.
[57] Chiu AT, Herblin WF, McCall DE, Ardecky RJ, Carini DJ, Duncia JV, Pease LJ, Wong PC, Wexler RR, Johnson AL, et al. Identification of angiotensin II receptor subtypes. *Biochem. Biophys. Res. Commun.* 1989;165:196-203.
[58] Bumpus FM, Catt KJ, Chiu AT, DeGasparo M, Goodfriend T, Husain A, Peach MJ, Taylor DG Jr, Timmermans PB. Nomenclature for angiotensin receptors. A report of the Nomenclature Committee of the Council for High Blood Pressure Research. *Hypertension* 1991;17:720-721.
[59] Griendling KK, Ushio-Fukai M, Lassegue B, Alexander RW. Angiotensin II signaling in vascular smooth muscle: New concepts. *Hypertension* 1997;29:366-373.
[60] Berk BC. Angiotensin II signal transduction in vascular smooth muscle: Pathways activated by specific tyrosine kinases. *J. Am. Soc. Nephrol.* 1999;10:S62-S68.
[61] Inagami T. Molecular biology and signaling of angiotensin receptors: An overview. *J. Am. Soc. Nephrol.* 1999;10:S2-S7.
[62] Blume A, Herdegen T, Unger T. Angiotensin peptides and inducible transcription factors. *J. Mol. Med.* 1999;77:339-357.
[63] Haendeler J, Berk BC. Angiotensin II mediated signal transduction: Important role of tyrosine kinases. *Regul. Pept.* 2000;95:1-7.
[64] Lewis EJ, Hunsicker LG, Clarke WR, Berl T, Pohl MA, Lewis JB, Ritz E, Atkins RC, Rohde R, Raz I; Collaborative Study Group. Renoprotective effect of the angiotensin-receptor antagonist irbesartan in patients with nephropathy due to type 2 diabetes. *N. Engl. J. Med.* 2001;345:851-860.
[65] Parving HH, Lehnert H, Bröchner-Mortensen J, Gomis R, Andersen S, Arner P; Irbesartan in Patients with Type 2 Diabetes and Microalbuminuria Study Group. The effect of irbesartan on the development of diabetic nephropathy in patients with type 2 diabetes. *N. Engl. J. Med.* 2001;345:870-878.
[66] Viberti G, Wheeldon NM; MicroAlbuminuria Reduction With VALsartan (MARVAL) Study Investigators. Microalbuminuria reduction with valsartan in patients with type 2 diabetes mellitus: a blood pressure-independent effect. *Circulation* 2002;106:672-678.

[67] Madrid AH, Bueno MG, Rebollo JM, Marín I, Peña G, Bernal E, Rodriguez A, Cano L, Cano JM, Cabeza P, Moro C. Use of irbesartan to maintain sinus rhythm in patients with long-lasting persistent atrial fibrillation: a prospective and randomized study. *Circulation* 2002;106:331-336.

[68] Schneider AW, Kalk JF, Klein CP. Effect of losartan, an angiotensin II receptor antagonist, on portal pressure in cirrhosis. *Hepatology* 1999;29:334-339.

[69] Anderson JL, Adams CD, Antman EM, Bridges CR, Califf RM, Casey DE Jr, Chavey WE 2nd, Fesmire FM, Hochman JS, Levin TN, Lincoff AM, Peterson ED, Theroux P, Wenger NK, Wright RS, Smith SC Jr, Jacobs AK, Adams CD, Anderson JL, Antman EM, Halperin JL, Hunt SA, Krumholz HM, Kushner FG, Lytle BW, Nishimura R, Ornato JP, Page RL, Riegel B; American College of Cardiology; American Heart Association Task Force on Practice Guidelines (Writing Committee to Revise the 2002 Guidelines for the Management of Patients With Unstable Angina/Non-ST-Elevation Myocardial Infarction); American College of Emergency Physicians; Society for Cardiovascular Angiography and Interventions; Society of Thoracic Surgeons; American Association of Cardiovascular and Pulmonary Rehabilitation; Society for Academic Emergency Medicine. ACC/AHA 2007 guidelines for the management of patients with unstable angina/non-ST-Elevation myocardial infarction: a report of the American College of Cardiology/American Heart Association Task Force on Practice Guidelines (Writing Committee to Revise the 2002 Guidelines for the Management of Patients With Unstable Angina/Non-ST-Elevation Myocardial Infarction) developed in collaboration with the American College of Emergency Physicians, the Society for Cardiovascular Angiography and Interventions, and the Society of Thoracic Surgeons endorsed by the American Association of Cardiovascular and Pulmonary Rehabilitation and the Society for Academic Emergency Medicine. *J. Am. Coll. Cardiol.* 2007;50:e1-e157.

[70] ISIS-4: a randomised factorial trial assessing early oral captopril, oral mononitrate, and intravenous magnesium sulphate in 58,050 patients with suspected acute myocardial infarction. ISIS-4 (Fourth International Study of Infarct Survival) Collaborative Group. *Lancet* 1995;345:669-685.

[71] Oral captopril versus placebo among 14,962 patients with suspected acute myocardial infarction: a multicenter, randomized, double-blind, placebo controlled clinical trial. Chinese Cardiac Study (CCS-1) Collaborative Group. *Chin. Med. J. (Engl)* 1997;110:834-838.

[72] Rutherford JD, Pfeffer MA, Moyé LA, Davis BR, Flaker GC, Kowey PR, Lamas GA, Miller HS, Packer M, Rouleau JL, et al. Effects of captopril on ischemic events after myocardial infarction. Results of the Survival and Ventricular Enlargement trial. SAVE Investigators. *Circulation* 1994;90:1731-1738.

[73] Gustafsson I, Torp-Pedersen C, Køber L, Gustafsson F, Hildebrandt P. Effect of the angiotensin-converting enzyme inhibitor trandolapril on mortality and morbidity in diabetic patients with left ventricular dysfunction after acute myocardial infarction. Trace Study Group. *J. Am. Coll. Cardiol.* 1999;34:83-89.

[74] Buch P, Rasmussen S, Abildstrom SZ, Køber L, Carlsen J, Torp-Pedersen C; TRACE investigators. The long-term impact of the angiotensin-converting enzyme inhibitor trandolapril on mortality and hospital admissions in patients with left ventricular

dysfunction after a myocardial infarction: follow-up to 12 years. *Eur. Heart J.* 2005;26:145-152.

[75] Yusuf S, Sleight P, Pogue J, Bosch J, Davies R, Dagenais G. Effects of an angiotensin-converting-enzyme inhibitor, ramipril, on cardiovascular events in high-risk patients. The Heart Outcomes Prevention Evaluation Study Investigators. *N. Engl. J. Med.* 2000;342:145-153.

[76] Yusuf S, Pepine CJ, Garces C, Pouleur H, Salem D, Kostis J, Benedict C, Rousseau M, Bourassa M, Pitt B. Effect of enalapril on myocardial infarction and unstable angina in patients with low ejection fractions. *Lancet* 1992;340:1173-1178.

[77] Sigurdsson A, Swedberg K. Left ventricular remodelling, neurohormonal activation and early treatment with enalapril (CONSENSUS II) following myocardial infarction. *Eur. Heart J.* 1994;15 Suppl B:14-19.

[78] GISSI-3: effects of lisinopril and transdermal glyceryl trinitrate singly and together on 6-week mortality and ventricular function after acute myocardial infarction. Gruppo Italiano per lo Studio della Sopravvivenza nell'infarto Miocardico. *Lancet* 1994;343:1115-1122.

[79] Ambrosioni E, Borghi C, Magnani B. The effect of the angiotensin-converting-enzyme inhibitor zofenopril on mortality and morbidity after anterior myocardial infarction. The Survival of Myocardial Infarction Long-Term Evaluation (SMILE) Study Investigators. *N. Engl. J. Med.* 1995;332:80-85.

[80] Pfeffer MA, McMurray JJ, Velazquez EJ, Rouleau JL, Køber L, Maggioni AP, Solomon SD, Swedberg K, Van de Werf F, White H, Leimberger JD, Henis M, Edwards S, Zelenkofske S, Sellers MA, Califf RM; Valsartan in Acute Myocardial Infarction Trial Investigators. Valsartan, captopril, or both in myocardial infarction complicated by heart failure, left ventricular dysfunction, or both. *N. Engl. J. Med.* 2003;349:1893-1906.

[81] Pfeffer MA, Swedberg K, Granger CB, Held P, McMurray JJ, Michelson EL, Olofsson B, Ostergren J, Yusuf S, Pocock S; CHARM Investigators and Committees. Effects of candesartan on mortality and morbidity in patients with chronic heart failure: the CHARM-Overall programme. *Lancet* 2003;362:759-766.

[82] Pitt B, Remme W, Zannad F, Neaton J, Martinez F, Roniker B, Bittman R, Hurley S, Kleiman J, Gatlin M; Eplerenone Post-Acute Myocardial Infarction Heart Failure Efficacy and Survival Study Investigators. Eplerenone, a selective aldosterone blocker, in patients with left ventricular dysfunction after myocardial infarction. *N. Engl. J. Med.* 2003;348:1309-1321.

[83] Pitt B, Zannad F, Remme WJ, Cody R, Castaigne A, Perez A, Palensky J, Wittes J. The effect of spironolactone on morbidity and mortality in patients with severe heart failure. Randomized Aldactone Evaluation Study Investigators. *N. Engl. J. Med.* 1999;341:709-717.

[84] Chaitman BR, Skettino SL, Parker JO, Hanley P, Meluzin J, Kuch J, Pepine CJ, Wang W, Nelson JJ, Hebert DA, Wolff AA; MARISA Investigators. Anti-ischemic effects and long-term survival during ranolazine monotherapy in patients with chronic severe angina. *J. Am. Coll. Cardiol.* 2004;43:1375-1382.

[85] Antzelevitch C, Belardinelli L, Zygmunt AC, Burashnikov A, Di Diego JM, Fish JM, Cordeiro JM, Thomas G. Electrophysiological effects of ranolazine, a novel antianginal agent with antiarrhythmic properties. *Circulation* 2004;110:904-910.

[86] Morrow DA, Scirica BM, Karwatowska-Prokopczuk E, Murphy SA, Budaj A, Varshavsky S, Wolff AA, Skene A, McCabe CH, Braunwald E; MERLIN-TIMI 36 Trial Investigators. Effects of ranolazine on recurrent cardiovascular events in patients with non-ST-elevation acute coronary syndromes: the MERLIN-TIMI 36 randomized trial. *JAMA* 2007;297:1775-1783.

[87] Patel DJ, Purcell HJ, Fox KM. Cardioprotection by opening of the K(ATP) channel in unstable angina. Is this a clinical manifestation of myocardial preconditioning? Results of a randomized study with nicorandil. CESAR 2 investigation. Clinical European studies in angina and revascularization. *Eur. Heart J.* 1999;20:51-57.

[88] Teo KK, Yusuf S, Collins R, Held PH, Peto R. Effects of intravenous magnesium in suspected acute myocardial infarction: overview of randomised trials. *BMJ* 1991;303:1499-1503.

[89] Woods KL, Fletcher S. Long-term outcome after intravenous magnesium sulphate in suspected acute myocardial infarction: the second Leicester Intravenous Magnesium Intervention Trial (LIMIT-2). *Lancet* 1994;343:816-819.

[90] Magnesium in Coronaries (MAGIC) Trial Investigators. Early administration of intravenous magnesium to high-risk patients with acute myocardial infarction in the Magnesium in Coronaries (MAGIC) Trial: a randomised controlled trial. *Lancet* 2002;360:1189-1196.

[91] Melidonis A, Stefanidis A, Tournis S, Manoussakis S, Handanis S, Zairis M, Dadiotis L, Foussas S. The role of strict metabolic control by insulin infusion on fibrinolytic profile during an acute coronary event in diabetic patients. *Clin. Cardiol.* 2000;23:160-164.

[92] Iwakura K, Ito H, Ikushima M, Kawano S, Okamura A, Asano K, Kuroda T, Tanaka K, Masuyama T, Hori M, Fujii K. Association between hyperglycemia and the no-reflow phenomenon in patients with acute myocardial infarction. *J Am Coll Cardiol* 2003;41:1-7.

In: Drugs in Cardiopulmonary Resuscitation
Editor: Theodoros Xanthos
ISBN: 978-1-61122-512-9

Chapter 6

Antithrombotic Therapy in Acute Coronary Syndromes - Anticoagulants

Konstantinos A. Ekmektzoglou
University of Athens, Medical School

Abstract

The goals of antithrombotic therapy for patients with ST-segment elevation myocardial infarction (STEMI) are to establish and maintain patency of the infarct-related artery, limit the consequences of myocardial ischemia, enhance myocardial healing, and reduce the likelihood of recurrent events. For patients with unstable angina/non-ST-segment elevation myocardial infarction (UA/NSTEMI), antithrombotic therapy has 2 components: *1)* anticoagulant therapy, which targets the clotting cascade to prevent the deposition of fibrin strands in the clot and is categorized into i) intravenous (IV), subcutaneous (SC) and oral anticoagulants ii) direct thrombin inhibitors, iii) factor Xa inhibitors and *2)* antiplatelet therapy, which reduces platelet activation and aggregation, integral steps in the formation of a thrombus after plaque disruption, which will be discussed in detail in the following chapter.

Introduction

Blood coagulates by the transformation of soluble fibrinogen into insoluble fibrin. Following vascular injury, several circulating proteins interact in a cascading series of limited proteolytic reactions. The main initiator of blood coagulation is the tissue factor (TF)/factor VIIa pathway, as exposure of TF on damaged endothelium binds and activates circulating factor VII. At each step, a clotting factor zymogen (eg, factor VII, IX, X and II) undergoes limited proteolysis and becomes an active protease (eg, factor VIIa, IXa, Xa and IIa, respectively). Thus, each protease factor activates the next clotting factor until finally a solid fibrin clot is formed. Although, the details of coagulation are still not fully understood, a proposed model of blood coagulation is described in Figure 1 [1,2].

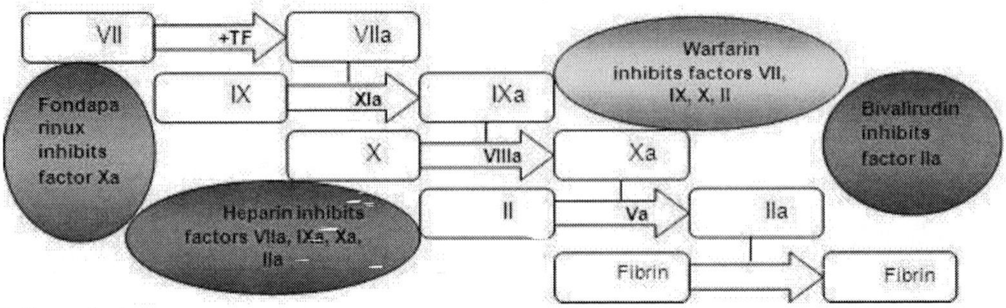

TF: tissue factor

Figure 1. The steps of blood coagulation and sites of action of anticoagulant drugs.

The anticoagulant drugs discussed below (that are part of the ACS therapeutic protocol) are categorized into i) IV or SC anticoagulants (unfractioned heparin - UFH - and low-molecular weight heparins - LMWHs - ii) direct thrombin inhibitors (DTIs) like bivalirudin, iii) factor Xa Inhibitors (fondaparinux) and iv) oral anticoagulants (warfarin).

UFH

Heparin is a glycosaminoglycan found in the secretory granules of mast cells. It is synthesized from uridine diphosphate (UDP)-sugar precursors as a polymer of alternating D-glucuronic acid and *N*-acetyl-D-glucosamine residues [1,3]. Heparin (Figure 2) exerts its anticoagulant effect by accelerating the action of circulating antithrombin, a proteolytic enzyme that inactivates factor IIa (thrombin), factor IXa, and factor Xa. Heparin binds tightly to antithrombin and causes a conformational change in this inhibitor, which, in turn, exposes its active site for more rapid interaction with the proteases. Heparin catalyzes the antithrombin-protease reaction without being consumed. Once the antithrombin-protease complex is formed, heparin is released. It prevents thrombus propagation but does not lyse existing thrombi [4].

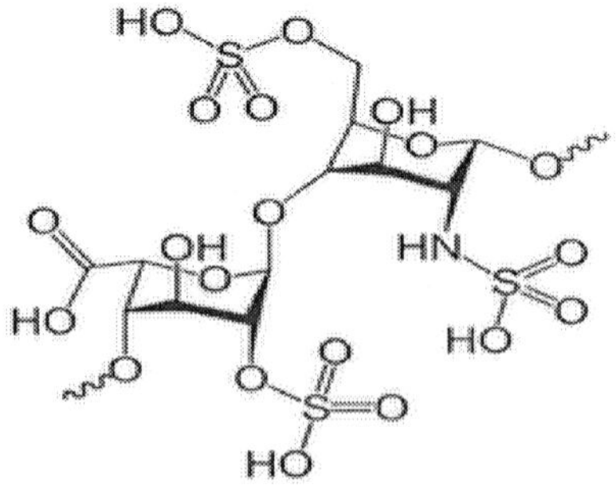

Figure 2. Structure of heparin.

UFH is a heterogeneous mixture of polysaccharide chains of molecular weights that range from 5,000 to 30,000 Daltons and have varying effects on anticoagulant activity. The antithrombin binding region of UFH consists of repeating sulfated disaccharide units composed of D-glucosamine-L-iduronic acid and D-glucosamine-D-glucuronic acid. UFH binds to a number of plasma proteins, blood cells, and endothelial cells [2].

Pharmacokinetics

UFH is not absorbed through the gastrointestinal mucosa and therefore is given by continuous IV infusion or SC injection. UFH has an immediate onset of action when given IV. In contrast, there is considerable variation in the bioavailability of heparin given SC, and the onset of action is delayed 1 to 2 hours.

The half-life of UFH in plasma depends on the dose administered. When doses of 100, 400, or 800 units/kg of heparin are injected IV, the half-lives of the anticoagulant activities are approximately 1, 2.5 and 5 hours, respectively.

UFH appears to be cleared and degraded primarily by the reticuloendothelial system; a small amount of undegraded heparin also appears in the urine. The half-life of heparin may be shortened in patients with pulmonary embolism and prolonged in patients with hepatic cirrhosis or end-stage renal disease [1].

Effects, Toxicity and Clinical Use

The anticoagulant effects of UFH are variable due to the variable binding of UFH to plasma proteins which, in turn, may limit optimal antithrombotic therapy and constitutes a potential advantage of direct antithrombin blockade with bivalirudin (discussed later) [5,6].

As a consequence of these pharmacokinetic limitations, the anticoagulant effect of UFH requires monitoring with the activated partial thromboplastin time (aPTT), a test that is sensitive to the inhibitory effects of UFH on thrombin (factor IIa), factor Xa, and factor IXa.

Many clinicians have traditionally prescribed a fixed initial dose of UFH (e.g., 5,000 U bolus, 1,000 U/h initial infusion); clinical trials have indicated that a weight-adjusted dosing regimen can provide more predictable anticoagulation than the fixed-dose regimen [7-9].

The American College of Chest Physicians Consensus conferencc has therefore recommended dosage adjustments of the nomograms to correspond to a therapeutic range equivalent to heparin levels of 0.3 to 0.7 U/ml by anti-factor Xa determinations, which correlates with aPTT values between 60 and 80 s [10].

In addition to body weight, other clinical factors that affect the response to UFH include age and sex, which are associated with higher aPTT values, and smoking history and diabetes mellitus, which are associated with lower aPTT values [9].

Going one step further, we should point out that the anticoagulant effects of UFH are not only variable but most of the benefits of the various anticoagulants are short term and not maintained on a long-term basis.

Reactivation of the disease process after the discontinuation of anticoagulants may contribute to this loss of early gain among medically treated patients (with acute coronary syndromes - ACS -) that has been described with UFH [11].

The combination of UFH and aspirin (ASA) appears to mitigate this reactivation in part, although there is hematologic evidence of increased thrombin activity after the cessation of IV UFH ("rebound") even in the presence of ASA [12].

Uncontrolled observations suggested a reduction in the “heparin rebound” by switching from IV to SC UFH for several days before the drug is stopped. The major adverse effect of heparin is bleeding. Levels for UFH may thus be determined by protamine titration (therapeutic levels 0.2-0.4 U/mL) or anti-Xa units (therapeutic levels 0.3-0.7 U/mL).

Elderly women and patients with renal failure are more prone to hemorrhage. Increased loss of hair and reversible alopecia have been reported. Long-term heparin therapy is associated with osteoporosis and spontaneous fractures [2].

Also, high doses of UFH can interfere with platelet aggregation and thereby prolong bleeding time. It is unclear to what extent the antiplatelet effect of heparin contributes to the hemorrhagic complications of treatment with the drug.

UFH "clears" lipemic plasma *in vivo* by causing the release of lipoprotein lipase into the circulation, which hydrolyzes triglycerides to glycerol and free fatty acids. The clearing of lipemic plasma may occur at concentrations of heparin below those necessary to produce an anticoagulant effect.

Rebound hyperlipemia may occur after UFH administration is stopped [1]. Mild thrombocytopenia may occur in 10% to 20% of patients who are receiving heparin, whereas significant thrombocytopenia (platelet count less than 100,000) occurs in 1% to 5% of patients and typically appears after 4 to 14 d of therapy [13-16].

Autoimmune heparin-induced thrombocytopenia (HIT) in association with thrombosis is a rare but dangerous complication of UFH administration (incidence is <0.2%) [1,2]. The points that should be considered in all patients receiving UFH are described in Table 1.

UFH is contraindicated in patients with established allergy, those that are actively bleeding, or have hemophilia, significant thrombocytopenia, purpura, severe hypertension, intracranial hemorrhage, infective endocarditis, active tuberculosis, gastrointestinal tract ulcers, threatened abortion, visceral carcinoma, or advanced hepatic or renal disease. Administration of warfarin alone is contraindicated since it may exacerbate the prothrombotic state associated with HIT [1,2].

Although, the anticoagulant effect of UFH disappears within hours of discontinuation of the drug, mild bleeding due to heparin usually can be controlled without the administration of an antagonist. If life-threatening hemorrhage occurs, the effect of heparin can be reversed quickly by the slow IV infusion of protamine sulfate.

Protamine binds tightly to UFH and thereby neutralizes its anticoagulant effect. Protamine also interacts with platelets and fibrinogen and may cause an anticoagulant effect of its own [1,2]. As for the clinical uses of UFH, they are summarized in Table 2 [17].

Table 1. Physician’s concerns in all patients receiving UFH

Platelet counts should be performed frequently
Thrombocytopenia should be considered to be heparin-induced
Any new thrombus can be the result of heparin
Thromboembolic disease thought to be heparin-induced should be treated by discontinuance of UFH and administration of an alternative drug

UFH: unfractioned heparin

Table 2. Clinical uses of UFH

- Venous thrombosis (treatment and prophylaxis)*
- Pulmonary embolism (treatment and prophylaxis)*
- ACS treatment
- CABG surgery
- Anticoagulation during pregnancy**

* An oral anticoagulant should be started concurrently, with UFH being continued for at least 4 to 5 days to allow the oral anticoagulant to achieve its full therapeutic effect

** If possible, the drug should be discontinued 24 h before delivery to minimize the risk of postpartum bleeding

ACS: acute coronary syndromes; CABG: coronary artery bypass grafting

UFH in ACS

The 2007 ACC/AHA UA/NSTEMI and STEMI guidelines recommend the initiation of anticoagulant therapy with UFH for all patients (without contraindications) as soon as possible after presentation (class I recommendation).

The same guidelines recommend weight-adjusted dosing of UFH (60 U/kg bolus and 12 U/kg/hr infusion), frequent monitoring of aPTT (every 6 hours until 2 consecutive values are within the target range, and every 24 hours thereafter), and titration of UFH according to a standardized nomogram with a target range of aPTT between 1.5 and 2.0 times that of control, or approximately 50 to 70 sec [18,19]. This strategy was implemented due to the positive results of several randomized trials.

Théroux *et al.*, when studying the usefulness of ASA, heparin and a combination of the two in the early management of acute UA, showed that heparin treatment was associated with a reduced incidence of myocardial infarction, with a trend favoring heparin over ASA.

Heparin treatment was also associated with a reduced incidence of refractory angina [20,21]. The same held true for the RISC Group where the patients with UA/NSTEMI, treated with ASA and heparin, had the lowest number of cardiovascular events during the initial 5 days that followed [22].

The ASSENT-2 and ASSENT-3 Investigators supported the use of smaller dose, weight-adjusted heparin in patients with STEMI treated with fibrinolysis, as these patients exhibited less major bleeding than patients who had received heparin stratified by weight [23].

The GUSTO-I trial showed that aPTT within a range of 50 to 70 sec was associated with the lowest 30-day rates of mortality, stroke and bleeding and with fewer instances of refractory ischemia than was an aPTT higher than 70 sec [24].

Administration of UFH should continue for at least 48 hours after presentation with ACS and start of fibrinolysis due to the limited evidence supporting the benefits of prolonged infusions of UFH and because of the progressive increase in the risk of HIT (both rapid- and delayed onset presentations) [25,26].

For patients with ACS, the physician should administer additional boluses of UFH as needed to support the procedure of percutaneous coronary intervention (PCI), taking into account whether glycoprotein (GP) IIb/IIIa receptor antagonists have been administered [19].

LMWHs

Because the rates of recurrence of ischemic events remain high even when UFH is administered, LMWHs were developed with the goal of providing improved anticoagulation. LMWHs bind to antithrombin and enhance its inactivation of factor Xa. LMWHs, although to a lesser extent than UFH, also enhance antithrombin's inactivation of thrombin (IIa). Numerous pharmaceutical agents are encompassed in the group (enoxaparin, dalteparin, tinzaparin, etc.) out of which only enoxaparin (Figure 3) plays a role in the management of ACS patients and will be dicussed here [2].

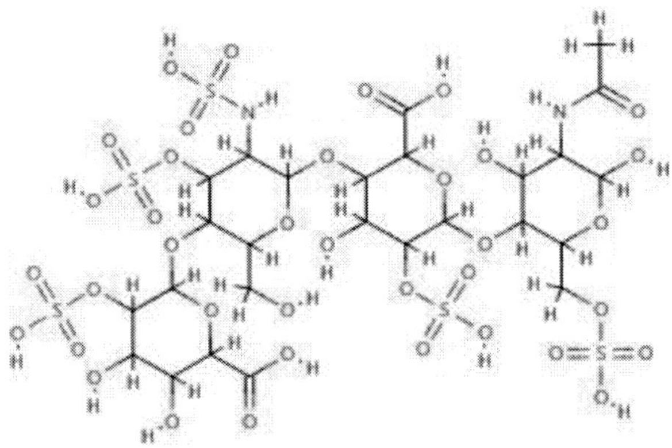

Figure 3. Structure of enoxaparin.

The LMWHs are obtained through chemical or enzymatic depolymerization of the polysaccharide chains of heparin to provide chains with different molecular weight distributions. Approximately 25% to 50% of the pentasaccharide-containing chains of LMWH preparations contain more than 18 saccharide units, with chains with fewer than 18 saccharide units retaining their ability to inactivate factor Xa but not thrombin, as noted above. Except from their equal efficacy with UFH, distinct advantages of LMWHs over UFH include decreased binding to plasma proteins and endothelial cells and dose-independent clearance, with a longer half-life that results in more predictable (increased bioavailability) and sustained anticoagulation with once- or twice-a-day SC administration. An advantage of LMWHs is that they do not usually require laboratory monitoring of activity. Furthermore, the LMWHs stimulate platelets less than UFH and are less frequently associated with HIT. Other advantages of enoxaparin include possibly lower risks of bleeding and osteopenia [27].

The pharmacodynamic and pharmacokinetic profiles of the different commercial preparations of LMWHs vary, with their mean molecular weights ranging from 4,200 to 6,000 Daltons [27]. Weight-based dosing of the enoxaparin results in predictable pharmacokinetics and plasma levels in patients with normal renal function. Therefore, enoxaparin levels are not generally measured (determined by anti-Xa units) except in the setting of renal insufficiency, obesity, and pregnancy. Peak therapeutic levels are 0.5-1 U/mL for twice daily dosing, determined 4 hours after administration, and approximately 1.5 U/mL for once daily dosing [2,28].

The clinical indications for the use of enoxaparin are the same as for UFH. However, the safety and efficacy of LMWH use during pregnancy have not been adequately evaluated.

LMWH preparations were first approved for prevention of venous thromboembolism. They are also effective in the treatment of venous thrombosis, pulmonary embolism, and ACS [17]. The anticoagulant effect of enoxaparin is less effectively reversed with protamine than that of UFH [1].

Enoxaparin in ACS

Various LMWHs (dalteparin, enoxaparin, nadroparin, tinzaparin) have been compared with UFH for the treatment of UA/NSTEMI, but only enoxaparin has been found to have a clear benefit. When LMWHs were compared between them, enoxaparin showed a cleared advantage. For example, in the EVET trial, 2 LMWHs, enoxaparin and tinzaparin, administered for 7 days, were compared in patients with UA/NSTEMI. Enoxaparin was associated with a lower rate of death/myocardial ischemia/recurrent angina at 7 and 30 days compared with tinzaparin, while the bleeding rates were similar [29].

The TIMI 11B-ESSENSE trial meta-analysis showed that enoxaparin should be considered as a replacement for UFH for the acute phase of management of patients with high-risk UA/NSTEMI [30]. The SYNERGY study showed that enoxaparin was a safe and effective alternative to UFH for the treatment of high-risk patients with NSTEMI.

However, more bleeding was observed with enoxaparin, a result not validated by the TIMI 11B study (mentioned above), in which enoxaparin was superior to UFH for reducing a composite of death and serious cardiac ischemic events during the acute management of UA/NSTEMI patients without causing a significant increase in the rate of major hemorrhage [31,32].

Not only that, but when a conservative approach to catheterization and PCI was planned for NSTEMI patients receiving tirofiban and ASA, enoxaparin was associated with superior efficacy and similar bleeding when compared to UFH [33].

Finally, in the ACUTE II study, UFH and enoxaparin were compared in patients with UA/NSTEMI receiving tirofiban. The incidence of major and minor bleeding was similar, and there was a trend to fewer adverse events in patients receiving enoxaparin [34].

The 2007 ACC/AHA guidelines clearly state that enoxaparin is preferable to UFH as anticoagulant therapy for UA/NSTEMI patients who will be treated conservatively, unless coronary artery bypass grafting (CABG) is planned within 24 hours (class IIa recommendation). In that case, the physician should discontinue enoxaparin 12 to 24 h before CABG and dose with UFH per institutional practice [18].

The benefit of enoxaparin is greater for patients at higher risk, such as those with elevated troponin concentrations, and high thrombolysis in myocardial infarction (TIMI) risk scores [35].

For patients with STEMI, which are less than 75 years of age, enoxaparin (provided the serum creatinine is <2.5 mg/dL in men and 2.0 mg/dL in women), an initial 30 mg IV bolus is given, followed 15 minutes later by SC injections of 1.0 mg/kg every 12 hours. For patients at least 75 years of age, the initial IV bolus is eliminated and the SC dose is reduced to 0.75 mg/ kg every 12 hours.

Regardless of age, if the creatinine clearance during the course of treatment is estimated to be <30 mL/min, the SC regimen is 1.0 mg/kg every 24 hours. Maintenance dosing with enoxaparin should be continued for the duration of the index hospitalization, up to 8 days [19].

For patients undergoing PCI after having received an anticoagulant regimen with enoxaparin, if the last SC dose was administered within the prior 8 hours, no additional enoxaparin should be given; if the last SC dose was administered at least 8 to 12 hours earlier, an IV dose of 0.3 mg per kg of enoxaparin should be given [19].

The CREATE trial revealed than, in STEMI patients, reviparin (although not currently approved in the United States) reduced mortality and reinfarction, without a substantive increase in overall stroke rates. However, a small absolute excess of life-threatening bleeding was observed [36].

In the CLARITY-TIMI 28 trial, which compared LMWH and UFH, in patients with STEMI receiving fibrinolytic therapy, the use of LMWH with other standard therapies, including clopidogrel and ASA, was associated with improved angiographic outcomes and lower rates of major adverse cardiovascular events. The rates of intracerebral hemorrhage and of major bleeding through 30 days were similar in the 2 groups [37].

When the ASSENT-3 trial investigators compared the efficacy and safety of tenecteplase plus enoxaparin or abciximab, with that of tenecteplase plus weight-adjusted UFH in patients with AMI, enoxaparin plus full-dose tenecteplase achieved a significantly better outcome than UFH plus full-dose tenecteplase regarding the rate of mortality, in-hospital reinfarction, or in-hospital refractory ischemia [38].

In patients with STEMI treated with ASA and thrombolysis, 14 trials involving a total of 25,280 patients were reviewed in a meta-analysis involving 25,280 patients with STEMI. UFH did not show to prevent reinfarction or death. LMWH given for 4 to 8 days compared with placebo reduced reinfarction by approximately one quarter and death by approximately 10%. When directly compared with UFH, LMWH reduced reinfarction by almost one half [39].

In a large trial (EXTRACT-TIMI 25) which randomly assigned 20,506 patients with STEMI, who were scheduled to undergo fibrinolysis to receive either enoxaparin or weight-based UFH for at least 48 hours, treatment with enoxaparin proved superior to treatment with UFH but was associated with an increase in major bleeding episodes. However, the net clinical benefit clearly favored enoxaparin over UFH [40].

DTIs

The DTIs are agents that exert their anticoagulant effect by directly binding to the active site of thrombin, thereby inhibiting thrombin's downstream effects. The DTIs bind thrombin without additional binding proteins, such as antithrombin and can thus directly inhibit clot-bound thrombin; Bivalirudin, hirudin, argatroban, melagatran are all DTIs. However, since only the former has an established role in ACS patients, this section of anticoagulant therapy pertains only to bivalirudin [1,3]. Bivalirudin (Figure 4), a 20-amino-acid polypeptide, is a bivalent synthetic analog of hirudin (a powerful and specific thrombin inhibitor found in leeches - *Hirudo medicinalis* -, which were used by physicians and surgeons for many years) that binds at both the catalytic or active site of thrombin as well as at a substrate recognition site and has a molecular weight of 2180 daltons. Bivalirudin contains the sequence Phe^1-Pro^2-Arg^3-Pro^4, which occupies the catalytic site of thrombin, followed by a polyglycine linker and a hirudin-like sequence that binds to exosite I (an additional substrate-binding site on a protease distinct from the catalytic core). Thrombin slowly cleaves the Arg^3-Pro^4 peptide bond and thus regains activity [1,3,41-43].

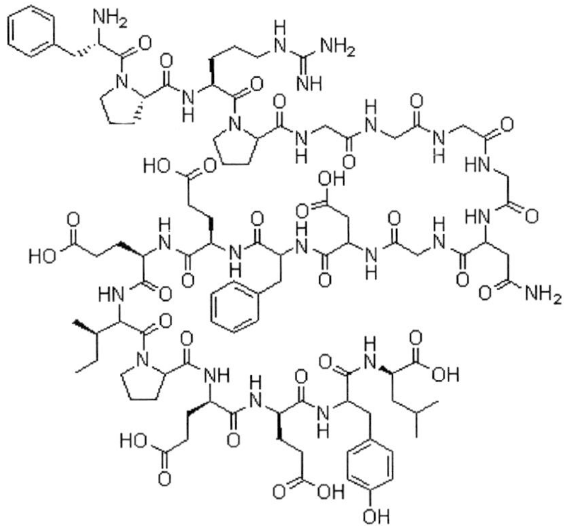

Figure 4. Structure of bivalirudin.

Pharmacokinetics

Bivalirudin is administered IV, with a rapid onset and offset of action. The drug has a short half-life with clearance that is 20% renal and the remainder metabolic (proteolytic cleavage). The half-life in patients with normal renal function is 25 min. Bivalirudin exhibits linear dose- and concentration-dependent anticoagulant activity as evidenced by prolongation of the activated clotting time (ACT), aPTT, prothrombin time (PT) and thrombin time (TT). IV administration produces an immediate anticoagulant effect, with coagulation times returning to baseline approximately 1 hour following cessation of bivalirudin administration [41-43].

Toxicity and Clinical Effects

Bivalirudin patients exhibit statistically significantly lower rates of bleeding, transfusions, and thrombocytopenia when compared to other anticoagulants. As a whole, other (rare) complications are included in Table 3. Bivalirudin should be used with caution in patients with disease states associated with an increased risk of bleeding. It is contraindicated in patients with active major bleeding or established hypersensitivity to the drug. For patients with renal impairment, the ACT should be monitored. In these patients, dosage reductions are recommended [1,3,41-43]. The clinical uses of bivalirudin are discussed immediately below in the section of ACS patients.

Table 3. Rare adverse effects of bivalirudin excluding bleeding and thrombocytopenia

Cardiovascular system
Hypotension
Syncope
Vascular anomaly
VF
Nervous system
Cerebral ischemia
Confusion
Facial paralysis
Respiratory system
Pulmonary edema
Urogenital system
Renal failure
Oliguria
General
Fever
Infection
Sepsis

VF: ventricular fibrillation

Bivalirudin in ACS

For patients with UA/NSTEMI in whom an invasive strategy is selected, bivalirudin is included in the regimens with established efficacy. The guidelines further state that it is reasonable to omit the administration of an IV GP IIb/IIIa antagonist if a thienopyridine (at least 300 mg of clopidogrel administered at least 6 h earlier than planned catheterization or PCI) is administered simultaneously with bivalirudin (class IIa recommendation). The physician should discontinue bivalirudin 3 h before CABG and dose with UFH per institutional practice. Bivalirudin has not been tested in a noninvasive strategy and hence cannot be recommended currently [18]. The ACUITY trial evaluated the role of thrombin-specific anticoagulation with bivalirudin in 13,819 patients with moderate- or high-risk ACS. Patients were assigned to one of three antithrombotic regimens: i) UFH or enoxaparin plus a GP IIb/IIIa inhibitor, ii) bivalirudin plus a GP IIb/IIIa inhibitor, or iii) bivalirudin alone, with the primary end points being a composite ischemia end point (death, myocardial infarction, or unplanned revascularization for ischemia), major bleeding and the net clinical outcome, defined as the combination of composite ischemia or major bleeding. No differences in the rates of the primary end point were observed between the group receiving UFH plus a GP IIb/IIIa inhibitor and the group receiving bivalirudin plus a GP IIb/IIIa inhibitor. However, the net clinical outcomes were significantly better for the group receiving bivalirudin alone than for the group receiving UFH plus a GP IIb/IIIa inhibitor due primarily to a substantially reduced rate of major bleeding [44].

The REPLACE 2 investigators compared bivalirudin (with provisional GP IIb/IIIa inhibition) with UFH with planned GP IIb/IIIa inhibition in patients undergoing urgent or elective PCI. Bivalirudin was statistically not inferior to heparin with regard to suppression of acute ischemic end points and was associated with less bleeding. Follow-up through 1 year also suggested similar mortality for the 2 approaches [45,46]. The 2007 ACC/AHA guidelines recommend the use of other direct thrombin inhibitors, such as lepirudin (recombinant hirudin) and argatroban, only for patients with HIT [18]. For patients with STEMI who are undergoing primary PCI, administering bivalirudin alone appears to reduce major bleeding complications, decrease cardiac mortality rates, and improve overall survival rates. This was shown in the HORIZONS-AMI trial which randomly assigned 3,602 patients with STEMI who presented within 12 hours after the onset of symptoms and who were undergoing primary PCI to treatment with heparin plus a GP IIb/IIIa inhibitor or to treatment with bivalirudin alone. Anticoagulation with bivalirudin alone resulted in significantly reduced 30-day rates of major bleeding and net adverse clinical events (death, myocardial iscemiA, ischemic target-vessel revascularization, stroke) [47].

Encouraging data had already emerged some years ago. The HERO-2 trial investigators randomly assigned 17,073 patients with acute STEMI to receive either bivalirudin or heparin, together with a standard dose of streptokinase. Although bivalirudin did not reduce mortality compared with UFH, it did, however, reduce the rate of adjudicated reinfarction within 96 h by 30%. The frequency of moderate and mild bleeding was also greater with bivalirudin [48]. Likewise, a meta-analysis, based on individual patients' data from randomised trials comparing a direct thrombin inhibitor (hirudin, bivalirudin, argatroban, efegatran, or inogatran) with heparin, reviewd 35,970 patients assigned up to 7 days treatment with a direct thrombin inhibitor or heparin and followed up for at least 30 days. The Direct Thrombin Inhibitor Trialists' Collaborative Group showed that direct thrombin inhibitors were associated with a lower risk of death or myocardial infarction at the end of treatment [49].

Factor Xa Inhibitors

Fondaparinux is a synthetic pentasaccharide (Figure 5) that is an indirect factor Xa inhibitor and requires antithrombin for its action. It is based on the structure of the antithrombin binding region of heparin and acts more upstream in the coagulation cascade (more proximally so as to inhibit the multiplier effects of the downstream coagulation reactions and, thereby, reduce the amount of thrombin generated). Fondaparinux does not have any action against thrombin that is already formed. This could possibly explain the observation of an increased rate of catheter thrombosis when factor Xa inhibitors such as fondaparinux are used alone to support PCI procedures [1,3].

Pharmacokinetics

Fondaparinux is administered by SC injection, reaches peak plasma levels in 2 hours, and is excreted in the urine with a half-life of 17 to 21 hours. Because it does not interact significantly with blood cells or plasma proteins other than antithrombin, fondaparinux can be given once a day at a fixed dose without coagulation monitoring (unlike UFH). Protamine will not reverse the activity of fondaparinux because they lack a protamine-binding domain; reversal of their action in the event of bleeding requires discontinuation of their administration and, if needed, transfusion of coagulation factors (e.g., fresh-frozen plasma, FFP). It should not be used in patients with renal failure [50-52].

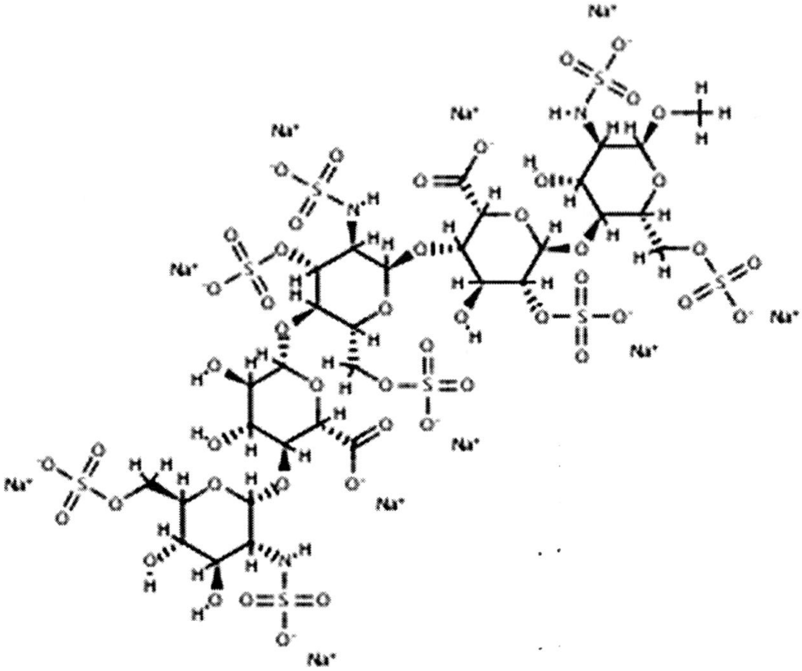

Figure 5. Structure of fondaparinux.

Toxicity and Clinical Use

Fondaparinux appears to be much less likely than heparin or LMWH to trigger the syndrome of HIT. Fondaparinux is approved for thromboprophylaxis of patients undergoing hip or knee surgery and for the therapy of pulmonary embolism and deep venous thrombosis [50-53]. Its role in ACS patients is analyzed in the section below.

Fondaparinux in ACS

The OASIS-5 trial, which involved 20,078 patients with high risk UA/NSTEMI, compared fondaparinux with standard-dose enoxaparin. Fondaparinux was found to be similar to enoxaparin in reducing the risk of ischemic events at nine days (death, myocardial infarction, or refractory ischemia), but it substantially reduced major bleeding (by almost 50%) and improved long term mortality. As for the subset of patients undergoing PCI, the authors concluded that supplemental UFH at the time of catheterization appeared to minimize the risk of catheter-related thrombi, which was more than 3 times higher in the fondaparinux arm than in the enoxaparin arm [54].

Fondaparinux is another anticoagulant that has been given a Class I recommendation in the management of UA/NSTEMI who will be managed by either a conservative or an early invasive strategy, unless CABG is planned within 24 hours. In the latter case, fondaparinux must be discontinued 24 h before CABG and UFH should be administered, because the anticoagulant effect of UFH can be more readily reversed than that of fondaparinux. Also, in patients in whom a conservative strategy is selected and who have an increased risk of bleeding, fondaparinux is preferable over other anticoagulants. Fondaparinux can replace UFH after the first 48 h of hospitalization for up to 8 days. After that, the physican should discontinue anticoagulant therapy [18].

As for patients with STEMI, the effects of fondaparinux on mortality and reinfarction of fondaparinux was evaluated in the OASIS-6 trial where 12,092 patients with STEMI were randomly assigned to receive either treatment with fondaparinux or placebo according to the original randomized assignment (placebo for those for whom UFH was not indicated, or UFH for up to 48 hours followed by placebo for up to 8 days). In patients with STEMI, particularly those not undergoing primary PCI, fondaparinux significantly reduced mortality and reinfarction without increasing bleeding and strokes [55].

Encouraging results had emerged some years ago. A total of 333 patients with evolving STEMI were treated with ASA and alteplase and randomized to UFH given IV for 48 to 72 hours or to a low, medium, or high dose of fondaparinux. The percentage of patients achieving TIMI grade 3 flow (restoring coronary artery patency) at 90 minutes was 68% in the UFH control group and ranged between 60% and 69% with fondaparinux, rendering the selective factor Xa inhibition with fondaparinux an attractive therapeutic concept in patients presenting with STEMI, as there was a trend towards less reocclusion and fewer revascularizations [56].

The 2007 update of the ACC/AHA guidelines states that fondaparinux should not be used as the sole anticoagulant during PCI but should be coupled with an additional agent, such as UFH or bivalirudin, so that the risk of catheter complications can be ameliorated. For patients with STEMI who do not undergo reperfusion therapy, fondaparinux can be used as the anticoagulant therapy of choice. The initial dose is 2.5 mg IV with subsequent SC injections of 2.5 mg once daily [19].

Oral Anticoagulants

It was more than 70 years ago that that the ingestion of spoiled sweet clover silage was responsible for the appearance of hemorrhage (due to a deficiency of plasma prothrombin) in cattle.

Campbell and Link, in 1939, identified the hemorrhagic agent as bishydroxycoumarin (dicoumarol). In 1948, a more potent synthetic congener of the coumarin family was introduced as an extremely effective rodenticide; this compound was named warfarin.

Since then, anticoagulants based on warfarin have become a mainstay for prevention of thromboembolic disease. Other coumarin anticoagulants are almost never used in the USA because they have less favorable pharmacologic properties or greater toxicity [1,3].

Warfarin (Figure 6) used clinically is a racemic mixture composed of equal amounts of two enantiomorphs with the levorotatory S-warfarin being four times more potent than the dextrorotatory R-warfarin. These enantiomorphs differ in anticoagulant potency, metabolism, elimination, and interactions with other drugs [1,3].

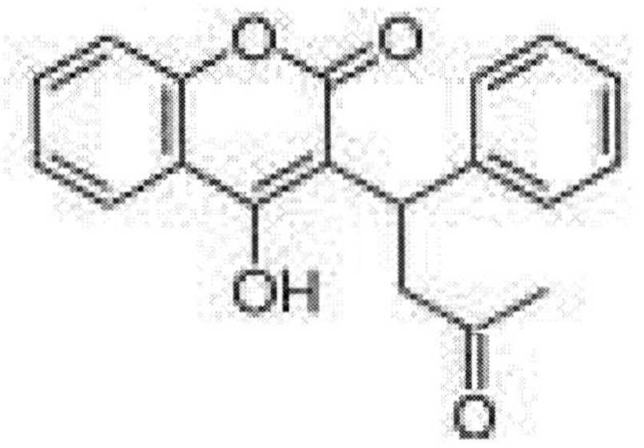

Figure 6. Structure of warfarin.

Pharmacokinetics

Warfarin is generally administered as the sodium salt and has 100% bioavailability (when given orally, IV, or rectally). Food in the gastrointestinal tract can decrease the rate of absorption. Over 99% of racemic warfarin is bound to plasma albumin, which may contribute to its small volume of distribution (the albumin space), its long half-life in plasma (mean 40 hours), its long duration of action (2 to 5 days) and the lack of urinary excretion of unchanged drug. Warfarin usually is detectable in plasma within 1 hour of its oral administration, and concentrations peak in 2 to 8 hours. The S-warfarin is transformed into inactive metabolites by CYP2C9 and the R-warfarin is transformed mostly by CYP1A2 and to a lesser extent by CYP2C19 and CYP3A4. The inactive metabolites of warfarin are excreted in urine and stool [1,3]. Treatment with warfarin should be initiated with standard doses of 5-10 mg/day for 2 to 4 days orally (except for elderly patients as well those with an increased risk of bleeding), followed by 2 to 10 mg/day as indicated by measurements of the international normalized ratio (INR), which defines the therapeutic range for oral anticoagulant therapy. Warfarin also can be given IV without modification of the dose [1,3].

Pharmacodynamics and Mechanism of Action

The oral anticoagulants are antagonists of vitamin K. Warfarin blocks the γ-carboxylation of several glutamate residues in prothrombin and factors II, VII, IX, and X as well as the endogenous anticoagulant proteins C and S, which are synthesized mainly in the liver and are biologically inactive otherwise. This carboxylation is directly coupled to the oxidation of vitamin K to its corresponding epoxide, a reaction catalyzed by vitamin K epoxide reductase, which, in its own turn, is inhibited by therapeutic doses of warfarin. Vitamin K can also be converted to the corresponding hydroquinone by a second reductase, DT-diaphorase. This enzyme requires high concentrations of vitamin K and is less sensitive to coumarin drugs, which may explain why administration of sufficient vitamin K can counteract even large doses of oral anticoagulants. Also, mutational change of vitamin K epoxide reductase can give rise to genetic resistance (discussed below) to warfarin in humans [1,3]. There is an 8- to 12-hour delay in the action of warfarin. The resulting inhibition of coagulation is dependent on the degradation rate of the clotting factors mentioned above in the circulation. Therapeutic doses of warfarin decrease by 30% to 50% the total amount of each clotting factor; in addition, the secreted molecules are not fully carboxylated, resulting in diminished biological activity. The time required for the activity of each factor in plasma to reach a new steady state after warfarin is administered depends on its individual rate of clearance. The approximate half-lives are, for factor VII, 6 hours, for factor IX, 24 hours, for factor X, 36 hours, for factor II, 50 hours, for protein C, 8 hours and for protein S, 30 hours. Because of the long half-lives of some of the coagulation factors, the full antithrombotic effect of warfarin is not achieved for several days. Larger initial doses of warfarin hasten the onset of the anticoagulant effect. Beyond this dosage, the speed of onset is independent of the dose size. The only effect of a larger loading dose is to prolong the time that the plasma concentration of drug remains above that required for suppression of clotting factor synthesis [1,3,57]. On one hand, some patients require large doses (>20 mg/day) of warfarin to achieve a therapeutic INR. These patients often have excessive vitamin K intake from the diet or parenteral supplementation. A few patients with hereditary warfarin resistance have been reported, in whom very high plasma concentrations of warfarin are associated with minimal depression of vitamin K-dependent coagulation factor biosynthesis [58]. On the other, approximately 10% of patients require small doses (<1.5 mg/day) to reach a therapeutic INR. These patients are more likely to possess one or two variant alleles of CYP2C9. In comparison with the wild-type CYP2C9*1 allele, the variant alleles CYP2C9*2 and CYP2C9*3 have been shown to inactivate S-warfarin much less efficiently *in vitro* [3,59].

Toxicity and Drug Interactions

Bleeding is the major adverse effect of warfarin. The risk of bleeding increases with the intensity and duration of anticoagulant therapy, the use of other medications that interfere with hemostasis, and the presence of a potential anatomical source of bleeding [60]. Intracranial, pericardial, nerve sheath, spinal cord, gastrointestinal, intraperitoneal, or retroperitoneal bleeding can occur. Although the reported incidence of major bleeding episodes varies considerably, it is generally less than 5% per year in patients treated with a target INR of 2 to 3 [1,3]. If the INR is above the therapeutic range but < than 5 and the patient is not bleeding or in need of a surgical procedure, warfarin can be discontinued temporarily. If the INR is > than 5, vitamin K_1 can be given orally (the INR falls within 24 to 48 hours without rendering the patient resistant to further warfarin therapy). One should note that this reduction in the INR is delayed, because reversal of anticoagulation requires synthesis of fully carboxylated coagulation factors. If the INR is > than 20, FFP should be transfused by the physician (10 to 20 ml/kg), supplemented with 10 mg of vitamin K_1, given by slow IV infusion. Transfusion of FFP may need to be repeated, since the transfused factors (particularly factor VII) are cleared from the circulation more rapidly than the residual oral anticoagulant. The physician should be cautious when administering IV vitamin K_1 due to the risk of anaphylactoid reactions. Patients who receive high doses of vitamin K_1 may become unresponsive to warfarin for several days, but heparin can be used if continued anticoagulation is required [60]. Finally, excessive anticoagulant effect and bleeding from warfarin can be reversed by administering prothrombin complex concentrates (PCC) and recombinant factor VIIa (rFVIIa) [3].

Warfarin-induced skin necrosis is a rare complication. Skin lesions typically seen on the extremities, as well as on adipose tissue, intestine, the penis, and the female breast also appear

3 to 10 days after treatment is initiated. These lesions are characterized by widespread thrombosis of the microvasculature and can spread rapidly, sometimes becoming necrotic and requiring disfiguring debridement or occasionally amputation. It has been proposed that the dermal necrosis is a manifestation of a temporal imbalance between the anticoagulant protein C and one or more of the procoagulant factors and is exaggerated in patients who are partially deficient in protein C or protein S, as cases have been reported in subjects heterozygous for protein C or protein S deficiency. Patients with normal activities of these proteins can also be affected. Morphologically similar lesions can occur in patients with vitamin K deficiency. Warfarin also appears to precipitate the syndromes of venous limb gangrene and multicentric skin necrosis that sometimes are associated with HIT [61].

Warfarin crosses the placenta readily and can cause not only a hemorrhagic disorder in the fetus but, also serious birth defects (nasal hypoplasia, stippled epiphyseal calcifications, central nervous system abnormalities) up to intrauterine death and abortion, making warfarin administration prohibited during pregnancy. Other toxicities include a reversible, sometimes painful, blue-tinged discoloration of the plantar surfaces and sides of the toes that blanches with pressure and fades with elevation of the legs (purple toe syndrome), alopecia, urticaria, dermatitis, fever, nausea, diarrhea, abdominal cramps and anorexia [1,3].

Many drugs and other factors can affect the action of warfarin. These interactions can be broadly divided into pharmacokinetic (enzyme induction, enzyme inhibition, and reduced plasma protein binding) and pharmacodynamic (synergism, competitive antagonism and altered physiologic control loop for vitamin K) effects [3]. The most serious interactions are those that increase the anticoagulant effect and the risk of bleeding (Table 4).

Table 4. Drugs and disease states that promote bleeding in patients taking warfarin

Drugs and other factors	Action (increase the risk of bleeding)
Amiodarone Fluconazole Cimetidine Clopidogrel Cotrimoxazole Disulfiram Fluoxetine, Isoniazid Metronidazole Sulfinpyrazone Tolcapone Zafirlukast Trimethoprim-sulfamethoxazole	Decreased metabolism due to CYP2C9 inhibition
Loop diuretics Valproate	Displacement from protein binding sites
Inadequate diet (postoperative patients on parenteral fluids) Elimination of intestinal flora (antibiotics) Inhibition in the vitamin K cycle (cephalosporins)	Vitamin K deficiency
Renal failure CHF Hypermetabolic states (hyperthyroidism)	Low concentrations of coagulation factors
Aspirin	Antiplatelet effect
Heparin	Inhibition of the activity of clotting factors

CHF: congestive heart failure

A decreased effect of oral anticoagulants include could be due to a variety of reasons;

i) reduced absorption of warfarin (e.g. cholestyramine binding in the gastrointestinal tract)
ii) increased volume of distribution and a short half-life secondary to hypoproteinemia (e.g. nephrotic syndrome)
iii) increased metabolic clearance of warfarin secondary to induction of hepatic enzymes (e.g. barbiturates, carbamazepine, rifampin
iv) increased vitamin K dietary intake
v) increased levels of coagulation factors (e.g. pregnancy)
vi) decreased clotting factor concentration (e.g. diuretics chlorthalidone and spironolactone)
vii) decreased turnover rate of clotting factors (e.g. hypothyroidism) and
viii) mutation of vitamin K reactivation cycle molecules (e.g. hereditary resistance) [1,3].

Drugs with no significant effect on anticoagulant therapy include ethanol, phenothiazines, benzodiazepines, acetaminophen, opioids, indomethacin and most antibiotics [1,3].

Clinical Use

As far as the indications of warfarin are concerned, the physician should bear in mind to undertake laboratory tests (in conjunction with the patient's history and physical examination) to uncover hemostatic defects that might make the use of oral anticoagulant drugs more dangerous (i.e. vascular abnormalities, thrombocytopenia, etc.).

Therapeutic ranges of the INR, for various clinical indications, have been established empirically and reflect dosages that reduce the morbidity from thromboembolic disease while minimally increasing the risk of serious hemorrhage.

For most indications the target INR is between 2.0 to 3.0 [60]. When treating patients with acute venous thromboembolism, heparin should be administered along with warfarin for at least 4 to 5 days and until the INR is in the therapeutic range on 2 consecutive days so as to allow for adequate depletion of the vitamin K-dependent coagulation factors with long half-lives, especially factor II [3].

The clinical uses of warfarin are shown on Table 5.

Oral Anticoagulation in ACS

Although the benefit of oral anticoagulants in patients with ACS, when combined with ASA over ASA alone, is well demonstrated through numerous trials, warfarin is not the preferred medication of choice. It has a limited clinical use since a similar degree of benefit is seen with clopidogrel plus ASA rather than with ASA alone, without the drawback of monitoring the INR, as is necessary with warfarin therapy.

Therefore, use of warfarin in conjunction with ASA and/or clopidogrel is associated with an increased risk of bleeding and should be monitored closely. In addition, the use of clopidogrel is well established for patients with ACS who undergo PCI and stenting [62-64].

Table 5. The clinical aplications of warfarin and optimal INR targets

Prevention of venous thromboembolism (INR between 2.0 and 3.0)
Treatment of DVT or PE (INR between 2.0 and 3.0)
Primary prevention of ischemic coronary events (INR between 1.3 and 1.8)
Prophylaxis and/or treatment of the thromboembolic complications in patients with prosthetic heart valves
• mechanical prosthetic valves (INR between 2.5 to 3.5)
• bioprosthetic valves (INR between 2.0 to 3.0)
Prophylaxis and/or treatment of the thromboembolic complications in patients with AF (INR between 2.0 and 3.0)
Treatment of ACS patients (discussed below)

INR: international normalized ratio; DVT: deep venous thrombosis; PE: pulmonary embolism; AF: atrial fibrillation; ACS: acute coronary syndrome

Warfarin either without (INR 2.5 to 3.5) or with low-dose ASA (75 to 81 mg/day; INR 2.0 to 2.5) may be reasonable for patients at high coronary artery disease (CAD) risk and low bleeding risk who do not require or are intolerant of clopidogrel.

The physician should manage warfarin to INR 2.5 to 3.5 in post-STEMI patients when clinically indicated (patients with atrial fibrillation, or left ventricular thrombus) or for those not able to take ASA or clopidogrel.

In patients requiring triple-anticoagulant therapy with warfarin, clopidogrel, and ASA, i.e. those with mechanical heart valve, an INR of 2.0 to 2.5 is recommended with low dose ASA (75 mg to 81 mg) and a 75 mg dose of clopidogrel [19]. Low- or moderate-intensity anticoagulation with fixed-dose warfarin is not recommended for routine use after hospitalization for UA/NSTEMI [18].

Since the long-term administration of warfarin has been evaluated in a few, mostly small studies, and by few observational data, with, sometimes, conflicting results, when triple-combination therapy is selected for clear indications and is based on clinical judgment that benefit will outweigh the incremental risk of bleeding, then therapy should be given for the minimum time and at the minimally effective doses necessary to achieve protection.

More studies are needed so as to expand evidence base [65-71].

Conclusion

Anticoagulant therapy, which targets the clotting cascade to prevent the deposition of fibrin strands in the clot is categorized into i) IV, SC and oral anticoagulants ii) direct thrombin inhibitors and iii) factor Xa Inhibitors. It remains an integral part of the therapeutic protocol in ACS patients, both for those with STEMI and UA/NSTEMI.

Inhibition of coagulation factors (II, IIa, VII, VIIa, IX, IXa, X, Xa) by the aforementioned drugs maintains the patency of the infarct-related artery, limits the consequences of myocardial ischemia, enhances myocardial healing, and reduces the likelihood of recurrent events.

References

[1] Majerus PW, Tollefsen DM. Blood Coagulation and Anticoagulant, Thrombolytic, and Antiplatelet Drugs. In: *Goodman and Gilman's The Pharmacological Basis of Therapeutics*, Brunton LL, Lazo JS, Parker KL, eds. *11th edition*, New York: McGraw-Hill, *2006, 1467-1488.*

[2] Sugahara K, Kitagawa H. Heparin and heparan sulfate biosynthesis. *IUBMB Life* 2002;54:163-175.

[3] Zehnder JL. Drugs Used in Disorders of Coagulation. In: *Basic and clinical pharmacology*, Katzung BG ed. 10th edition, Boston: 2006, 542-559.

[4] Hirsh J. Heparin. *N. Engl. J. Med.* 1991;324:1565-1574.

[5] Rich JD, Maraganore JM, Young E, Lidon RM, Adelman B, Bourdon P, Charenkavanich S, Hirsh J, Theroux P, Cannon CP. Heparin resistance in acute coronary syndromes. *J. Thromb Thrombolysis* 2007;23:93-100.

[6] Hirsh J, Warkentin TE, Raschke R, Granger C, Ohman EM, Dalen JE. Heparin and low-molecular-weight heparin: mechanisms of action, pharmacokinetics, dosing considerations, monitoring, efficacy, and safety. *Chest* 1998;114:489S-510S.

[7] Hassan WM, Flaker GC, Feutz C, Petroski GF, Smith D. Improved anticoagulation with a weight-adjusted heparin nomogram in patients with acute coronary syndromes: a randomized trial. *J. Thromb Thrombolysis* 1995;2:245-249.

[8] Becker RC, Ball SP, Eisenberg P, Borzak S, Held AC, Spencer F, Voyce SJ, Jesse R, Hendel R, Ma Y, Hurley T, Hebert J. A randomized, multicenter trial of weight-adjusted intravenous heparin dose titration and point of- care coagulation monitoring in hospitalized patients with active thromboembolic disease: Antithrombotic Therapy Consortium Investigators. *Am. Heart J.* 1999;137:59-71.

[9] Hochman JS, Wali AU, Gavrila D, Sim MJ, Malhotra S, Palazzo AM, De La Fuente B. A new regimen for heparin use in acute coronary syndromes. *Am. Heart J.* 1999;138:313-318.

[10] Hirsh J, Raschke R. Heparin and low-molecular-weight heparin: the Seventh ACCP Conference on Antithrombotic and Thrombolytic Therapy. *Chest* 2004;126:188S-203S.

[11] Theroux P, Waters D, Lam J, Juneau M, McCans J. Reactivation of unstable angina after the discontinuation of heparin. *N. Engl. J. Med.* 1992;327:141-145.

[12] Granger CB, Miller JM, Bovill EG, Gruber A, Tracy RP, Krucoff MW, Green C, Berrios E, Harrington RA, Ohman EM, et al. Rebound increase in thrombin generation and activity after cessation of intravenous heparin in patients with acute coronary syndromes. *Circulation* 1995;91:1929-1935.

[13] Oliveira GB, Anstrom KJ, Honeycutt EF, et al. Intravenous unfractionated heparin, patient profile, and the magnitude of thrombocytopenia are associated with heparin-induced thrombocytopenia (HIT) antibodies: insights from the CATCH Registry (abstr). *Eur. Heart J.* 2005;725.

[14] Oliveira GB, Anstrom KJ, Honeycutt EF, et al. Prolonged heparin exposure, development of thrombocytopenia, use of GP IIb/IIIa inhibitors, and history of renal dysfunction predict moderate or severe bleeding: a report from the Complications After Thrombocytopenia Caused by Heparin (CATCH) registry (abstr). *J. Am. Coll. Cardiol.* 2006;251A.

[15] Ohman EM, Granger CB, Rice L, Abrams CS, Becker RC, Berger PB, Kleiman NS, Moliterno D, Moll S, Rodgers JE, Steinhubl SS, Tapson VF, Sinnaeve P, Anstrom KJ; Complication After Thrombocytopenia Caused by Heparin (CATCH) Registry. Identification, diagnosis and treatment of heparin-induced thrombocytopenia and thrombosis: a registry of prolonged heparin use and thrombocytopenia among hospitalized patients with and without cardiovascular disease. The Complication After Thrombocytopenia Caused by Heparin (CATCH) Registry Steering Committee. *J. Thromb Thrombolysis* 2005;19:11-19.

[16] Warkentin TE, Levine MN, Hirsh J, Horsewood P, Roberts RS, Gent M, Kelton JG. Heparin-induced thrombocytopenia in patients treated with low-molecular-weight heparin or unfractionated heparin. *N. Engl. J. Med.* 1995;332:1330-1335.

[17] Hirsh J, Anand SS, Halperin JL, Fuster V; American Heart Association. Guide to anticoagulant therapy: Heparin : a statement for healthcare professionals from the American Heart Association. *Circulation* 2001;103:2994-3018.

[18] Anderson JL, Adams CD, Antman EM, Bridges CR, Califf RM, Casey DE Jr, Chavey WE 2nd, Fesmire FM, Hochman JS, Levin TN, Lincoff AM, Peterson ED, Theroux P, Wenger NK, Wright RS, Smith SC Jr, Jacobs AK, Adams CD, Anderson JL, Antman EM, Halperin JL, Hunt SA, Krumholz HM, Kushner FG, Lytle BW, Nishimura R, Ornato JP, Page RL, Riegel B; American College of Cardiology; American Heart Association Task Force on Practice Guidelines (Writing Committee to Revise the 2002 Guidelines for the Management of Patients With Unstable Angina/Non-ST-Elevation Myocardial Infarction); American College of Emergency Physicians; Society for Cardiovascular Angiography and Interventions; Society of Thoracic Surgeons; American Association of Cardiovascular and Pulmonary Rehabilitation; Society for Academic Emergency Medicine. ACC/AHA 2007 guidelines for the management of patients with unstable angina/non-ST-Elevation myocardial infarction: a report of the American College of Cardiology/American Heart Association Task Force on Practice Guidelines (Writing Committee to Revise the 2002 Guidelines for the Management of Patients With Unstable Angina/Non-ST-Elevation Myocardial Infarction) developed in collaboration with the American College of Emergency Physicians, the Society for Cardiovascular Angiography and Interventions, and the Society of Thoracic Surgeons endorsed by the American Association of Cardiovascular and Pulmonary Rehabilitation and the Society for Academic Emergency Medicine. *J. Am. Coll. Cardiol.* 2007;50:e1-e157.

[19] Antman EM, Hand M, Armstrong PW, Bates ER, Green LA, Halasyamani LK, Hochman JS, Krumholz HM, Lamas GA, Mullany CJ, Pearle DL, Sloan MA, Smith SC Jr; 2004 Writing Committee Members, Anbe DT, Kushner FG, Ornato JP, Jacobs AK, Adams CD, Anderson JL, Buller CE, Creager MA, Ettinger SM, Halperin JL, Hunt SA, Lytle BW, Nishimura R, Page RL, Riegel B, Tarkington LG, Yancy CW. 2007 Focused Update of the ACC/AHA 2004 Guidelines for the Management of Patients With ST-Elevation Myocardial Infarction: a report of the American College of Cardiology/American Heart Association Task Force on Practice Guidelines: developed in collaboration With the Canadian Cardiovascular Society endorsed by the American Academy of Family Physicians: 2007 Writing Group to Review New Evidence and Update the ACC/AHA 2004 Guidelines for the Management of Patients With ST-

Elevation Myocardial Infarction, Writing on Behalf of the 2004 Writing Committee. *Circulation* 2008;117:296-329.

[20] Théroux P, Ouimet H, McCans J, Latour JG, Joly P, Lévy G, Pelletier E, Juneau M, Stasiak J, deGuise P, et al. Aspirin, heparin, or both to treat acute unstable angina. *N Engl. J. Med.* 1988;319:1105-1111.

[21] Théroux P, Waters D, Qiu S, McCans J, de Guise P, Juneau M. Aspirin versus heparin to prevent myocardial infarction during the acute phase of unstable angina. *Circulation* 1993;88:2045-2048.

[22] Anonymous. Risk of myocardial infarction and death during treatment with low dose aspirin and intravenous heparin in men with unstable coronary artery disease. The RISC Group. *Lancet* 1990;336:827-830.

[23] Curtis JP, Alexander JH, Huang Y, Wallentin L, Verheugt FW, Armstrong PW, Krumholz HM, Van de Werf F, Danays T, Cheeks M, Granger CB; ASSENT-2 and ASSENT-3 Investigators. Efficacy and safety of two unfractionated heparin dosing strategies with tenecteplase in acute myocardial infarction (results from Assessment of the Safety and Efficacy of a New Thrombolytic Regimens 2 and 3). *Am. J. Cardiol.* 2004;94:279-283.

[24] Granger CB, Hirsch J, Califf RM, Col J, White HD, Betriu A, Woodlief LH, Lee KL, Bovill EG, Simės RJ, Topol EJ. Activated partial thromboplastin time and outcome after thrombolytic therapy for acute myocardial infarction: results from the GUSTO-I trial. *Circulation* 1996;93:870-878.

[25] Smythe MA, Stephens JL, Mattson JC. Delayed-onset heparin-induced thrombocytopenia. *Ann. Emerg. Med.* 2005;45:417-419.

[26] Warkentin TE. Heparin-induced thrombocytopenia. *Hematol. Oncol. Clin. North Am.* 2007;21:589-607.

[27] Weitz JI. Low-molecular-weight heparins. *N. Engl. J. Med.* 1997;337:688-698.

[28] Xiao Z, Theroux P. Platelet activation with unfractionated heparin at therapeutic concentrations and comparisons with a low-molecular weight heparin and with a direct thrombin inhibitor. *Circulation* 1998;97:251-256.

[29] Michalis LK, Katsouras CS, Papamichael N, Adamides K, Naka KK, Goudevenos J, Sideris DA. Enoxaparin versus tinzaparin in non-ST-segment elevation acute coronary syndromes: the EVET trial. *Am. Heart J.* 2003;146:304-310.

[30] Antman EM, Cohen M, Radley D, McCabe C, Rush J, Premmereur J, Braunwald E. Assessment of the treatment effect of enoxaparin for unstable angina/non-Q-wave myocardial infarction. TIMI 11B-ESSENCE meta-analysis. *Circulation* 1999;100:1602-1608.

[31] Ferguson JJ, Califf RM, Antman EM, Cohen M, Grines CL, Goodman S, Kereiakes DJ, Langer A, Mahaffey KW, Nessel CC, Armstrong PW, Avezum A, Aylward P, Becker RC, Biasucci L, Borzak S, Col J, Frey MJ, Fry E, Gulba DC, Guneri S, Gurfinkel E, Harrington R, Hochman JS, Kleiman NS, Leon MB, Lopez-Sendon JL, Pepine CJ, Ruzyllo W, Steinhubl SR, Teirstein PS, Toro-Figueroa L, White H; SYNERGY Trial Investigators. Enoxaparin vs unfractionated heparin in high-risk patients with non-ST-segment elevation acute coronary syndromes managed with an intended early invasive strategy: primary results of the SYNERGY randomized trial. *JAMA* 2004;292:45-54.

[32] Antman EM, McCabe CH, Gurfinkel EP, Turpie AG, Bernink PJ, Salein D, Bayes De Luna A, Fox K, Lablanche JM, Radley D, Premmereur J, Braunwald E. Enoxaparin

prevents death and cardiac ischemic events in unstable angina/non-Q-wave myocardial infarction. Results of the thrombolysis in myocardial infarction (TIMI) 11B trial. *Circulation* 1999;100:1593-601.

[33] de Lemos JA, Blazing MA, Wiviott SD, Brady WE, White HD, Fox KA, Palmisano J, Ramsey KE, Bilheimer DW, Lewis EF, Pfeffer M, Califf RM, Braunwald E; A to Z Investigators. Enoxaparin versus unfractionated heparin in patients treated with tirofiban, aspirin and an early conservative initial management strategy: results from the A phase of the A-to-Z trial. *Eur. Heart J.* 2004;25:1688-1694.

[34] Cohen M, Théroux P, Borzak S, Frey MJ, White HD, Van Mieghem W, Senatore F, Lis J, Mukherjee R, Harris K, Bigonzi F; ACUTE II Investigators. Randomized double-blind safety study of enoxaparin versus unfractionated heparin in patients with non-ST-segment elevation acute coronary syndromes treated with tirofiban and aspirin: the ACUTE II study. The Antithrombotic Combination Using Tirofiban and Enoxaparin. *Am. Heart J.* 2002;144:470-477.

[35] Kumar A, Cannon CP. Acute coronary syndromes: diagnosis and management, part I. *Mayo. Clin. Proc.* 2009;84:917-938.

[36] Yusuf S, Mehta SR, Xie C, Ahmed RJ, Xavier D, Pais P, Zhu J, Liu L; CREATE Trial Group Investigators. Effects of reviparin, a low-molecular-weight heparin, on mortality, reinfarction, and strokes in patients with acute myocardial infarction presenting with ST-segment elevation. *JAMA* 2005;293:427-435.

[37] Sabatine MS, Morrow DA, Montalescot G, Dellborg M, Leiva-Pons JL, Keltai M, Murphy SA, McCabe CH, Gibson CM, Cannon CP, Antman EM, Braunwald E; Clopidogrel as Adjunctive Reperfusion Therapy (CLARITY)-Thrombolysis in Myocardial Infarction (TIMI) 28 Investigators. Angiographic and clinical outcomes in patients receiving low-molecular-weight heparin versus unfractionated heparin in ST-elevation myocardial infarction treated with fibrinolytics in the CLARITY-TIMI 28 Trial. *Circulation* 2005;112:3846-3854.

[38] Assessment of the Safety and Efficacy of a New Thrombolytic Regimen (ASSENT)-3 Investigators. Efficacy and safety of tenecteplase in combination with enoxaparin, abciximab, or unfractionated heparin: the ASSENT-3 randomised trial in acute myocardial infarction. *Lancet* 2001;358:605-613.

[39] Eikelboom JW, Quinlan DJ, Mehta SR, Turpie AG, Menown IB, Yusuf S. Unfractionated and low-molecular-weight heparin as adjuncts to thrombolysis in aspirin-treated patients with ST-elevation acute myocardial infarction: a meta-analysis of the randomized trials. *Circulation* 2005;112:3855-3867.

[40] Antman EM, Morrow DA, McCabe CH, Murphy SA, Ruda M, Sadowski Z, Budaj A, López-Sendón JL, Guneri S, Jiang F, White HD, Fox KA, Braunwald E; ExTRACT-TIMI 25 Investigators. Enoxaparin versus unfractionated heparin with fibrinolysis for ST-elevation myocardial infarction. *N. Engl. J. Med.* 2006;354:1477-1488.

[41] Carswell CI, Plosker GL. Bivalirudin: a review of its potential place in the management of acute coronary syndromes. *Drugs* 2002;62:841-870.

[42] Gladwell TD. Bivalirudin: a direct thrombin inhibitor. *Clin. Ther.* 2002;24:38-58.

[43] Sciulli TM, Mauro VF. Pharmacology and clinical use of bivalirudin. *Ann. Pharmacother.* 2002;36:1028-1041.

[44] Stone GW, McLaurin BT, Cox DA, Bertrand ME, Lincoff AM, Moses JW, White HD, Pocock SJ, Ware JH, Feit F, Colombo A, Aylward PE, Cequier AR, Darius H, Desmet

W, Ebrahimi R, Hamon M, Rasmussen LH, Rupprecht HJ, Hoekstra J, Mehran R, Ohman EM; ACUITY Investigators. Bivalirudin for patients with acute coronary syndromes. *N. Engl. J. Med.* 2006;355:2203-2216.

[45] Lincoff AM, Bittl JA, Harrington RA, Feit F, Kleiman NS, Jackman JD, Sarembock IJ, Cohen DJ, Spriggs D, Ebrahimi R, Keren G, Carr J, Cohen EA, Betriu A, Desmet W, Kereiakes DJ, Rutsch W, Wilcox RG, de Feyter PJ, Vahanian A, Topol EJ; REPLACE-2 Investigators. Bivalirudin and provisional glycoprotein IIb/IIIa blockade compared with heparin and planned glycoprotein IIb/IIIa blockade during percutaneous coronary intervention: REPLACE-2 randomized trial. *JAMA* 2003;289:853-863.

[46] Lincoff AM, Kleiman NS, Kereiakes DJ, Feit F, Bittl JA, Jackman JD, Sarembock IJ, Cohen DJ, Spriggs D, Ebrahimi R, Keren G, Carr J, Cohen EA, Betriu A, Desmet W, Rutsch W, Wilcox RG, de Feyter PJ, Vahanian A, Topol EJ; REPLACE-2 Investigators. Long-term efficacy of bivalirudin and provisional glycoprotein IIb/IIIa blockade vs heparin and planned glycoprotein IIb/IIIa blockade during percutaneous coronary revascularization: REPLACE-2 randomized trial. *JAMA* 2004;292:696-703.

[47] Stone GW, Witzenbichler B, Guagliumi G, Peruga JZ, Brodie BR, Dudek D, Kornowski R, Hartmann F, Gersh BJ, Pocock SJ, Dangas G, Wong SC, Kirtane AJ, Parise H, Mehran R; HORIZONS-AMI Trial Investigators. Bivalirudin during primary PCI in acute myocardial infarction. *N. Engl. J. Med.* 2008;358:2218-2230.

[48] White H; Hirulog and Early Reperfusion or Occlusion (HERO)-2 Trial Investigators. Thrombin-specific anticoagulation with bivalirudin versus heparin in patients receiving fibrinolytic therapy for acute myocardial infarction: the HERO-2 randomised trial. *Lancet* 2001;358:1855-1863.

[49] Direct Thrombin Inhibitor Trialists' Collaborative Group. Direct thrombin inhibitors in acute coronary syndromes: principal results of a meta-analysis based on individual patients' data. *Lancet* 2002;359:294-302.

[50] Büller HR, Davidson BL, Decousus H, Gallus A, Gent M, Piovella F, Prins MH, Raskob G, van den Berg-Segers AE, Cariou R, Leeuwenkamp O, Lensing AW; Matisse Investigators. Subcutaneous fondaparinux versus intravenous unfractionated heparin in the initial treatment of pulmonary embolism. *N. Engl. J. Med.* 2003;349:1695-1702.

[51] Sharma T, Mehta P, Gajra A. Update on Fondaparinux: Role in Management of Thromboembolic and Acute Coronary Events. *Cardiovasc. Hematol. Agents Med. Chem*. 2010 [Epub ahead of print].

[52] Samama MM, Gerotziafas GT. Evaluation of the pharmacological properties and clinical results of the synthetic pentasaccharide (fondaparinux). *Thromb. Res.* 2003;109:1-11.

[53] Turpie AG. Fondaparinux: a Factor Xa inhibitor for antithrombotic therapy. *Expert Opin. Pharmacother.* 2004;5:1373-1384.

[54] Fifth Organization to Assess Strategies in Acute Ischemic Syndromes Investigators, Yusuf S, Mehta SR, Chrolavicius S, Afzal R, Pogue J, Granger CB, Budaj A, Peters RJ, Bassand JP, Wallentin L, Joyner C, Fox KA. Comparison of fondaparinux and enoxaparin in acute coronary syndromes. *N. Engl. J. Med.* 2006;354:1464-1476.

[55] Yusuf S, Mehta SR, Chrolavicius S, Afzal R, Pogue J, Granger CB, Budaj A, Peters RJ, Bassand JP, Wallentin L, Joyner C, Fox KA; OASIS-6 Trial Group. Effects of fondaparinux on mortality and reinfarction in patients with acute ST-segment elevation myocardial infarction: the OASIS-6 randomized trial. *JAMA* 2006;295:1519-1530.

[56] Coussement PK, Bassand JP, Convens C, Vrolix M, Boland J, Grollier G, Michels R, Vahanian A, Vanderheyden M, Rupprecht HJ, Van de Werf F; PENTALYSE investigators. A synthetic factor-Xa inhibitor (ORG31540/SR9017A) as an adjunct to fibrinolysis in acute myocardial infarction. The PENTALYSE study. *Eur. Heart* . 2001;22:1716-1724.

[57] Zivelin A, Rao LV, Rapaport SI. Mechanism of the anticoagulant effect of warfarin as evaluated in rabbits by selective depression of individual procoagulant vitamin K-dependent clotting factors. *J. Clin. Invest.* 1993;92:2131-2140.

[58] Rost S, Fregin A, Ivaskevicius V, Conzelmann E, Hörtnagel K, Pelz HJ, Lappegard K, Seifried E, Scharrer I, Tuddenham EG, Müller CR, Strom TM, Oldenburg J. Mutations in VKORC1 cause warfarin resistance and multiple coagulation factor deficiency type 2. *Nature* 2004;427:537-541.

[59] Daly AK, King BP. Pharmacogenetics of oral anticoagulants. *Pharmacogenetics* 2003;13:247-252.

[60] Hirsh J, Fuster V, Ansell J, Halperin JL; American Heart Association/American College of Cardiology Foundation. American Heart Association/American College of Cardiology Foundation guide to warfarin therapy. *J. Am. Coll. Cardiol.* 2003;41:1633-1652.

[61] Warkentin TE. Heparin-induced thrombocytopenia: pathogenesis and management. *Br. J. Haematol.* 2003;121:535-555.

[62] Anonymous. Effects of long-term, moderate-intensity oral anticoagulation in addition to aspirin in unstable angina. The Organization to Assess Strategies for Ischemic Syndromes (OASIS) Investigators. *J. Am. Coll. Cardiol.* 2001;37:475-484.

[63] van Es RF, Jonker JJ, Verheugt FW, Deckers JW, Grobbee DE; Antithrombotics in the Secondary Preventionof Events in Coronary Thrombosis-2 (ASPECT-2) Research Group. Aspirin and coumadin after acute coronary syndromes (the ASPECT-2 study): a randomised controlled trial. *Lancet* 2002;360:109-113.

[64] Hurlen M, Abdelnoor M, Smith P, Erikssen J, Arnesen H. Warfarin, aspirin, or both after myocardial infarction. *N. Engl. J. Med.* 2002;347:969-974.

[65] Williams DO, Kirby MG, McPherson K, Phear DN. Anticoagulant treatment of unstable angina. *Br. J. Clin. Pract.* 1986;40:114-116.

[66] Cohen M, Adams PC, Parry G, Xiong J, Chamberlain D, Wieczorek I, Fox KA, Chesebro JH, Strain J, Keller C, et al. Combination antithrombotic therapy in unstable rest angina and non-Q-wave infarction in nonprior aspirin users. Primary end points analysis from the ATACS trial. Antithrombotic Therapy in Acute Coronary Syndromes Research Group. *Circulation* 1994;89:81-88.

[67] Williams MJ, Morison IM, Parker JH, Stewart RA. Progression of the culprit lesion in unstable coronary artery disease with warfarin and aspirin versus aspirin alone: preliminary study. *J. Am. Coll. Cardiol.* 1997;30:364-369.

[68] Anonymous. Randomised double-blind trial of fixed low-dose warfarin with aspirin after myocardial infarction. Coumadin Aspirin Reinfarction Study (CARS) Investigators. *Lancet* 1997;350:389-396.

[69] Fiore LD, Ezekowitz MD, Brophy MT, Lu D, Sacco J, Peduzzi P; Combination Hemotherapy and Mortality Prevention (CHAMP) Study Group. Department of Veterans Affairs Cooperative Studies Program Clinical Trial comparing combined

warfarin and aspirin with aspirin alone in survivors of acute myocardial infarction: primary results of the CHAMP study. *Circulation* 2002;105:557-563.

[70] Hurlen M, Abdelnoor M, Smith P, Erikssen J, Arnesen H.Warfarin, aspirin, or both after myocardial infarction. *N. Engl. J. Med.* 2002;347:969-974.

[71] Kushner FG, Antman EM. Oral anticoagulation for atrial fibrillation after ST-elevation myocardial infarction: new evidence to guide clinical practice. *Circulation* 2005; 112:3212-3214.

In: Drugs in Cardiopulmonary Resuscitation
Editor: Theodoros Xanthos
ISBN: 978-1-61122-512-9

Chapter 7

Antithrombotic Therapy in Acute Coronary Syndromes - Antiplatelets

Konstantinos A. Ekmektzoglou
University of Athens, Medical School

Abstract

Clinical outcomes for patients with Acute Coronary Syndromes (ACS) can be optimized by revascularization coupled with aggressive medical therapy that includes, amongst others (anti-ischemic, anticoagulant, lipid-lowering) antiplatelet drugs. Antiplatelet therapy includes aspirin, clopidogrel, ticlopidine and newer $P2Y_{12}$ adenosine diphosphate (ADP) inhibitors, as well as glycoprotein (GP) IIb/IIIa inhibitors.

Since platelets play a crucial role in ACS, newer antiplatelet drugs continue to be developed with the goal of maximizing the reduction in atherothrombotic events while minimizing bleeding complications.

Introduction

Antiplatelet drugs act by inhibiting arachidonic acid (AA) production, GP IIb/IIIa receptor expression or ADP release (all crucial steps for platelet aggregation). The sites of action of all antiplatelet agents used in patients with ACS are depicted in Figure 1.

Aspirin

Aspirin (Figure 2), a non-opioid analgesic, belongs to the family of nonsteroidal anti-inflammatory drugs (NSAIDs). Aspirin (acetylsalicylic acid, ASA), along with similar agents, suppresses the signs and symptoms of inflammation and has antipyretic and analgesic effects [1].

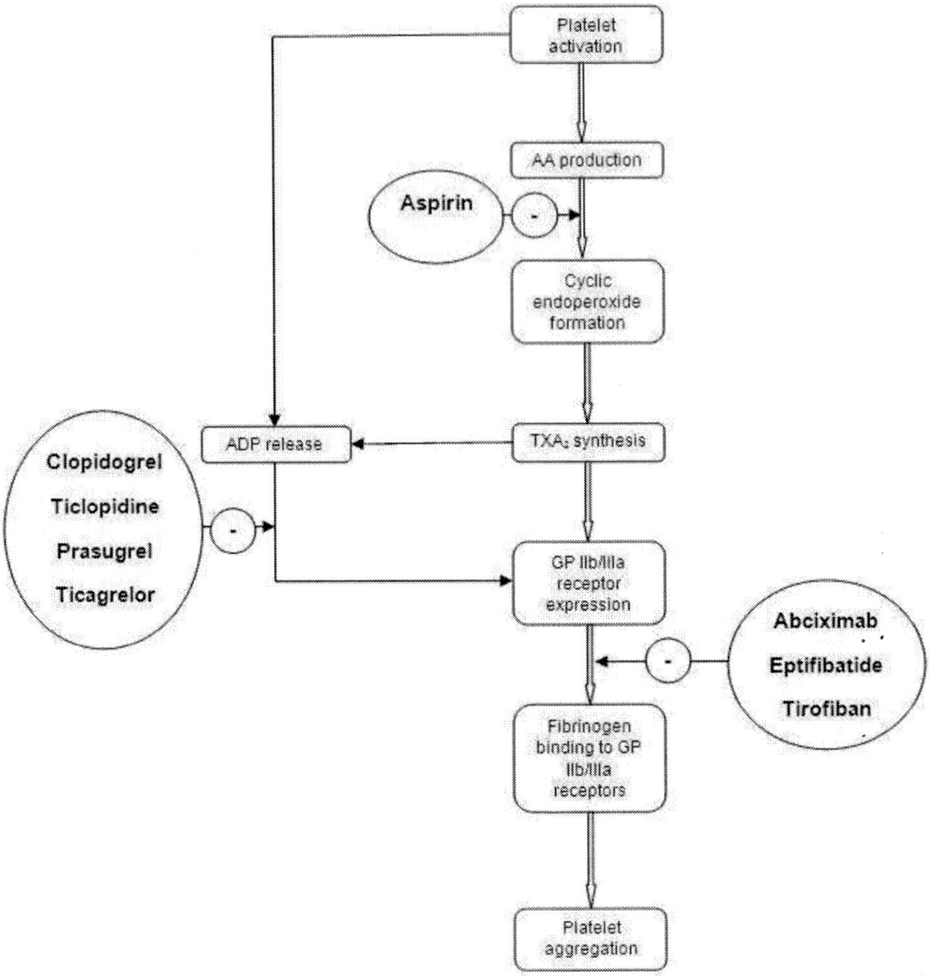

Figure 1. The sites of action of all antiplatelet agents in ACS.

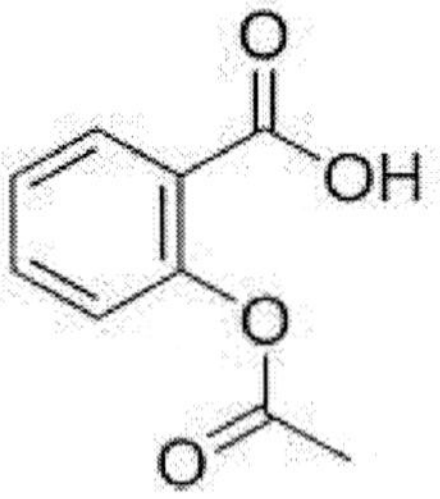

Figure 2. Structure of aspirin.

Pharmacokinetics

ASA is rapidly absorbed from the stomach and upper small intestine and hydrolyzed (serum half-life 15 minutes) to acetic acid and salicylate by esterases in tissue and blood. Its peak plasma concentration is within 1-2 hours. Salicylate is bound to albumin, but the binding is saturable so that the unbound fraction increases as total concentration increases. Although salicylate may be excreted unchanged, especially when urine become alkalized, the metabolic pathways for salicylate disposition become saturated when the total body load of salicylate exceeds 600 mg. Beyond this amount, increases in salicylate dosage increase salicylate concentration disproportionately and, therefore, salicylate elimination half-life (up to 12-16 hours [1,2].

Pharmacodynamics and Effects

ASA exerts its anti-inflammatory and antiplatelet effects by diminishing platelet aggregation, via the blockage of the synthesis of thromboxane A_2 (TXA_2) through the irreversible inhibition of the enzyme cyclooxygenase (COX) - mainly the constitutive form COX-1 by irreversibly acetylating a serine residue in its active site [1-3]. TXA_2, a prostaglandin, is an arachidonate product that causes platelets to change shape, release their granules, and aggregate. Drugs that antagonize this pathway (like ASA) interfere with platelet aggregation in vitro and prolong the bleeding time in vivo. Single low doses of ASA produce a slightly prolonged bleeding time, which doubles if administration is continued for a week. Since platelets do not synthesize new proteins, the action of ASA on platelet COX is permanent, lasting for the life of the platelet (7 to 10 days). Thus, repeated doses of ASA produce a cumulative effect on platelet function. Complete inactivation of platelet COX-1 is achieved when 160 mg of ASA is taken daily [1,2]. Salicylate, also, acts as an oxygen radical scavenger. ASA, also, interferes with the chemical mediators of the kallikrein system thus inhibiting granulocyte adherence to damaged vasculature, stabilizing lysosomes, and inhibiting the chemotaxis of polymorphonuclear leukocytes and macrophages [1]. As far as its analgesic effects, ASA is most effective in reducing pain of mild to moderate intensity through its effects on inflammation and because it, probably, inhibits pain stimuli at a subcortical site. ASA exhibits antipyretic effects as well, by reducing elevated temperature, probably mediated by both COX inhibition in the central nervous system and inhibition of interleukin-1 (IL-1), which is released from macrophages during episodes of inflammation [1].

Clinical Uses and Toxicity

ASA is used for the treatment of mild to moderate pain of varied origin but is not effective for severe visceral pain. ASA and other NSAIDs have been also combined with opioid analgesics for treatment of cancer pain. High-dose salicylates are effective for treatment of rheumatic fever, rheumatoid arthritis and other inflammatory joint conditions. ASA are indicated in patients with transient ischemic attacks (TIAs), unstable angina (UA), acute myocardial infarction (AMI) and thrombosis after coronary artery bypass grafting (CABG). Epidemiologic studies suggest that long-term use of ASA at low dosage is associated with a lower incidence of colon cancer, possibly related to its COX-inhibiting effects [1]. ASA's adverse effects are summarized in Table 1. Small doses of ASA increase serum uric acid levels, whereas higher doses ($>$ 4 g daily) decrease urate levels. ASA should not be administered in patients with hemophilia [1,2].

Table 1. Adverse effects of aspirin

Gastrointestinal system
Gastric intolerance
Gastritis
Gastric and duodenal ulcers and bleeding
Hepatotoxicity
Renal system
Nephrotoxicity
Salicylism
Vomiting
Tinnitus
Decreased hearing
Vertigo
Respiratory system
Asthma
Hyperpnea
Respiratory alkalosis
Respiratory depression
Cardiovascular system
Cardiotoxicity
Others
Rash
Metabolic acidosis
Glucose intolerance

Aspirin in ACS

According to the current American College of Cardiology/American Heart Association (ACC/AHA) guidelines, ASA should be given as early as possible in all patients with suspected ACS, as long as they have not taken any beforehand, as it has been shown, through multiple studies, to reduce mortality rates by as far as 50%. The recommended dose is between 162 and 325 mg. The ASA tablet should be chewed and, thereafter, a daily dose of 75 to 162 mg should be initiated indefinitely [3-9]. While data from clinical studies suggested that there was no difference in the rate of thrombotic events according to the ASA dose, a dose-dependent increase in bleeding was observed. This is why the ACC/AHA recommend these relative low doses [3]. The ISIS-2 Collaborative Group showed emphatically more than 20 years ago that ASA administration in more than 17,000 patients with suspected AMI reduced vascular deaths (absolute risk difference in 35-day mortality of 2.4%). The same study revealed that when ASA was combined with streptokinase, the absolute risk difference in mortality was even higher (5.2%) [10]. ASA has been also shown to reduce coronary reocclusion and recurrent ischemic events after fibrinolytic therapy [11]. The use of ASA is contraindicated in those with a hypersensitivity to salicylates, active bleeding or known platelet disorder. Clopidogrel or ticlopidine can be used instead. ASA has been said to have an anti-inflammatory effect as well, which could have a potential benefit for patients with UA and non-ST-elevation myocardial infarction (NSTEMI). However, the relative low doses used in the therapeutic protocol make this formulation most unlikely [12].

Clopidogrel

Clopidogrel, a thienopyridine derivative (Figure 3), decreases platelet activation and aggregation, increasing bleeding time and reducing blood viscosity [1].

Pharmacokinetics

Clopidogrel is rapidly absorbed after oral administration of repeated doses of 75 mg with peak plasma levels of the main circulating metabolite occurring approximately 1 hour after dosing [13]. Its absorption is unaffected by the presence of food or antacids [14]. Since clopidogrel is extensively metabolized by the hepatic cytochrome P450 enzyme to its active metabolite, its plasma concentrations are very low beyond 2 hours of dosing even after repeated oral doses. The main circulating metabolite is its carboxylic acid derivative, which, however, has no effect on platelet aggregation. Clopidogrel and its metabolite bind reversibly and to a high extent to human plasma proteins and are excreted in both urine and feces. The elimination half-life of clopidogrel is 8 hours [13]. Dose dependent inhibition of platelet aggregation can be seen 2 hours after a single oral dose of 75 mg of clopidogrel or within 5 hours after an oral loading dose of 300 mg. This inhibition reaches a steady state between day 3 and day 7 with repeated doses. Platelet aggregation and bleeding time gradually return to baseline values after treatment is discontinued, generally in about 5 days [14].

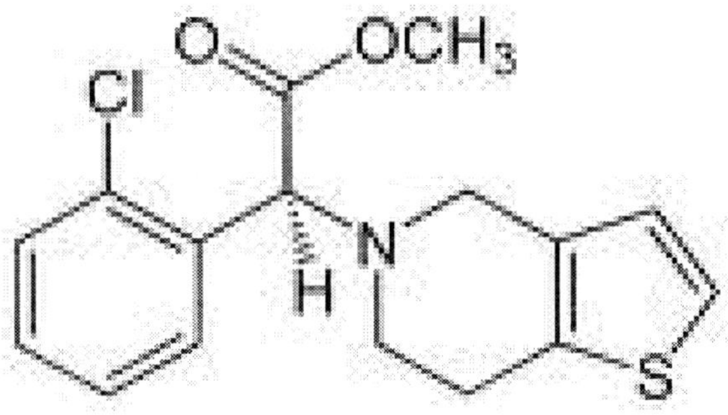

Figure 3. Strucure of Clopidogrel.

Pharmacodynamics

Clopidogrel irreversibly blocks the $P2Y_{12}$ ADP receptor (one out of the two purinergic receptors found on platelets). The $P2Y_{12}$ receptor couples to G_i and, when activated by ADP, inhibits adenylyl cyclase, resulting in lower levels of cyclic adenosine monophosphate (AMP) and, thereby, less cyclic AMP-dependent inhibition of platelet activation. Based on pharmacological studies, it appears that both receptors must be stimulated to result in platelet activation and inhibition of either receptor is sufficient to block platelet activation [15]. It permanently inhibits the $P2Y_{12}$ receptor by forming a disulfide bridge between the thiol on the drug and a free cysteine residue in the extracellular region of the receptor and thus has a prolonged effect [1,2]. Unlike ASA, clopidogrel has no effect on prostaglandin metabolism.

Effects, Toxicity and Clinical Uses

Clopidogrel treatment, through the decrease in platelet activation, is associated with a lower incidence in overall risk reduction, a decrease in all-cause mortality and all-cause strokes in patients with established cardiovascular disease. In patients after a stroke or an AMI, the incidence of subsequent events is lower after administration of clopidogrel. The benefits of clopidogrel appear to be strongest in patients with peripheral vascular disease (especially those who also had a history of myocardial infarction) and weaker in stroke patients [1,2].

Clopidogrel has few adverse effects and so is preferred over other agents (discussed below). Clopidogrel is, rarely, associated with neutropenia and thrombotic thrombocytopenic purpura (TTP). Other adverse reactions include gastrointestinal hemorrhage, abdominal pain, dyspepsia, gastritis, diarrhea, constipation and skin disorders (rash). Clopidogrel is contraindicated if there is hypersensitivity to the drug or any component of the product and active pathological bleeding.

It should be used with caution in patients at risk of increased bleeding from trauma, surgery, or other pathological conditions. If a patient is to undergo elective surgery and an antiplatelet effect is not desired, it should be discontinued 7 days prior to surgery [1,2].

Clopidogrel is indicated for the reduction of atherosclerotic events (myocardial infarction, stroke, and vascular death) in patients with atherosclerosis documented by recent stroke, recent myocardial infarction, or established peripheral arterial disease [16,17].

Use of clopidogrel to prevent thrombosis is now considered standard practice in patients undergoing placement of a coronary stent. Its specific role in patients with ACS is analyzed below.

Clopidogrel in ACS

According to the most recent guidelines, clopidogrel at a dose of 75 mg/day should be administered to patients with ST-elevation myocardial infarction (STEMI), regardless of whether they undergo reperfusion with fibrinolytic therapy or not (class I recommendation). ACC/AHA suggest that not only a loading dose of 300 mg orally should be given to all patients up to the age of 75 but that clopidogrel should be added to the long-term maintenance therapy, although no data are available from clinical trials regarding long-term clopidogrel treatment in STEMI patients [18].

Since publication of the 2004 STEMI Guidelines, 2 trials have been reported that provide data supporting the use of clopidogrel to STEMI patients. The CLARITY-TIMI 28 trial enrolled 3,491 patients, who presented within 12 hours after the onset of an STEMI and randomly assigned them to receive clopidogrel or placebo. Patients received a fibrinolytic agent, ASA, and when appropriate, heparin and were scheduled to undergo angiography 48 to

192 hours after the start of study medication. While the rates of major bleeding and intracranial hemorrhage were similar in the two groups, the addition of clopidogrel improved the patency rate of the infarct-related artery and reduced ischemic complications by as high as 36% [19].

The second trial, the COMMIT/CCS-2 study, included 45,852 patients within 24 h of suspected AMI onset who were randomly allocated clopidogrel or matching placebo in addition to 162 mg of ASA daily. Treatment was to continue until discharge or up to 4 weeks in hospital. Allocation to clopidogrel produced a highly significant 9% proportional reduction in death, reinfarction, or stroke and a significant 7% proportional reduction in any death. Regarding its safety, no significant excess risk was noted with clopidogrel, either overall, or in patients aged older than 70 years or in those given fibrinolytic therapy [20].

While on the basis of the CLARITY-TIMI 28 study, the administration of clopidogrel, at the time of initial fibrinolytic therapy, appeared to be of benefit when primary coronary intervention (PCI) was performed subsequently, it was the PCI-CLARITY study (a prospectively planned analysis of the 1,863 patients undergoing PCI after mandated angiography in the CLARITY-TIMI 28 trial), that revealed that pretreatment with clopidogrel significantly reduced the incidence of cardiovascular death, myocardial infarction, or stroke before and after PCI without a significant increase in major or minor bleeding [21].

As far as UA/NSTEMI, the CURE trial randomly assigned 12,562 patients to receive either ASA alone or ASA plus clopidogrel [22,23]. The incidence of the primary end point of cardiovascular death, myocardial infarction, or stroke was 20% lower for both low-risk and high risk patients with UA/NSTEMI who received ASA plus clopidogrel than for those who received ASA alone. Benefit was seen as early as 24 hours after the initiation of treatment and continued throughout the trial's 1-year treatment period. Although there were significantly more patients with major bleeding in the clopidogrel group than in the placebo group, there were not significantly more patients with episodes of life-threatening bleeding or hemorrhagic strokes. Taken into consideration the CREDO trial where the effectiveness of antiplatelet therapy with 300 mg of clopidogrel before PCI and 75 mg daily for one year afterward in reducing the combined risk of death, myocardial infarction, and stroke was validated, combined with the CLARITY-TIMI 28 study, the current ACC/AHA and Society for Coronary Angiography and Interventions (SCAI) guidelines clearly state that PCI should follow clopidogrel pretreatment [24-26]. After PCI, clopidogrel at a dose of 75 mg daily should be continued ideally for at least 1 year, as long as patients are not at a high risk of bleeding [3]. In patients taking clopidogrel in whom CABG is planned, the drug should be withheld for at least 5 days, and preferably for 7 days, unless the urgency for revascularization outweighs the risks of excess bleeding [4,27].

Ticlopidine

Ticlopidine (Figure 4) belongs to the family of thienopyridines (like clopidogrel) that is approved for antiplatelet therapy and has been used successfully for the secondary prevention of stroke and myocardial infarction [28,29].

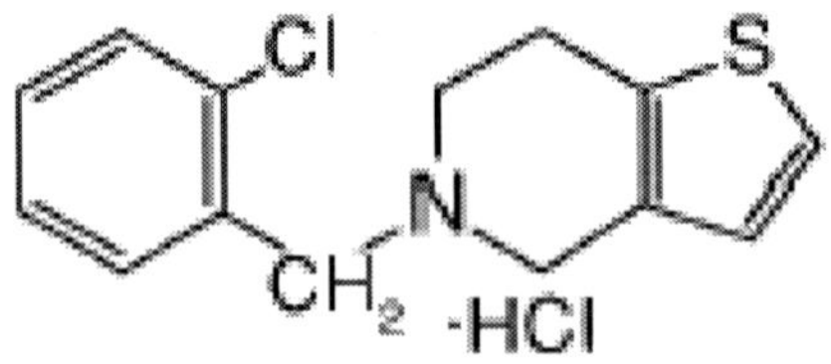

Figure 4. Strucure of Ticlopidine.

Pharmacokinetics

Absorption of ticlopidine after oral administration is rapid and improved when the drug is administered with food, but reduced by the co-administration of antacids. Ticlopidine is extensively metabolized, with little unchanged drug present in the plasma. After administration of a single dose, unchanged ticlopidine can be detected for up to 96 hours. Repeated administration of ticlopidine 250 mg twice daily results in 3- to 4-fold accumulation of the drug after 2 weeks. The terminal elimination half-life is between 20 and 50 hours. Dosage selection is not determined by the pharmacokinetic profile of the drug, but rather by determination of the effect of the drug on bleeding time [30].

Pharmacodynamics

The mechanism of action of ticlopidine is the same as that of clopidogrel discussed above [1].

Effects, Toxicity and Clinical Use

The adverse effects of ticlopidine appear more often than when clopidogrel is used (diarrhea, abdominal pain, nausea, vomiting, neutropenia and agranulocytosis, TTP), thereby limiting its usefulness; therefore, monitoring of ticlopidine therapy requires a complete blood count that includes a differential count every 2 weeks for the first 3 months of therapy [3]. This, along with the fact that clopidogrel inhibits platelets more rapidly, make the later the drug of choice.

The clearance of theophylline and phenazone (antipyrine) are reduced by ticlopidine, resulting in increased plasma drug concentrations. In contrast, the plasma concentration of cyclosporin is reduced. ASA increases the bleeding time in patients receiving ticlopidine concurrently, while corticosteroids reduce bleeding time. Furthermore, ticlopidine should be discontinued 2 weeks before surgery and dental intervention [1,2].

Ticlopidine is approved to reduce the risk of thrombotic stroke in patients who have experienced stroke precursors, and in patients who have had a completed thrombotic stroke. Since ticlopidine (as well as clopidogrel) has a mechanism of action distinct from that of ASA, combining the drugs might be expected to provide additive or even synergistic effects.

This appears to be the case, and the combination has been used in patients undergoing angioplasty and stenting for coronary artery disease (CAD), as discussed below [1,2].

Ticlopidine in ACS

A study showed that after the placement of coronary-artery stents in unselected patients, antiplatelet therapy with ASA and clopidogrel seemed to be comparably safe and effective as ASA and ticlopidine. However, noncardiac events (noncardiac death, stroke, severe peripheral vascular or hemorrhagic events) were significantly reduced with clopidogrel [31]. The CLASSICS study randomized 1,020 patients after successful stent placement and initiated them on a 28-day regimen of either (1) 300 mg clopidogrel loading dose and 325 mg/day ASA on day 1, followed by 75 mg/day clopidogrel and 325 mg/day ASA; (2) 75 mg/day clopidogrel and 325 mg/day ASA; or (3) 250 mg twice daily ticlopidine and 325 mg/day ASA, marking the superiority of the safety/tolerability spectrum of clopidogrel (plus ASA) to that of ticlopidine (plus ASA). However, overall rates of major adverse cardiac events (cardiac death, myocardial infarction, target lesion revascularization) were low and comparable between treatment groups [32]. In the therapeutic protocol of ACS, ticlopidine can be used in clopidogrel-allergic patients at a loading dose of 500 mg orally or a maintenance dose of 250 mg orally twice daily either as part of the initial medical treatment or at a loading dose of 500 mg orally during PCI for patients who did not receive initial medical treatment [3,4].

Newer $P2Y_{12}$ ADP Inhibitors

Prasugrel (Figure 5) is a new thienopyridine that is more potent than standard-dose clopidogrel in healthy subjects and patients with stable CAD. The PRINCIPLE-TIMI 44 trial was a randomized, double-blind, 2-phase crossover study of prasugrel compared with high-dose clopidogrel in patients undergoing cardiac catheterization for planned PCI, among which, not only the loading dose but, also, the maintenance dose with prasugrel resulted in a greater antiplatelet effect when compared to clopidogrel [33]. The TRITON-TIMI 38 investigators compared prasugrel with clopidogrel, by randomly assigned 13,608 patients with moderate-to-high-risk ACS with scheduled PCI to receive prasugrel (a 60 mg loading dose and a 10 mg daily maintenance dose) or clopidogrel (a 300 mg loading dose and a 75 mg daily maintenance dose) for 6 to 15 months. Taking death from cardiovascular causes, nonfatal myocardial infarction, or nonfatal stroke as the primary efficacy end point and major bleeding as the key safety end point, the study showed that, although overall mortality did not differ significantly between treatment groups, prasugrel therapy was associated with significantly reduced rates of ischemic events, including stent thrombosis, but with an increased risk of major bleeding [34].

Ticagrelor (Figure 6), an oral, reversible, direct-acting inhibitor of the ADP receptor $P2Y_{12}$, has a more rapid onset and more pronounced platelet inhibition than clopidogrel. The PLATO study showed that in patients who have an ACS with or without ST-segment elevation, treatment with ticagrelor as compared with clopidogrel significantly reduced the rate of death from major cardiovascular causes without an increase in the rate of overall major bleeding but with an increase in the rate of non-procedure-related bleeding [35].

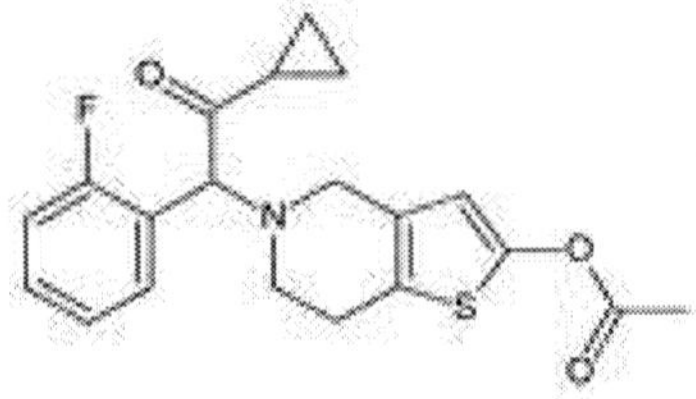

Figure 5. Structure of Prasugrel.

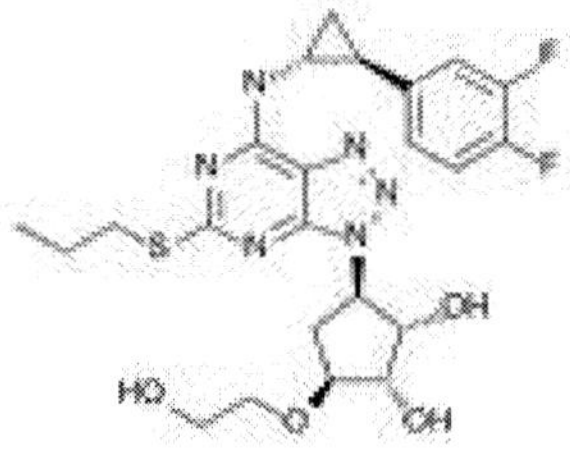

Figure 6. Structure of Ticagrelor.

Glycoprotein Iib/Iiia Inhibitors

GP IIb/IIIa is a platelet-surface integrin. This dimeric GP is a receptor for fibrinogen and von Willebrand factor which anchor platelets to foreign surfaces and to each other, thereby mediating aggregation. When platelets are activated, the GP IIb/IIIa receptor that is abundant on the platelet surface undergoes a change in conformation that increases its affinity for binding to fibrinogen and other ligands. The binding of molecules of fibrinogen to receptors on different platelets results in platelet aggregation. The platelet GP IIb/IIIa inhibitors act by occupying the receptors, preventing fibrinogen from binding and, thereby, preventing platelet aggregation [36]. Investigators have shown that 80% occupancy of the receptor population and inhibition of platelet aggregation by at least 80% results in potent antithrombotic effects [37]. However, each GP IIb/IIIa inhibitor has different pharmacokinetic and pharmacodynamic properties [38].Three agents are currently available for use: abciximab, eptifibatide, and tirofiban (Figures 7,8). Abciximab is a Fab fragment of a humanized murine antibody that has a short plasma half-life but strong affinity for the receptor, resulting in some receptor occupancy that persists in part for weeks. It also binds to the vitronectin receptor on platelets, vascular endothelial cells, and smooth muscle cells. Platelet aggregation gradually returns to normal 24 to 48 hours after discontinuation of the drug. The unbound antibody is cleared from the circulation with a half-life of about 30 minutes [2]. The major side effect of abciximab is bleeding, and the contraindications (as with all the GP IIb/IIIa inhibitors) to its use are shown in Table 2. The frequency of major hemorrhage in clinical trials varies from 1% to 10%, depending on the intensity of anticoagulation with heparin. Thrombocytopenia is seen in about 2% of patients and may be due to development of neo-epitopes induced by bound antibody. Since the duration of action is long, if major bleeding or emergency surgery occurs, platelet transfusions can reverse the aggregation defect. Re-administration of antibody has been performed in a small number of patients without evidence of decreased efficacy or allergic reactions. The expense of the antibody limits its use [2].

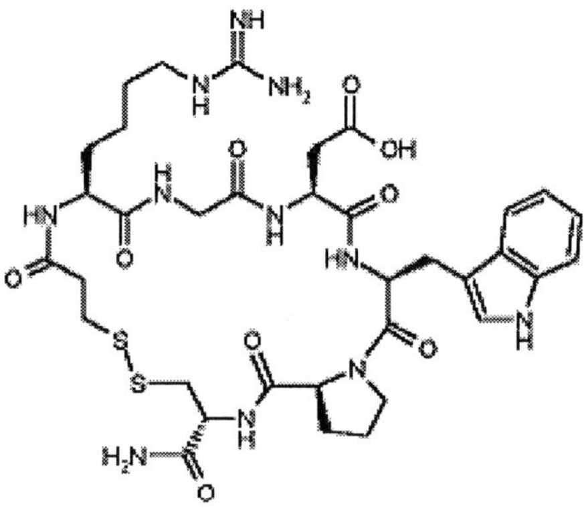

Figure 7. Structure of eptifibatide.

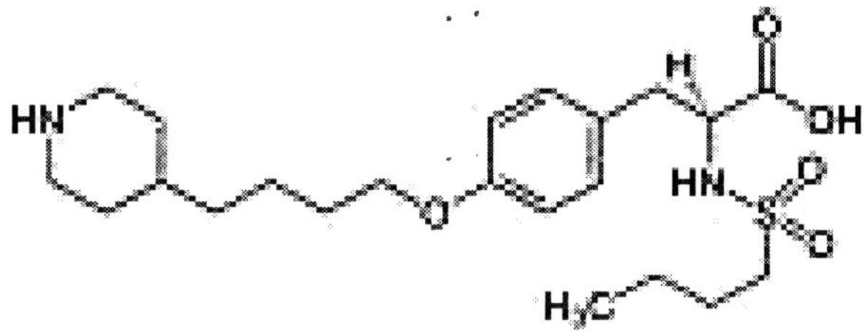

Figure 8. Strucure of tirofiban.

Abciximab is indicated only if angiography will not be appreciably delayed and PCI is likely to be performed.

Table 2. Contraindications to abciximab use

Active bleeding or hemorrhagic disorder
Serious gastrointestinal bleeding within 3 months
Previous cerebrovascular accident or active intracranial process
Aortic dissection
Surgery within 10 days, including organ biopsy, puncture of noncompressible vessels, cardiopulmonary resuscitation
Trauma
History of hypertension (diastolic pressure >110 mm Hg)
Acute pericarditis

Eptifibatide is a cyclic heptapeptide that contains the KGD (Lys-Gly-Asp) sequence and is an inhibitor of the fibrinogen binding site. Eptifibatide blocks platelet aggregation *in vitro* after intravenous infusion into patients. Although the drug has not been compared directly to abciximab, it appears that its benefit is somewhat less than that obtained with the antibody, perhaps because eptifibatide does not react with the vitronectin receptor. The duration of action of the drug is relatively short and platelet aggregation is restored within 6 to 12 hours after cessation of infusion. Eptifibatide generally is administered in conjunction with ASA and heparin. Tirofiban is a nonpeptide mimetic of the RGD (Arg-Gly-Asp) sequence of fibrinogen that appears to have a similar mechanism of action as eptifibatide. Tirofiban has a short duration of action. It is used in conjunction with heparin [2].

Receptor occupancy with these 2 synthetic antagonists is, in general, in equilibrium with plasma levels. They have half-lives of 2 to 3 hours and are highly specific for the GP IIb/IIIa receptor. Platelet aggregation returns to normal in 4 to 8 hours after their discontinuation [3]. Eptifibatide or tirofiban administerd intravanously are the medications of choice. The main risk when using a GP IIb/IIIa inhibitor is the increased bleeding rate. Therefore, patients should be monitored closely for hemorrhage, most often, at the site of vascular intervention, and complete blood cell counts should be determined regularly [1]. Lamifiban, is an experimental drug under evaluation [39,40].

GP IIB/IIIa Iinhibitors in ACS

Although GP IIb/IIIa inhibitors have been combined with fibrinolytic agents (usually at half the dose) in an effort to improve the likelihood of achieving Thrombolysis in Myocardial Infarction (TIMI) 3 flow (i.e. complete recanalization and unimpeded perfusion of distal vasculature in the coronary vessel), the current American College of Cardiology/American Heart (ACA/AHA) guidelines do not recommend combination pharmacological reperfusion with GP IIb/IIIa inhibitors and a fibrinolytic agent in STEMI patients. This is because despite that phase 2 angiographic studies, like the TIMI-14 and SPEEDl, have demonstrated higher TIMI 3 flow rates at 60 to 90 minutes [41,42], various other published studies revealed no benefit in mortality rates. The GUSTO V investigators did a randomised, open-label trial to compare the effect of reteplase (a fibrilnolytic agent) alone with reteplase plus abciximab in patients with AMI (16,588 patients in the first 6 hours of evolving STEMI). There were fewer deaths or non-fatal reinfarctions with the combination than with fibrinolytic agent alone, and there was less need for urgent revascularisation and fewer major non-fatal ischaemic complications of AMI. On the other hand, there were more non-intracranial bleeding complications in the combination group. The rates of intracranial haemorrhage and non-fatal disabling stroke were similar [43]. Likewise, the ASSENT-3 trial randomly assigned more than 6,000 patients with STEMI to i) fulldose tenecteplase with unfractioned heparin (UFH), ii) full-dose tenecteplase with enoxaparin, or iii) half-dose tenecteplase plus abciximab plus weight-adjusted, reduced-dose UFH. The study showed that the combination of abciximab and half-dose tenecteplase was not associated with lower mortality rates than was full-dose tenecteplase; however, this combination was associated with substantially lower rates of in-hospital infarction and refractory ischemia. Notably, the rate of major bleeding was substantially higher in the abciximab group [44].

A few words regarding the role of GP IIb/IIIa inhibitors in facilitated PCI; facilitated PCI refers to a strategy of planned immediate PCI after administration of an initial pharmacological regimen intended to improve coronary patency before the procedure (in our case, the combination of a GP IIb/IIIa inhibitor with a 50% reduced-dose of a fibrinolytic agent). Facilitated PCI bares great expectations: earlier time to reperfusion, smaller infarct size, improved patient stability, higher TIMI flow rates, and improved survival rates. Despite the potential advantages of this strategy, clinical trials of facilitated PCI involving the use of a GP IIb/IIIa inhibitor have not shown any benefit in improving outcomes. The largest of these, the ASSENT-4 PCI trial, was terminated prematurely because of a higher in-hospital mortality rate in the facilitated PCI group [45]. Keeley *et al.*, in a quantitative review of 17 trials comparing facilitated PCI with primary PCI, out of which most involved administration of GP IIb/IIIa inhibitors alone and only 2 combination of a fibrinolytic agent plus a GP IIb/IIIa inhibitor, reported no differences in efficacy or safety when facilitated PCI with a GP IIb/IIIa inhibitor was compared with primary PCI [46]. Therefore, facilitated PCI using a GP IIb/IIIa inhibitor with a 50% reduced-dose of a fibrinolytic agent might be considered as a reperfusion strategy when all of the following are present: a) patients are at high risk, b) PCI is not immediately available within 90 minutes, and c) bleeding risk is low (younger age, absence of poorly controlled hypertension, normal body weight) [3].

As far as patients with UA/NSTEMI are concerned, the 2007 ACC/AHA guidelines recommend that, for patients who will be treated initially according to an invasive strategy, an intravenous GP IIb/IIIa inhibitor should be added to ASA and anticoagulant therapy before diagnostic angiography is performed (class I recommendation). Boersma *et al.* in a meta-analysis of GP IIb/IIIa antagonists in the setting of large, randomized, placebo-controlled trials suggested that GP IIb/IIIa inhibitors are of substantial benefit in patients with UA/NSTEMI who undergo PCI, are of modest benefit in patients who are not routinely scheduled to undergo revascularization (but who may do so), and are of questionable benefit in patients who do not undergo revascularization [3,47].

GP IIb/IIIa administration has shown even greater benefit for patients who are at higher risk of complications. In the CAPTURE trial, the rates of death or nonfatal MI, when cardiac troponin was elevated, were 23.9% with placebo versus 9.5% with abciximab. The same result was validated by the PRISM Study investigators as far as tirofiban was concerned [48,49]. GP IIb/IIIa receptor blockade with tirofiban, as analysed in the PRISM-PLUS trial, has been shown to improves outcomes in diabetic patients presenting with UA/NSTEMI as well as in patients with recurrent angina or in those with a TIMI risk score >4 [50-52]. Reduction of recurrent ischemia with abciximab during continuous electrocardiography (ECG)-ischemia monitoring in patients with UA refractory to standard treatment has also been validated [53]. Eptifibatide, studied in the PURSUIT trial, gave promising results to NSTEMI patients with prior ASA use [54]. Abciximab in patients with ACS undergoing PCI after clopidogrel pretreatment, as evaluated in the ISAR-REACT 2 randomized trial, showed also a distinct benefit [55]. Very recently, the EARLY ACS trial, that involved 9,492 patients and randomly assigned them either to early eptifibatide or to provisional eptifabatide administration after angiography, showed that the former exerted no statistically significant benefit in reducing the composite end point of adverse cardiovascular events but were associated with a statistically significant increase in bleeding rates, raising the question of the optimal timing of GP IIa/IIIb initiation in the ACS therapeutic protocol [56].

Conclusion

The ACC/AHA guidelines recommend tailoring the specific antithrombotic agents to the treatment strategy selected. Antiplatelet therapy includes ASA, clopidogrel, ticlopidine and newer $P2Y_{12}$ ADP inhibitors, as well as GP IIb/IIIa inhibitors. Since platelets play a crucial role in ACS, newer antiplatelet drugs continue to be developed with the goal of maximizing the reduction in atherothrombotic events while minimizing bleeding complications.

References

[1] Furst DE, Ulrich RW. Non Steroidal Anti-inflammatory Drugs, Disease-Modifying Antirheumatic Drugs, Nonopioid analgesics and Drugs Used in Gout. In: *Basic and clinical pharmacology*, Katzung BG ed. 10th edition, Boston: 2006, 573-598.

[2] Majerus PW, Tollefsen DM. Blood Coagulation and Anticoagulant, Thrombolytic, and Antiplatelet Drugs. In: *Goodman and Gilman's The Pharmacological Basis of Therapeutics*, Brunton LL, Lazo JS, Parker KL, eds. *11th edition*, New York: McGraw-Hill, *2006, 1467-1488.*

[3] Anderson JL, Adams CD, Antman EM, Bridges CR, Califf RM, Casey DE Jr, Chavey WE 2nd, Fesmire FM, Hochman JS, Levin TN, Lincoff AM, Peterson ED, Theroux P, Wenger NK, Wright RS, Smith SC Jr, Jacobs AK, Adams CD, Anderson JL, Antman EM, Halperin JL, Hunt SA, Krumholz HM, Kushner FG, Lytle BW, Nishimura R, Ornato JP, Page RL, Riegel B; American College of Cardiology; American Heart Association Task Force on Practice Guidelines (Writing Committee to Revise the 2002 Guidelines for the Management of Patients With Unstable Angina/Non-ST-Elevation Myocardial Infarction); American College of Emergency Physicians; Society for Cardiovascular Angiography and Interventions; Society of Thoracic Surgeons; American Association of Cardiovascular and Pulmonary Rehabilitation; Society for Academic Emergency Medicine. ACC/AHA 2007 guidelines for the management of patients with unstable angina/non-ST-Elevation myocardial infarction: a report of the American College of Cardiology/American Heart Association Task Force on Practice Guidelines (Writing Committee to Revise the 2002 Guidelines for the Management of Patients With Unstable Angina/Non-ST-Elevation Myocardial Infarction) developed in collaboration with the American College of Emergency Physicians, the Society for Cardiovascular Angiography and Interventions, and the Society of Thoracic Surgeons endorsed by the American Association of Cardiovascular and Pulmonary Rehabilitation and the Society for Academic Emergency Medicine. *J. Am. Coll. Cardiol.* 2007;50:e1-e157.

[4] Antman EM, Anbe DT, Armstrong PW, Bates ER, Green LA, Hand M, Hochman JS, Krumholz HM, Kushner FG, Lamas GA, Mullany CJ, Ornato JP, Pearle DL, Sloan MA, Smith SC Jr; American College of Cardiology; American Heart Association; Canadian Cardiovascular Society. ACC/AHA guidelines for the management of patients with ST-elevation myocardial infarction--executive summary. A report of the American College of Cardiology/American Heart Association Task Force on Practice Guidelines (Writing Committee to revise the 1999 guidelines for the management of patients with acute myocardial infarction). *J. Am. Coll. Cardiol.* 2004;44:671-719.

[5] Antithrombotic Trialists' Collaboration. Collaborative meta-analysis of randomised trials of antiplatelet therapy for prevention of death, myocardial infarction, and stroke in high risk patients. *BMJ* 2002;324:71-86.

[6] Lewis HD Jr, Davis JW, Archibald DG, Steinke WE, Smitherman TC, Doherty JE 3rd, Schnaper HW, LeWinter MM, Linares E, Pouget JM, Sabharwal SC, Chesler E, DeMots H. Protective effects of aspirin against acute myocardial infarction and death in men with unstable angina. Results of a Veterans Administration Cooperative Study. *N. Engl. J. Med.* 1983;309:396-403.

[7] Cairns JA, Gent M, Singer J, Finnie KJ, Froggatt GM, Holder DA, Jablonsky G, Kostuk WJ, Melendez LJ, Myers MG, et al. Aspirin, sulfinpyrazone, or both in unstable angina. Results of a Canadian multicenter trial. *N. Engl. J. Med.* 1985;313:1369-1375.

[8] Risk of myocardial infarction and death during treatment with low dose aspirin and intravenous heparin in men with unstable coronary artery disease. The RISC Group. *Lancet* 1990;336:827-830.

[9] Although enteric coated aspirin for initial dosing has also been studied, aspirin ahould be chewed so as to be more rapidly absorbed. Sagar KA, Smyth MR. A comparative bioavailability study of different aspirin formulations using on-line multidimensional chromatography. *J. Pharm. Biomed. Anal.* 1999;21:383-392.

[10] Randomised trial of intravenous streptokinase, oral aspirin, both, or neither among 17,187 cases of suspected acute myocardial infarction: ISIS-2. ISIS-2 (Second International Study of Infarct Survival) Collaborative Group. *Lancet* 1988;2:349-360.

[11] Roux S, Christeller S, Lüdin E. Effects of aspirin on coronary reocclusion and recurrent ischemia after thrombolysis: a meta-analysis. *J. Am. Coll. Cardiol.* 1992;19:671-677.

[12] Ridker PM, Cushman M, Stampfer MJ, Tracy RP, Hennekens CH. Inflammation, aspirin, and the risk of cardiovascular disease in apparently healthy men. *N. Engl. J. Med.* 1997;336:973-979.

[13] Guillin MC, Bonnet G, Sissmann J, Necciari J, Dickinson JP. Pharmacodynamics and pharmacokinetics of the novel antiplatelet agent, clopidogrel, in the young and the elderly with and without symptomatic atherosclerosis. *Eur. Heart J.* 1996;17:161.

[14] McEwen J, Strauch G, Perles P, Pritchard G, Moreland TE, Necciari J, Dickinson JP. Clopidogrel bioavailability: absence of influence of food or antacids. *Semin. Thromb. Hemost.* 1999;25:47-50.

[15] Jin J, Kunapuli SP. Coactivation of two different G protein-coupled receptors is essential for ADP-induced platelet aggregation. *Proc. Natl. Acad. Sci. U S A* 1998;95:8070-8074.

[16] CAPRIE Steering Committee. A randomised, blinded, trial of clopidogrel versus aspirin in patients at risk of ischaemic events (CAPRIE). *Lancet* 1996;348:1329-1339.

[17] Easton JD. Clinical aspects of the use of Clopidogrel, a new antiplatelet agent. *Semin. Thromb. Haemost.* 1999;25:69-75.

[18] Antman EM, Hand M, Armstrong PW, Bates ER, Green LA, Halasyamani LK, Hochman JS, Krumholz HM, Lamas GA, Mullany CJ, Pearle DL, Sloan MA, Smith SC Jr; 2004 Writing Committee Members, Anbe DT, Kushner FG, Ornato JP, Jacobs AK, Adams CD, Anderson JL, Buller CE, Creager MA, Ettinger SM, Halperin JL, Hunt SA, Lytle BW, Nishimura R, Page RL, Riegel B, Tarkington LG, Yancy CW. 2007 Focused Update of the ACC/AHA 2004 Guidelines for the Management of Patients With ST-Elevation Myocardial Infarction: a report of the American College of Cardiology/American Heart Association Task Force on Practice Guidelines: developed in collaboration With the Canadian Cardiovascular Society endorsed by the American Academy of Family Physicians: 2007 Writing Group to Review New Evidence and

Update the ACC/AHA 2004 Guidelines for the Management of Patients With ST-Elevation Myocardial Infarction, Writing on Behalf of the 2004 Writing Committee. *Circulation* 2008;117:296-329.

[19] Sabatine MS, Cannon CP, Gibson CM, López-Sendón JL, Montalescot G, Theroux P, Claeys MJ, Cools F, Hill KA, Skene AM, McCabe CH, Braunwald E; CLARITY-TIMI 28 Investigators. Addition of clopidogrel to aspirin and fibrinolytic therapy for myocardial infarction with ST-segment elevation. *N. Engl. J. Med.* 2005;352:1179-1189.

[20] Chen ZM, Jiang LX, Chen YP, Xie JX, Pan HC, Peto R, Collins R, Liu LS; COMMIT (ClOpidogrel and Metoprolol in Myocardial Infarction Trial) collaborative group. Addition of clopidogrel to aspirin in 45,852 patients with acute myocardial infarction: randomised placebo-controlled trial. *Lancet* 2005;366:1607-1621.

[21] Sabatine MS, Cannon CP, Gibson CM, López-Sendón JL, Montalescot G, Theroux P, Lewis BS, Murphy SA, McCabe CH, Braunwald E; Clopidogrel as Adjunctive Reperfusion Therapy (CLARITY)-Thrombolysis in Myocardial Infarction (TIMI) 28 Investigators. Effect of clopidogrel pretreatment before percutaneous coronary intervention in patients with ST-elevation myocardial infarction treated with fibrinolytics: the PCI-CLARITY study. *JAMA* 2005;294:1224-1232.

[22] Mehta SR, Yusuf S; Clopidogrel in Unstable angina to prevent Recurrent Events (CURE) Study Investigators. The Clopidogrel in Unstable angina to prevent Recurrent Events (CURE) trial programme; rationale, design and baseline characteristics including a meta-analysis of the effects of thienopyridines in vascular disease. *Eur. Heart J.* 2000;21:2033-2041.

[23] Yusuf S, Zhao F, Mehta SR, Chrolavicius S, Tognoni G, Fox KK; Clopidogrel in Unstable Angina to Prevent Recurrent Events Trial Investigators. Effects of clopidogrel in addition to aspirin in patients with acute coronary syndromes without ST-segment elevation. *N. Engl. J. Med.* 2001;345:494-502.

[24] Beinart SC, Kolm P, Veledar E, Zhang Z, Mahoney EM, Bouin O, Gabriel S, Jackson J, Chen R, Caro J, Steinhubl S, Topol E, Weintraub WS. Long-term cost effectiveness of early and sustained dual oral antiplatelet therapy with clopidogrel given for up to one year after percutaneous coronary intervention results: from the Clopidogrel for the Reduction of Events During Observation (CREDO) trial. *J. Am. Coll. Cardiol.* 2005;46:761-769.

[25] Smith SC Jr, Feldman TE, Hirshfeld JW Jr, Jacobs AK, Kern MJ, King SB 3rd, Morrison DA, O'Neill WW, Schaff HV, Whitlow PL, Williams DO, Antman EM, Adams CD, Anderson JL, Faxon DP, Fuster V, Halperin JL, Hiratzka LF, Hunt SA, Nishimura R, Ornato JP, Page RL, Riegel B; American College of Cardiology/American Heart Association Task Force on Practice Guidelines; American College of Cardiology/American Heart Association/Society for Cardiovascular Angiography and Interventions Writting Committee to Update the 2001 Guidelines for Percutaneous Coronary Intervention. ACC/AHA/SCAI 2005 Guideline Update for Percutaneous Coronary Intervention--summary article: a report of the American College of Cardiology/American Heart Association Task Force on Practice Guidelines (ACC/AHA/SCAI Writing Committee to Update the 2001 Guidelines for Percutaneous Coronary Intervention). *Circulation* 2006;113:156-175.

[26] King SB 3rd, Smith SC Jr, Hirshfeld JW Jr, Jacobs AK, Morrison DA, Williams DO; 2005 WRITING COMMITTEE MEMBERS, Feldman TE, Kern MJ, O'Neill WW, Schaff HV, Whitlow PL, Adams CD, Anderson JL, Buller CE, Creager MA, Ettinger SM, Halperin JL, Hunt SA, Krumholz HM, Kushner FG, Lytle BW, Nishimura R, Page RL, Riegel B, Tarkington LG, Yancy CW. 2007 Focused Update of the ACC/AHA/SCAI 2005 Guideline Update for Percutaneous Coronary Intervention: a report of the American College of Cardiology/American Heart Association Task Force on Practice Guidelines: 2007 Writing Group to Review New Evidence and Update the ACC/AHA/SCAI 2005 Guideline Update for Percutaneous Coronary Intervention, Writing on Behalf of the 2005 Writing Committee. *Circulation* 2008;117:261-295.

[27] Eagle KA, Guyton RA, Davidoff R, Edwards FH, Ewy GA, Gardner TJ, Hart JC, Herrmann HC, Hillis LD, Hutter AM Jr, Lytle BW, Marlow RA, Nugent WC, Orszulak TA, Antman EM, Smith SC Jr, Alpert JS, Anderson JL, Faxon DP, Fuster V, Gibbons RJ, Gregoratos G, Halperin JL, Hiratzka LF, Hunt SA, Jacobs AK, Ornato JP; American College of Cardiology; American Heart Association Task Force on Practice Guidelines; American Society for Thoracic Surgery and the Society of Thoracic Surgeons. ACC/AHA 2004 guideline update for coronary artery bypass graft surgery: summary article: a report of the American College of Cardiology/American Heart Association Task Force on Practice Guidelines (Committee to Update the 1999 Guidelines for Coronary Artery Bypass Graft Surgery). *Circulation* 2004;110:1168-1176.

[28] Schror K. The basic pharmacology of ticlopidine and clopidogrel. *Platelets* 1993;4:252-261.

[29] Balsano F, Rizzon P, Violi F, Scrutinio D, Cimminiello C, Aguglia F, Pasotti C, Rudelli G. Antiplatelet treatment with ticlopidine in unstable angina. A controlled multicenter clinical trial. The Studio della Ticlopidina nell'Angina Instabile Group. *Circulation* 1990;82:17-26.

[30] Desager JP. Clinical pharmacokinetics of ticlopidine. *Clin. Pharmacokinet* 1994;26:347-355.

[31] Müller C, Büttner HJ, Petersen J, Roskamm H. A randomized comparison of clopidogrel and aspirin versus ticlopidine and aspirin after the placement of coronary-artery stents. *Circulation* 2000;101:590-593.

[32] Bertrand ME, Rupprecht HJ, Urban P, Gershlick AH; CLASSICS Investigators. Double-blind study of the safety of clopidogrel with and without a loading dose in combination with aspirin compared with ticlopidine in combination with aspirin after coronary stenting : the clopidogrel aspirin stent international cooperative study (CLASSICS). *Circulation* 2000;102:624-629.

[33] Wiviott SD, Trenk D, Frelinger AL, O'Donoghue M, Neumann FJ, Michelson AD, Angiolillo DJ, Hod H, Montalescot G, Miller DL, Jakubowski JA, Cairns R, Murphy SA, McCabe CH, Antman EM, Braunwald E; PRINCIPLE-TIMI 44 Investigators. Prasugrel compared with high loading- and maintenance-dose clopidogrel in patients with planned percutaneous coronary intervention: the Prasugrel in Comparison to Clopidogrel for Inhibition of Platelet Activation and Aggregation-Thrombolysis in Myocardial Infarction 44 trial. *Circulation* 2007;116:2923-2932.

[34] Wiviott SD, Braunwald E, McCabe CH, Montalescot G, Ruzyllo W, Gottlieb S, Neumann FJ, Ardissino D, De Servi S, Murphy SA, Riesmeyer J, Weerakkody G,

Gibson CM, Antman EM; TRITON-TIMI 38 Investigators. Prasugrel versus clopidogrel in patients with acute coronary syndromes. *N. Engl. J. Med.* 2007;357:2001-2015.

[35] Wallentin L, Becker RC, Budaj A, Cannon CP, Emanuelsson H, Held C, Horrow J, Husted S, James S, Katus H, Mahaffey KW, Scirica BM, Skene A, Steg PG, Storey RF, Harrington RA; PLATO Investigators, Freij A, Thorsén M. Ticagrelor versus clopidogrel in patients with acute coronary syndromes. *N. Engl. J. Med.* 2009;361:1045-1057.

[36] Lefkovits J, Plow EF, Topol EJ. Platelet glycoprotein IIb/IIIa receptors in cardiovascular medicine. *N. Engl. J. Med.* 1995;332:1553-1559.

[37] Coller BS. Monitoring platelet GP IIb/IIIa antagonist therapy. *Circulation* 1998;97:5-9.

[38] Topol EJ, Byzova TV, Plow EF. Platelet GPIIb-IIIa blockers. *Lancet* 1999;353:227-231.

[39] PARAGON investigators in ACS patients. International, randomized, controlled trial of lamifiban (a platelet glycoprotein IIb/IIIa inhibitor), heparin, or both in unstable angina. Platelet IIb/IIIa Antagonism for the Reduction of Acute coronary syndrome events in a Global Organization Network. *Circulation* 1998;97:2386-2395.

[40] The Platelet IIb/IIIa Antagonist for the Reduction of Acute Coronary Syndrome Events in a Global Organization Network (PARAGON)-B Investigators. Randomized, placebo-controlled trial of titrated intravenous lamifiban for acute coronary syndromes. *Circulation* 2002;105:316-321.

[41] Antman EM, Giugliano RP, Gibson CM, et al, for the TIMI 14 Investigators. Abciximab facilitates the rate and extent of thrombolysis: results of the thrombolysis in myocardial infarction (TIMI) 14 trial. *Circulation* 1999;99:2720-2732.

[42] Strategies for Patency Enhancement in the Emergency Department (SPEED) Group. Trial of abciximab with and without low-dose reteplase for acute myocardial infarction. *Circulation* 2000;101:2788-2794.

[43] Topol EJ; GUSTO V Investigators. Reperfusion therapy for acute myocardial infarction with fibrinolytic therapy or combination reduced fibrinolytic therapy and platelet glycoprotein IIb/IIIa inhibition: the GUSTO V randomised trial. *Lancet* 2001;357:1905-1914.

[44] Assessment of the Safety and Efficacy of a New Thrombolytic Regimen (ASSENT)-3 Investigators. Efficacy and safety of tenecteplase in combination with enoxaparin, abciximab, or unfractionated heparin: the ASSENT-3 randomised trial in acute myocardial infarction. *Lancet* 2001;358:605-613.

[45] Primary versus tenecteplase-facilitated percutaneous coronary intervention in patients with ST-segment elevation acute myocardial infarction (ASSENT-4 PCI): randomised trial. *Lancet* 2006;367:569-578.

[46] Keeley EC, Boura JA, Grines CL. Comparison of primary and facilitated percutaneous coronary interventions for ST-elevation myocardial infarction: quantitative review of randomised trials. *Lancet* 2006;367:579-588.

[47] Boersma E, Harrington RA, Moliterno DJ, et al. Platelet glycoprotein IIb/IIIa inhibitors in acute coronary syndromes: a meta-analysis of all major randomised clinical trials. *Lancet* 2002;359:189-198.

[48] Hamm CW, Heeschen C, Goldmann B, et al. Benefit of abciximab in patients with refractory unstable angina in relation to serum troponin T levels: c7E3 Fab Antiplatelet

Therapy in Unstable Refractory Angina (CAPTURE) Study Investigators. *N. Engl. J. Med.* 1999;340:1623-1629.

[49] Heeschen C, Hamm CW, Goldmann B, Deu A, Langenbrink L,White HD. Troponin concentrations for stratification of patients with acute coronary syndromes in relation to therapeutic efficacy of tirofiban. PRISM Study Investigators. Platelet Receptor Inhibition in Ischemic Syndrome Management. *Lancet* 1999;354:1757-1762.

[50] Inhibition of the platelet glycoprotein IIb/IIIa receptor with tirofiban in unstable angina and non-Q-wave myocardial infarction. Platelet Receptor Inhibition in Ischemic Syndrome Management in Patients Limited by Unstable Signs and Symptoms (PRISM-PLUS) Study Investigators. *N. Engl. J. Med.* 1998;338:1488-1497.

[51] Theroux P, Alexander J Jr, Pharand C, et al. Glycoprotein IIb/IIIa receptor blockade improves outcomes in diabetic patients presenting with unstable angina/non-ST-elevation myocardial infarction: results from the Platelet Receptor Inhibition in Ischemic Syndrome Management in Patients Limited by Unstable Signs and Symptoms (PRISM-PLUS) study. *Circulation* 2000;102:2466-2472.

[52] Morrow DA, Antman EM, Snapinn SM, McCabe CH, Theroux P, Braunwald E. An integrated clinical approach to predicting the benefit of tirofiban in non-ST elevation acute coronary syndromes: application of the TIMI Risk Score for UA/NSTEMI in PRISM-PLUS. *Eur. Heart J.* 2002;23:223-229.

[53] Klootwijk P, Meij S, Melkert R, Lenderink T, Simoons ML. Reduction of recurrent ischemia with abciximab during continuous ECG-ischemia monitoring in patients with unstable angina refractory to standard treatment (CAPTURE). *Circulation* 1998;98:1358-1364.

[54] Alexander JH, Harrington RA, Tuttle RH, et al. PURSUIT Investigators. Prior aspirin use predicts worse outcomes in patients with non-ST- elevation acute coronary syndromes. *Am. J. Cardiol.* 1999;83:1147-1151.

[55] Kastrati A, Mehilli J, Neumann FJ, et al. Intracoronary Stenting and Antithrombotic Regimen: Rapid Early Action for Coronary Treatment 2 (ISAR-REACT 2) Trial Investigators. Abciximab in patients with acute coronary syndromes undergoing percutaneous coronary intervention after clopidogrel pretreatment: the ISAR-REACT 2 randomized trial. *JAMA* 2006;295:1531-1538.

[56] Giugliano RP, White JA, Bode C, et al.; EARLY ACS Investigators. Early versus delayed, provisional eptifibatide in acute coronary syndromes. *N. Engl. J. Med.* 2009;360:2176-2190.

In: Drugs in Cardiopulmonary Resuscitation
Editors:, Theodoros Xanthos, pp.
ISBN: 978-1-61122-512-9

Chapter 8

Beta-Blockade in the Treatment of Periarrest Arrhythmias and Cardiac Arrest

Eleni Bassiakou
University of Athens, Medical School

Abstract

This chapter discusses the functions of β-adrenoreceptors in the intact and failing human heart, as well as the connection that seems to be between β-adrenergic stimulation and arrhythmiogenesis. Chronic beta-blockers usage has expanded over the last decades and indications now include hypertension, cardio-protection after myocardial infarction, angina, congestive heart failure, and rate control for arrhythmias. Beta-blockade is also independently associated with improved survival in patients with ventricular fibrillation (VF) or symptomatic ventricular tachycardia (VT). The anti-ischemic and anti-anginal actions of beta-blockers are discussed, as well as the beneficial outcomes of β-adrenergic blockade in experimental models and in human studies in the cardiopulmonary resuscitation (CPR) field.

Introduction

Beta-blockers are a heterogeneous group of aryloxypropanolamines that competitively bind to one or more β-subtype receptors, resulting in antagonism of β-adrenergic stimulation. Some of the pharmacologic actions possessed by β-blockers include blockade of β_1- and β_2-adrenergic receptors, intrinsic sympathomimetic activity, inverse agonism, guanine-nucleotide modulatable-binding, and ancillary properties such as α_1-receptor antagonism and vasodilatation [1,2].

β-Blockers inhibit both the short-term pharmacologic effects of endogenous or exogenous catecholamine stimulation, including inotropic- and chronotropic-induced ischemia [3]. Their effects on ion-current channels and susceptibility to arrhythmias may be direct, such as L-type calcium (Ca^{2+}) channel blocking and intracellular cyclic adenosine monophosphate (cAMP) accumulation, or may involve electrical remodelling by modulating channel protein expression [4]. Chronic β-blockers usage has expanded over the last one to two decades and indications now include hypertension, cardio-protection after myocardial infarction (MI), angina, congestive heart failure, and rate control for arrhythmias [5].

β-Blockers are the fourth most commonly prescribed medication for hypertension [6] and an average of approximately 60% of post-MI patients at all hospitals are discharged on beta-blockers [7].

β-Blockade is also independently associated with improved survival in patients with VF or symptomatic VT [8], and its use also appears to prevent shocks in patients with implanted defibrillators [9].

β -Adrenoceptors in the Non-Failing Human Heart

Three different β-adrenoceptor subtypes have been cloned so far and identified pharmacologically; they are designed β_1-, β_2-and β_3-adrenoceptors [10]. The non-failing human heart expresses β-adrenoceptors, of which approximately 80% are β_1 and 20% are β_2 [11].

It is now generally accepted that in the human heart, functional β_1- and β_2-adrenoceptors coexist and both regulate myocardial contractility, heart rate and peripheral vascular resistance [12]. Furthermore, both β_1- and β_2-adrenoceptors participate in the systemic response to stress [13]. Stimulation of both these receptors act through G stimulatory proteins (Gs) to activate adenylyl cyclase, and stimulation of both β_1- and β_2-adrenoceptor subtypes increases the intracellular level of cAMP (Figure 1).

This cAMP, in turn, causes protein kinase A (PKA) to phosphorylate and activate several key regulatory proteins, including the L-type Ca^{2+} channels, that modulate the cardiac inotropic and chronotropic responses to catecholamine stimulation through the elevation of intracellular calcium (Ca^{+2}_i); this ultimately leads to increases force of contraction and heart rate [14]. In the human heart, cAMP is preferentially activated by β_1-adrenoceptor stimulation [15].

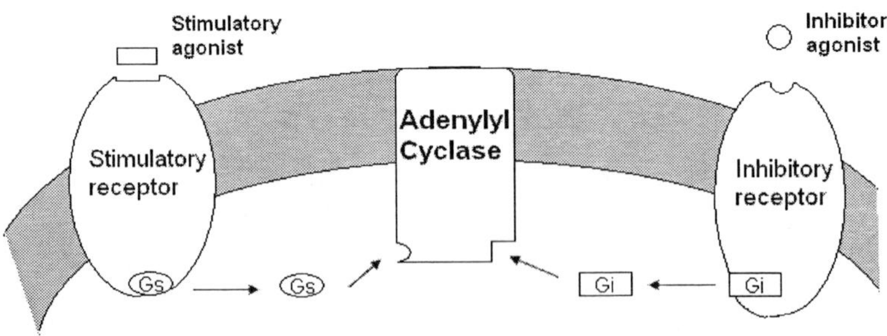

Figure 1. Stimulation of β_1- and β_2-adrenoceptors. Adenylyl cyclase may be stimulated or inhibited. Stimulatory agonists activate Gs, which interacts with adenylyl cyclase to stimulate it. Inhibitory agonists activate Gi, which interacts with adenylyl cyclase to inhibit it. (Modified from Berne RM, Levy MN. Physiology, Chapter 5 Fig 5.5, Mosby Year Book, Inc, USA 1993)

The mechanism behind these different coupling efficiencies of human myocardial β_1- and β_2-adrenoceptors to adenylyl cyclase is not known at present. In addition, although β_1-adrenoceptors increase $Ca^{+2}{}_i$ through the cAMP-dependent pathway, β_2- adrenoceptors can also increase Ca^{2+} influx through a non–cAMP-mediated mechanism, perhaps through the direct actions of G-protein on L-type channels [16-19].

Furthermore, although in *in vitro* experiments it has been shown that both adrenoceptors can mediate positive inotropic effects in atrial and ventricular preparations, in ventricles, only β_1-adrenoceptor stimulation can evoke maximum positive inotropic effects, and β_2-adrenoceptors only submaximal positive inotropic effects [15].

That is the reason why, the functional significance of mammalian ventricular β_2-adrenoceptors has been controversial, because for most normal hearts or myocytes, physiologically or therapeutically relevant concentrations of β_2-adrenoceptor agonists have surprisingly little effect on contractility [20].

Differences in β-Adrenoceptors between Non-Failing and Failing Human Heart

Preexisting coronary arterial disease and its consequences, such as acute myocardial ischaemia, scarring from previous MI and heart failure, are manifested in 80% of cardiac arrest victims [21].

Cardiac remodeling, following MI, can lead to hypertrophy, dilatation of the ventricles and eventually congestive heart failure. Cardiac hypertrophy and failure are characterized by some loss in the sensitivity of beta adrenergic stimulation [22]. The number of β_1-adrenoceptors declines, the amount of the adenylyl cyclase inhibitory G-protein (G_i) increases [23] (Figure 1) and, as a result, the failing heart is unable to adequately modulate its contractility. Paradoxically, the overall number of β_2-adrenoceptors remains stable in the failing heart [23].

A study by Bristow *et al.* (1986) [22] established that the positive inotropic effects of the highly selective β_2-adrenoceptor agonist zinterol were comparable in normal and failing trabaculae, despite the fact that failure was associated with pronounced depression in the response to isoproterenol. Consistent with these observations, the density of β_2-adrenoceptors was not reduced in failing hearts, but total β-adrenoceptor density was decreased by >50%. Furthermore, it has been shown that diseased ventricles exhibit a heightened response to β_2-adrenoceptor stimulation [16,18].

β_2-Adrenoceptor stimulation also appears to increase in patients with hypertension and in heart transplant recipients [24]. Aging has also been shown to alter the presence and function of β-adrenoceptor in the myocardium. Numerous studies, investigating *in vitro* age-dependent changes in β-adrenoceptors in the human heart, revealed a significant decline in β-adrenoceptor numbers predominately due to a loss of β_1-adrenoceptors [25]. In addition, ventricular cAMP responses to isoprenaline, which activates both β_1- and β_2-adrenoceptors, and to zinterol, decreased with aging [14].

Due to the significant selective β_1-adrenoceptor down-regulation in the failing and aging heart, β_2-adrenoceptors seem to be relatively more important in controlling myocardial responses to adrenergic stimulation.

β-Adrenergic Stimulation and Arrhythmiogenesis

There is good evidence that heightened beta adrenergic stimulation contributes to fatal arrhythmias [26,27]. The fact that higher incidence of sudden cardiac arrest in the morning hours was reduced in subjects receiving ß-adrenoceptor antagonists, gave support to the concept that beta adrenergic stimulation itself is an important trigger for the generation of lethal arrhythmias [28].

β-Adrenoceptor stimulation has been shown to affect ion currents that may influence the formation of arrhythmias, including VF. The inwardly rectifying potassium current (I_{Ki}), which is responsible for generating the resting membrane potential, is inhibited by PKA mediated phosphorylation through β-adrenoceptor activation, thereby prolonging action potential duration [29]. Furthermore, β-adrenoceptor stimulation has also been shown to increase the current density of the hyperpolarization activated cyclic nucleotide dependent current (I_f) in ventricular myocytes, allowing its activation at less-negative membrane potentials. This beta-mediated increase in I_f combined with the beta-mediated increase in resting membrane potential due to inhibition of I_{Ki} can lead to an increase in ectopic arrhythmias, especially in the setting of myocardial disease where I_{Ki} is already reduced and I_f is already increased [30]. As repolarization is delayed, multiple electrical activities are triggered from the ventricles, facilitating, thus, arrhythmiogenesis including VF [4,31].

Anti Ischemic and Anti Anginal Actions of Beta-Blockers

The discovery and development of the β-adrenoceptor antagonists represents one of the most significant advances in the history of cardiovascular pharmacology and therapeutics. Sir James Black is credited with leading the team that discovered the first clinically useful b-adrenoceptor antagonist, propranolol, which was developed specifically for the treatment of angina. Black proposed that pharmacologic blockade of cardiac β-adrenoceptors would reduce heart rate and myocardial oxygen demand and thereby prevent angina of effort associated with activation of the sympathetic nervous system (e.g., exercise, emotional stress, anxiety) [32]. This was a novel concept at that time (late 1950s, early 1960s) since the only effective antianginal drugs were the organic nitrates, such as nitroglycerin, whose therapeutic effects were attributed to vasodilation and increased coronary blood flow. Black was awarded the Nobel Prize in 1988, in part, for his role in the discovery of propranolol and the approach that he used. Since then, β-adrenoceptor antagonists are widely used in acute and long-term maintenance therapy in patients suffering from acute coronary syndromes (ACS) [33].

Their anti-ischemic effects are due primarily to a reduction in myocardial oxygen demand. By decreasing heart rate, myocardial contractility and afterload, β-adrenoceptor antagonists reduce myocardial workload and oxygen consumption at rest as well as during periods of exertion or stress [33]. Thus, the fundamental approach to reducing myocardial ischemia occurring in ACS and relieving anginal pain, is to restore the proper balance between myocardial oxygen supply and oxygen demand [34,35].

β-Adrenoceptor antagonists competitively inhibit the binding of endogenous catecholamines to β_1-adrenoceptors in the heart and most evidence strongly suggests that their anti-ischemic and anti-anginal effects are due to cardiac depression [32,36]. Furthermore, by inhibiting the actions of norepinephrine and epinephrine on the heart, β-adrenoceptor antagonists reduce myocardial oxygen demand via a reduction in both heart rate and cardiac contractility and, thereby, attenuate the myocardial response to sympathetic nervous system stimulation that occurs, for example, with increased stress or exercise [32,36].

Though most β-adrenoceptor antagonists lower resting heart rate to some extent, the effect on exercise-induced tachycardia is much more pronounced. It is important to note that the β-adrenoceptor antagonists do not change the point of imbalance between myocardial oxygen supply and consumption at which angina or MI occurs; rather, they reduce the likelihood that this point is reached [33].

By mechanisms that remain poorly understood, β-adrenoceptor antagonists also decrease peripheral vascular resistance, which leads to a reduction in arterial blood pressure and afterload [36,37]. Reduced afterload results in decreased left ventricular wall tension, which is another major determinant of myocardial oxygen demand. Furthermore, since β-adrenoceptor antagonists are not coronary vasodilators, they have little propensity to increase coronary blood flow and myocardial oxygen supply. If anything, β-adrenoceptor antagonists may increase coronary vascular resistance by inhibiting the β_2-adrenoceptor-mediated vasodilator effects of endogenous catecholamines and leaving a-adrenoceptor-mediated vasoconstriction unopposed [38,39].

Thus, the anti-ischemic and anti-anginal effects of the β-adrenoceptor antagonists are largely due to their ability to reduce myocardial workload and decrease oxygen consumption, rather than to improve myocardial oxygen supply.

β-Blockers in Stable Angina

β-Adrenoceptor antagonists are a mainstay in the treatment of chronic, stable angina [40]. While coronary blood flow (i.e., oxygen supply) may be sufficient to meet myocardial oxygen requirements at rest in patients with fixed atherosclerotic lesions, the obstruction prevents blood flow from increasing during periods of increased oxygen demand. Under these conditions, coronary blood flow is already at a maximal level in most patients; thus any increase in myocardial work can trigger an episode of acute angina [33].

Due to their effects in reducing myocardial workload and oxygen consumption, β-blockers are widely used in long-term maintenance therapy to prevent acute ischemic episodes.

β-Blockers in the Treatment of Acute Coronary Syndromes

It is well established that ACS in their different clinical presentations share a widely common pathophysiological substrate. Pathological, angioscopic, and biological observations have demonstrated that atherosclerotic plaque rupture or erosion, with differing degrees of superimposed thrombosis and distal embolization, resulting in myocardial underperfusion, represent the basic pathophysiological mechanisms in most ACS [41,42]. Many trials of intravenous β-blockade have been undertaken in the acute phase of MI, because of their potential to limit infarct size, reduce the incidence of fatal arrhythmias, and to relieve pain.

During the acute phase of ACS, relief of pain is of paramount importance, not only for humane reasons but because the pain is associated with sympathetic activation which causes vasoconstriction and increases the workload of the heart. If opioids fail to relieve the pain after repeated administration, intravenous β-blockers or nitrates are sometimes effective. Furthermore, β-blockers, unless contraindicated, are the first line of therapy in prolonged episodes of VT that may occur in the acute phase of ACS.

Evidence for the beneficial effects of β-blockers in unstable angina is based on limited randomized trial data, along with pathophysiological considerations and extrapolation from experience in stable angina and in ST-elevation myocardial infarction (STEMI). Two double-blind, randomized trials have compared β-blockers with placebo in unstable angina [43,44]. A meta-analysis suggested that β-blocker treatment was associated with a 13% relative reduction in risk of progression to STEMI [45]. β-Blockers are also recommended in non-ST elevation myocardial infarction (NSTEMI) in the absence of contraindications and are usually well tolerated. In most cases, oral treatment is sufficient. The target heart rate for a good treatment effect should be between 50 and 60 beats per minute. Meta-analysis and registry data have shown that long-term treatment with beta-blockers in patients suffering from NSTEMI may lead to a significant risk reduction for death [46]. Concerning STEMI and the acute phase of an episode, pooling of 28 trials of intravenous beta-blockade reveals an absolute reduction of mortality at 7 days from 4.3% to 3.7% [47]. These studies were conducted prior to the use of fibrinolytic agents or the performance of primary percutaneous coronary interventions. A post-hoc analysis on the other hand of the use of atenolol in the GUSTO-I trial and a systematic review do not support the routine early intravenous use of β-blockers [48,49]. There is a good case for the greater use of an intravenous β-blocker when there is tachycardia (in the absence of heart failure), relative hypertension, or pain unresponsive to opioids. In most patients, however, oral β-blockade will suffice [43].Concerning maintenance therapy, several trials and meta-analyses have demonstrated that β-adrenoreceptor blocking drugs reduce mortality and reinfarction by 20–25% even if fibrinolytic agents have been given or angiotensin-converting enzyme (ACE) inhibitors are co-administered [3,47,49-52]. The significant mortality reductions observed with β-blockers in heart failure in general, further support the use of these agents after MI. Evidence from all available studies suggests that beta-blockers should be used indefinitely in all patients who recovered from an acute MI [49,51,52].

β-Blockade In the Treatment of Atrial Fibrillation

In a typical patient with atrial fibrillation (AF) and no evidence of atrioventricular node disease, the ventricular rate ranges from 90 to 170 beats per minute. Excessively rapid ventricular rate is associated with increased morbidity and mortality and can contribute to symptoms such as developing embolic complications, hypertension, stroke and congestive heart failure [53]. Hence, there is need to control the ventricular rate in some patients when it is not intended to restore sinus rhythm. β-Blockers are one category of pharmacological agents used to achieve rate control [54]. Studies have shown that β-blockers can be effective both at rest and during activity in controlling heart rate [55,56]. Rapid acting esmolol, metoprolol, or propranolol are widely used intravenously to slow down the ventricular rate. Oral β-blockers are as well used widely as primary therapy for rate control in AF and they are the preferred therapy in patients with congestive heart failure, ischemic heart disease and depressed left ventricular function [54].

β- Adrenergic Stimulation and Ventricular Fibrillation

In the setting of VF, due to severe stress, sympathetic activity and, therefore, ß-adrenoceptor stimulation is increased. Observations in isolated heart muscle have shown that ß-adrenoceptor stimulation, especially when coronary perfusion pressure (CPP) is low, aggravates ischemic injury in the myocardium during VF [57]. Further evidence suggests that unusually heightened myocardial responsiveness to β_2-adrenoceptor agonists, such as epinephrine, increases susceptibility to VF [28] and may contribute to severe post-resuscitation myocardial dysfunction [58]. Furthermore, it is well known that states of severe stress, such as that occurring during VF and CPR, are associated with significant increases in sympathetic activity and circulating catecholamines; even without exogenous epinephrine administration, extremely high levels of plasma epinephrine concentrations have been measured during cardiac arrest and CPR [59-62]. For example, in an animal model of VF, adrenaline levels were elevated 170 times; therefore ß-adrenoceptors may have already been activated maximally, when adrenaline is administered [63]. Thus, whether it is from the repeated administration of exogenous epinephrine or from the high levels of circulating endogenous catecholamines, the fibrillating heart during CPR is subject to substantial β-adrenergic stimulation, along with its associated potential deleterious effects.

β-Blockade and Cardiopulmonary Resuscitation

Vasopressors are generally accepted to improve the outcome of cardiac arrest, by improving blood flow to the heart and brain in resuscitation attempts maximizing the possibility of return of spontaneous circulation (ROSC) [64,65]. Numerous studies have been performed in order to determine the minimal CPP that is required during CPR to meet the metabolic demands of the heart during VF [66-68]. A minimal CPP of about 30 mmHg seems to be required for ROSC in humans [69]. This minimum level during external standard CPR is usually not reached without the use of vasopressor agents [70].

Epinephrine has been preferred for almost 40 years as the adrenergic amine for increasing CPP during CPR in humans experiencing cardiac arrest and periodic intravenous administration has been recommended, if initial defibrillation has failed [71,72]. Epinephrine is a mixed adrenergic agonist, acting on α- and β-adrenergic receptors; its beneficial actions for ROSC are mostly mediated by its α-adrenergic properties. Epinephrine increases CPP via systemic arteriolar vasoconstriction, which maintains peripheral vascular tone and prevents arteriolar collapse [73]. Although this drug has been used as a standard first-line drug in cardiac arrest for many decades, currently, its role during CPR is controversial [74].

In contrast to the α-adrenergic stimulation, β-stimulation has been shown to have deleterious effects by increasing the oxygen consumption of the fibrillating myocardium, by augmenting the intrapulmonary shunting caused by hypoxic pulmonary vasoconstricion and by reducing subendocardial perfusion [75,76]. *A*ccordingly, epinephrine increases myocardial lactate concentration and decreases adenosine triphosphate (ATP) content even though coronary blood flow may be doubled [77], and is associated with poorer post-resuscitation myocardial function [78].

Interestingly, although VF accounted for approximately 40-60% of out-of-hospital cardiac arrests in the United States in the 1980s and early 1990s, at present, VF is estimated to account for approximately 25% of all out-of-hospital cardiac arrests [79,80]. A recent study suggested that there is an association between ß-adrenoceptor antagonists and the changing epidemiology of arrest rhythms, accounting for a decreasing incidence of VF [81]. Beta adrenergic blockade is also independently associated with improved survival in patients with VF [82], and its use also appears to reduce the number of shocks in patients with implanted defibrillators [9]. Several animal studies also suggest that ß-adrenoceptor antagonists during CPR are associated with increased rates of successful resuscitation and improved post-resuscitation myocardial function [63,83-87].

Evidence points to the beneficial use of ß-adrenoceptor antagonists in the setting of VF. ß-adrenoceptor antagonists have been shown to improve ROSC, initial successful defibrillation attempts and to increase duration of post-resuscitation survival in various experimental models [63,84,88]. It seems that ß-adrenergic blockade, by decreasing the force of contraction of the fibrillating heart, might decrease coronary vascular resistance enhancing thus coronary blood flow [86]. ß-Adrenergic blockade has also been associated with significantly greater post-resuscitation myocardial function [84,87,88]; this cardioprotective effect is thought to be mediated by a decrease in the oxygen requirements of the fibrillating heart, which reduces myocardial ischemic injury suffered during resuscitation, thereby improving post-resuscitation myocardial function [87]. Several animal studies have shown that ß-adrenoceptor antagonists increase the VF threshold [89-91] although the exact mechanism by which ß-adrenoceptor antagonists prevent VF is not entirely clear. Most studies agree that it is due to their antiadrenergic effects, but some authors believe that additional mechanisms are involved, including possible membrane stabilizing effects [90,91].

In the meantime, questions arise whether selective $ß_1$-, selective $ß_2$- or non selective ß adrenoceptor antagonists are the future in resuscitation field. In order to try to answer this question, one should first of all have in mind that both β_1- and β_2-adrenoceptors participate in the systemic response to stress [13].

According to these facts, one should logically conclude that non-selective beta adrenergic blockade should be applied. Evidence, on the other hand, suggests that only β_1-adrenoceptor stimulation can evoke maximum positive inotropic effects in ventricles, in contrast to β_2-adrenoceptors that exert only submaximal positive inotropic effects resulting in surprisingly little effect on contractility of physiologically or therapeutically relevant concentrations of β_2-adrenoceptor agonists [20].

Taking into consideration the fact that administered adrenaline in CPR increases the severity of myocardial dysfunction in the post-resuscitation period [77] and that $ß_1$-adrenoceptor action of catecholamines maximizes defibrillation's energy requirements, one should conclude that $ß_1$-adrenoceptor antagonists are beneficial in resuscitation. However, most of cardiac arrest victims suffer from coronary artery disease that leads to myocardial ischaemia. In cardiac hypertrophy and failure that could follow a MI, as well as in the aging heart, the number of β_1-adrenoceptors declines. In this same setting, paradoxically, the overall number of β_2-adrenoceptors remains stable [22] making thus β_2-adrenoceptors being relatively more important in controlling myocardial responses to beta adrenergic stimulation. Furthermore, it seems that in the intact human heart, cAMP is preferentially activated by β_2-adrenoceptor stimulation [15] and in diseased ventricles β_2- adrenoceptor stimulation exhibit a heightened response [16,18].

Although several cases relating the successful use of beta adrenergic blockade in the treatment of VF have been reported [92-94], to date high quality human trials are lacking. Unfortunately, we have no sufficient data of beta adrenergic blockade during VF in humans to compare the similarities and differences of its effects that may arise between human and non-human myocardium. Additional studies are necessary in order to comprehend and to assess more fully the effects of ß-adrenoceptor antagonists in the treatment of VF.

Beneficial Outcomes of β Adrenergic Blockade in Experimental Models

The mechanism, by which administered adrenaline in CPR, increases the severity of myocardial dysfunction in the post-resuscitation period is traditionally thought to point to its β_1-adrenoceptor stimulation, which elicits positive chronotropic and inotropic responses, thus increasing the oxygen needs in the fibrillating myocardium [77].

In addition, it has been suggested that the β_1-action of catecholamines maximizes defibrillation's energy requirements [76,95,96]. Many investigators co-administered selective β_1-adrenoceptor antagonists with epinephrine during resuscitation procedures in various animal models. β_1-Adrenoceptor antagonist esmolol has been shown to improve ROSC and survival in pigs [63] and resulted in improved initial cardiac resuscitation, minimized post-resuscitation myocardial impairment and increased duration of post-resuscitation survival in 2 studies of rat models [84,88]. Furthermore, co-administration of epinephrine and atenolol resulted in improved initial resuscitation success and increased blood and CPP during CPR in a swine model of VF [83].Further evidence suggested that the addition of a non-selective ß-adrenoceptor antagonist increases CPP during CPR and this raised the question of whether non-selective ß-adrenergic blockade can enhance vasoconstriction by allowing unopposed α-adrenergic stimulation [86]. Pre-treatment witha non-selective ß-adrenoceptor antagonist, before VF induction, followed by the suggested adrenaline doses seems to lead to myocardial injury reduction, without compromising the possibility of successful defibrillation, or left ventricular function in the post-resuscitation period. Propranolol was found to improve post-resuscitation myocardial dysfunction and short-term post-resuscitation survival in pretreated rats [87] and was associated with a greater increase in diastolic blood pressure than the tracheally administered adrenaline alone in a canine model [97]. This effect was attributed to its β_2-action [98]. Table 1 summarises the studies examining the effects of ß-adrenoceptor antagonists in animal models of cardiac arrest.

Table 1. Animal studies examining the effects of beta-blockade in models of cardiac arrest

Author	Animal Model	Minutes of untreated ventricular fibrillation	Drug study groups	Results
Ditchey et al 1994	Dogs	0 min	1) epinephrine 2) epinephrine+propranolol	Propranolol reduced myocardial injury during cardiopulmonary resuscitation
Ditchey et al. 1994	Dogs	cardiopulmonary resuscitation started immediately after ventricular fibrillation	1) epinephrine 2) phenylephrine 3)Phenylephrine+ propranolol	Balance between myocardial oxygen supply and demand improved in the phenylephrine+propranolol group
Tang et al. 1995	Sprague-Dawley rats.	4 min	1) Phenylephrine 2) epinephrine 3) epinephrine+esmolol	Post-resuscitation myocardial dysfunction was significantly improved in groups 1 and 3
Pellis et al. 2003	Swine	7 min	1) epinephrine 2) epinephrine + prazocin + propranolol 3) vasopressin	epinephrine + prazocin + propranolol group resulted in improved post-resuscitation cardiac and neurological recovery.
Huang et al. 2004	Sprague-Dawley rats.	cardiopulmonary resuscitation started immediately after ventricular fibrillation	1) epinephrine 2)epinephrine+Propranolol	Propranolol improved the outcome of cardiopulmonary resuscitation and post-resuscitation myocardial dysfunction
Cammarata et al. 2004	Sprague-Dawley rats.	6 min	1) saline as placebo 2) Esmolol	esmolol group minimized post-resuscitation myocardial dysfunction and increased duration of post-resuscitation survival
Killingsworth et al. 2004	Swine	8 min	1) saline placebo 2) esmolol	Esmolol improved return of spontaneous circulation and 4-hour survival
Bassiakou et al. 2008	Swine	8 min	1) epinephrine 2) epinephrine+atenolol	Atenolol improved initial resuscitation success and increased blood and coronary perfusion pressures during cardiopulmonary resuscitation

Human Studies

Several cases have been published relating the successful use of a ß-blocker in the treatment of refractory or recurrent VF/pulseless VT. In most instances, propranolol was the ß-blocking agent administered. In many of the cases reported, cardiac arrest from VF occurred in the context of MI. Propranolol and esmolol were found to be successful in terminating acute MI-associated refractory VF [94,99-102].

Propranolol has been also administered in cases of VF not associated with MI and has been reported effective in terminating this malignant arrhythmia. Propranolol has been successfully used to treat recurrent VF or pulseless VT in patients with isoprenaline [103] and synephrine overdoses [92], with digitalis intoxication [99], myocarditis [104], as well as in a patient with electrical storm after implantation of a cardioverter-defibrillator [93].

Although the aforementioned cases relate the successful use of ß-adrenergic blockade in the treatment of VF, to date, high quality human trials are lacking. Furthermore, no human prospective randomized trials examining the effects of ß-blocker administration during CPR from VF to date exist.

Conclusion

ß-Blockers are a heterogeneous group of aryloxypropanolamines that competitively bind to one or more β-subtype receptors, resulting in antagonism of β-adrenergic stimulation. Indications for the use of β-blockers include hypertension, cardio-protection after MI, angina, congestive heart failure, and rate control for arrhythmias. By decreasing heart rate, myocardial contractility and afterload, β-adrenoceptor antagonists reduce myocardial workload and oxygen consumption at rest as well as during periods of exertion or stress. That is why β-blockers are important antiarrhythmic and anti-anginal therapeutic agents used in AF, stable angina and ACS.

Furthermore, β-blockade is also independently associated with improved survival in patients with VF or symptomatic VT as it has been shown by several experimental studies and clinical cases. These facts, along with the evidence that heightened ß-adrenergic stimulation contributes to fatal arrhythmias, lead to the conclusion that β-blockers could be of some value in the resuscitation field.

Unfortunately, to date high quality human trials are lacking. Additional studies are necessary in order to comprehend and to assess more fully the effects of ß-adrenoceptor antagonists in the treatment of VF.

References

[1] Lombardi, W.L. and Gilbert, E.M. Carvedilol in the failing heart. *Clin. Cardiol.* 2001, *24*, 757–766.

[2] Baker, JG; Hall, IP; Hill, SJ. Agonist and inverse agonist actions of beta-blockers at the human beta 2-adrenoceptor provide evidence for agonist-directed signalling. *Mol. Pharmacol.* 2003, 64, 1357–1369.

[3] Anonymous. Effect of metoprolol CR/XL in chronic heart failure: Metoprolol CR/XL Randomised Intervention Trial in Congestive Heart Failure (MERIT-HF). *Lancet* 1999, 353, 2001–2007.

[4] Adamson, P.B. and Gilbert, E.M. (2006). Reducing the Risk of Sudden Death in Heart Failure With β-Blockers. *J. Card. Fail. 12*, 734-746.

[5] Youngquist, ST; Kaji, AH; Niemann, JT. Beta-blocker use and the changing epidemiology of out-of-hospital cardiac arrest rhythms. *Resuscitation* 2008, 76, 376-380.

[6] Stafford, RS; Monti, V; Furberg, CD; Ma, J. Long-term and shortterm changes in antihypertensive prescribing by office-based physicians in the United States. *Hypertension* 2006, 48, 196-197.

[7] Bradley, EH; Herrin, J; Mattera, JA; Holmboe, ES; Wang, Y; Frederick, P; Roumanis, SA; Radford, MJ; Krumholz, HM. Quality improvement efforts and hospital performance: rates of beta-blocker prescription after acute myocardial infarction. *Med. Care.* 2005, 43, 282-292.

[8] Exner, DV; Reiffel, JA; Epstein, AE; Ledingham, R; Reiter, MJ; Yao, Q; Duff, HJ; Follmann, D; Schron, E; Greene, HL; Carlson, MD; Brodsky, MA; Akiyama, T; Baessler, C; Anderson, JL. Beta-blocker use and survival in patients with ventricular fibrillation or symptomatic ventricular tachycardia: the antiarrhythmics versus implantable defibrillators (AVID) trial. *J. Am. Coll. Cardiol.* 1999, 34, 325-333.

[9] Connolly, SJ; Dorian, P; Roberts, RS; Gent, M; Bailin, S; Fain, ES; Thorpe, K; Champagne, J; Talajic, M; Coutu, B; Gronefeld, GC; Hohnloser, SH. Optimal Pharmacological Therapy in Cardioveter Defibrillator Patients (OPTIC) Investigators. Comparison of beta-blockers, amiodarone plus beta-blockers, or sotalol for prevention of shocks from implantable cardioverter defibrillators: the OPTIC study: a randomized trial. *JAMA* 2006, 295, 165-171.

[10] Bylund, DB; Eikenberg, DC; Hieble, JP; Langer, SZ; Lefkowitz, RJ; Minneman, KP; Molinoff, PB; Ruffolo, RRJr; Trendelenburg, U. International Union of pharmacology nomenclature of adrenoceptors. *Pharmacol. Rev.* 1994, 46, 121-136.

[11] Brodde, OE. Beta-adrenoceptors in cardiac disease. *Pharmacol. Ther.* 1994, 60, 405-430.

[12] Brodde, OE; Bruck, H; Leineweber, K; Seyfarth, T. Presence, distribution and physiological function of adrenergic and muscarinic receptor subtypes in the human heart. *Basic Res. Cardiol.* 2001, 96, 528-538.

[13] Lefkowitz, RJ; Hoffman, B; Taylor, P. Neurohumoral transmission: the autonomic and somatic motor nervous system. In: Gilman A. G, Rall T. W, Nies A. S, and Taylor P. editors. *The pharmacologic basis of Therapeutics.* New York: McGraw Hill; 1993; 84-121.

[14] Brodde, O.E. and Michel, M. (1999). Adrenergic and muscarinic receptors in the human heart. *Pharmacol. Rev. 51*, 651-690.

[15] Bristow, MR; Hershberger, RE; Port, JD; Minobe, W; Rasmussen, R. β_1- and β_2-adrenergic receptor-mediated adenylate cyclase stimulation in non-failing and failing human ventricular myocardioum. *Mol. Pharmacol,* 1989, 35, 295-303.

[16] Altschuld, RA; Starling, RC; Hamlin, RL; Billman, GE; Hensley, J; Castillo, L; Fertel, RH; Hohl, CM; Robitaille, PM; Jones, LR, et al. Response of failing canine heart and human heart cells to β2 adrenergic stimulation. *Circulation* 1995, 92, 1612-1618.

[17] Billman, GE; Castillo, LC; Hensley, J; Hohl, CM; Altschuld, RA. Beta 2-adrenergic receptor antagonists protect against ventricular fibrillation: in vivo and in vitro evidence for enhanced sensitivity to beta 2-adrenergic stimulation in animals susceptible to sudden death. *Circulation* 1997, 96, 1914–1922.

[18] Zhang, ZS; Cheng, HJ; Ukai, T; Tachibana, H; Cheng, CP. Enhanced cardiac L-type calcium current response to beta2-adrenergic stimulation in heart failure. *J. Pharmacol. Exp. Ther.* 2001, 298, 188–196.

[19] Xiao, RP; Ji, X; Lakatta, EG. Functional coupling of the beta 2-adrenoceptor to a pertussis toxin-sensitive G protein in cardiac myocytes. *Mol. Pharmacol.* 1995, 47, 322-329.

[20] Cui, Y; Shen, YT; Kalthof, B; Iwase, M; Sato, N; Uechi, M; Vatner, SF; Vatner, DE. Identification and functional role of β_1-adrenergic receptor subtypes in primate and rodent: in vivo versus isolated myocytes. *J. Mol. Cell Cardiol.* 1996, 28, 1307-1317.

[21] Huikuri, HV; Castellanos, A; Myerburg, RJ. Sudden death due to cardiac arrhythmias. *N. Engl. J. Med.* 2001, 345, 1473-1482.

[22] Bristow, MR; Ginsburg, R; Umans, V; Fowler, M; Minobe, W; Rasmussen, R; Zera, P; Menlove, R; Shah, P; Jamieson, S; et al. β_1- and β_2- adrenergic receptor subpopulations in nonfailing and failing human ventricular myocardium: coupling of both receptior subtypes to muscle contraction and selective β_1-receptor down-regulation in heart failure. *Circ. Res.* 1986, 59, 297-309.

[23] Kiuchi, K; Shannon, RP; Komamura, K; Cohen, DJ; Bianchi, C; Homcy, CJ; Vatner, SF; Vatner, DE. Myocardial β-adrenergic receptor function during the development of pacing-induced heart failure. *J. Clin. Invest.* 1993, 91, 907-914.

[24] Leenen, FHH; Davies, RA; Fourney, A. Catecholamines and heart function in heart transplant patients: Effects of beta-1 versus non-selective β-blockade. *Clin. Pharmacol. Ther.* 1998, 64, 522-535.

[25] White, M.and Leenen, F.H.H. (1994). Aging and cardiovascular responsivness to β-agonists in humans: Role of changes in β receptor responses versus baroreflex activity. *Clin. Pharmacol. Ther. 56*, 543-558.

[26] Chen, PS; Chen, LS; Cao, JM; Sharifi, B; Karagueuzian, HS; Fishbein, MC. Sympathetic nerve sprouting, electrical remodeling and the mechanisms of sudden cardiac death. *Cardiovasc. Res.* 2001, 50, 409–416.

[27] Tomaselli, G.F. and Zipes, D.P. (2004). What causes sudden death in heart failure? *Circ. Res. 95*, 754–763.

[28] Altschuld, R.A. and Billman, G.E. (2000). β_2-adrenoreceprors and ventricular fibrillation. *Pharmacol. Therap. 80*, 1-14.

[29] Koumi, S; Backer, CL; Arentzen, CE; Sato, R. Beta-adrenergic modulation of the inwardly rectifying potassium channel in isolated human ventricular myocytes. Alteration in channel response to beta-adrenergic stimulation in failing human hearts. *J. Clin. Invest.* 1995, 96, 2870–2881.

[30] Hoppe, UC; Jansen, E; Südkamp, M; Beuckelmann, DJ. Hyperpolarization-activated inward current in ventricular myocytes from normal and failing human hearts. *Circulation* 1998, 97, 55–65.

[31] Packer, M. Sudden unexpected death in patients with congestive heart failure: A second frontier. *Circulation* 1985, 72, 681-685.

[32] Black, J. Drugs from emasculated hormones: the principle of syntopic antagonism. *Science* 1989, 245, 486-493.

[33] O'Rourke, ST. Antianginal actions of beta-adrenoceptor antagonists. *Am. J. Pharm. Educ*. 2007, 71, 95.

[34] Abrams, J. Clinical practice. Chronic stable angina. *N. Engl. J. Med.* 2005, 352, 2524-2533.

[35] Michel, T. Treatment of myocardial ischemia. In: Brunton LL, Lazo JS, Parker KL, editors. *Goodman and Gilman's The Pharmacological Basis of Therapeutics.* New York: McGraw-Hill; 2006; 823-844.

[36] Opie, LH; Sonnenblick, EH; Frishman, W; Thadani, U. Beta blocking agents. In: Opie LH, editor. Drugs for the heart. Philadelphia: WB Saunders; 1995; 1-27.

[37] Hoffman, BB. Adrenoceptor antagonist drugs. In: Katzung BG, editor. *Basic and Clinical Pharmacology*. New York: McGraw-Hill; 2007; 141-158.

[38] Robertson, RM; Wood, AJJ; Vaughn, WK; Robertson, D. Exacerbation of vasotonic angina pectoris by propranolol. *Circulation* 1982, 65, 281-285.

[39] Nielsen, H; Egeblad, H; Mortensen, SA; Sandoe, E. Observations on increased susceptibility to coronary artery vasospasm during beta blockade. *Am. Heart J.* 1987, 114, 192-194.

[40] Thadani, U. Current medical management of chronic stable angina. *J. Cardiovasc. Pharmacol. Ther.* 2004, 9, S11-S29.

[41] Rapezzi, C; Biagini, E; Branzi, A. Guidelines for the diagnosis and treatment of non-ST-segment elevation acute coronary syndromes: the task force for the diagnosis and treatment of non-ST-segment elevation acute coronary syndromes of the European Society of Cardiology. *Eur. Heart J.* 2007, 28, 1598–1660.

[42] Van de Werf, F; Ardissino, D; Betriu, A; Cokkinos, DV; Falk, E; Fox, KA; Julian, D; Lengyel, M; Neumann, FJ; Ruzyllo, W; Thygesen, C; Underwood, SR; Vahanian, A; Verheugt, FW; Wijns, W. Management of acute myocardial infarction in patients presenting with ST-segment elevation. The task force on the management of acute myocardial infarction of the European Society of Cardiology. *Eur. Heart J.* 2003, 24, 28–66.

[43] Telford, A.M. and Wilson, C. (1981). Trial of heparin versus atenolol in prevention of myocardial infarction in intermediate coronary syndrome. *Lancet, 1*, 1225–1228.

[44] Lubsen, J. and Tijssen, J.G. (1987). Efficacy of nifedipine and metoprolol in the early treatment of unstable angina in the coronary care unit: findings from the Holland Interuniversity Nifedipine/metoprolol Trial (HINT). *Am. J. Cardiol. 60*, 18A–25A.

[45] Yusuf, S; Wittes, J; Friedman, L. Overview of results of randomized clinical trials in heart disease. II. Unstable angina, heart failure, primary prevention with aspirin, and risk factor modification. *JAMA* 1988, 260, 2259–2263.

[46] Lopez-Sendon, J; Swedberg, K; McMurray, J; Tamargo, J; Maggioni, AP; Dargie, H; Tendera, M; Waagstein, F; Kjekshus, J; Lechat, P; Torp-Pedersen, C. Expert consensus document on beta-adrenergic receptor blockers. *Eur. Heart J.* 2004, 25, 1341–1362.

[47] Yusuf, S; Lessem, J; Jha, P; Lonn, E. Primary and secondary prevention of myocardial infarction and strokes: an update of randomly allocated controlled trials. *J. Hypertens.* 1993, 11, S61–S73.

[48] Pfisterer, M; Cox, JL; Granger, CB; Brener, SJ; Naylor, CD; Califf, RM; van de Werf, F; Stebbins, AL; Lee, KL; Topol, EJ; Armstrong, PW. Atenolol use and clinical

outcomes after thrombolysis for acute myocardial infarction: the GUSTO-I experience. Global Utilization of Streptokinase and TPA (alteplase) for Occluded Coronary Arteries. *J. Am. Coll. Cardiol.* 1998, 32, 634–640.

[49] Freemantle, N; Cleland, J; Young, P; Mason, J; Harrison, J. Beta blockade after myocardial infarction: systematic review and meta regression analysis. *BMJ* 1999, 318, 1730–1737.

[50] Dargie, HJ. Effect of carvedilol on outcome after myocardial infarction in patients with left-ventricular dysfunction: the CAPRICORN randomised trial. *Lancet* 2001, 357, 1385–1390.

[51] Olsson, G; Oden, A; Johansson, L; Sjögren, A; Rehnqvist, N. Prognosis after withdrawal of chronic postinfarction metoprolol treatment: a 2 to 7 year follow-up. *Eur. Heart J.* 1988, 9, 365–372.

[52] Pedersen, TR. Six-year follow-up of the Norwegian multicenter study on timolol after acute myocardial infarction. *N. Engl. J. Med.* 1985, 313, 1055–1058.

[53] Benjamin, EJ; Wolf, PA; D'Agostino, RB; Silbershatz, H; Kannel, WB; Levy, D. Impact of atrial fibrillation on the risk of death: the Framingham Heart study. *Circulation* 1998, 98, 946-952.

[54] Hersi, A; Wyse, DG. Management of Atrial Fibrillation. *Curr. Probl. Cardiol.* 2005, 30, 175–234.

[55] Koh, KK; Song, JH; Kwon, KS; Park, HB; Baik, SH; Park, YS; In, HH; Moon, TH; Park, GS; Cho, SK; et al. Comparative study of efficacy and safety of low-dose diltiazem or betaxolol in combination with digoxin to control ventricular rate in chronic atrial fibrillation: randomized crossover study. *Int. J. Cardiol.* 1995, 52, 167-174.

[56] Farshi, R; Kistner, D; Sama, JS; Longmate, JA; Singh, BN. Ventricular rate control in atrial fibrillation during daily activity and programmed exercise: a crossover open-label study of five drug regimens. *J. Am. Coll. Cardiol.* 1999, 33, 304-310.

[57] Midei, MG; Sugiura, S; Maughan, WL; Sagawa, K; Weisfeldt, ML; Guerci, AD. Preservation of ventricular function by treatment of ventricular fibrillation with phenylephrine. *J. Am. Coll. Cariol.* 1990, 16, 489-494.

[58] Niemann, JT; Haynes, KS; Garner, D; Rennie, CJ 3rd; Jagels, G; Stormo, O. Post-countershock pulseless rhythms: Response to CPR, artificial cardiac pacing, and adrenergic agonists. *Ann. Emerg. Med.* 1986, 15, 112-120.

[59] Kern, KB; Elchisak, MA; Sanders, AB; Badylak, SF; Tacker, WA; Ewy, GA. Plasma catecholamines and resuscitation from prolonged cardiac arrest. *Crit. Care Med.* 1989, 17, 786-791.

[60] Lindner, KH; Haak, T; Keller, A; Bothner, U; Lurie, K.G. Release of endogenous vasopressors during and after cardiopulmonary resuscitation. *Heart* 1996, 75, 145-150.

[61] Little, RA; Frayn, KN; Randall, PE; Stoner, HB; Yates, DW; Laing, GS; Kumar, S; Banks, JM. Plasma catecholamines in patients with acute myocardial infarction and in cardiac arrest. *Q. J. Med.* 1985, 54, 133-140.

[62] Wortsman, J; Frank, S; Cryer, PE. Adrenomedullary response to maximal stress in humans. *Am. J. Med.* 1984, 77, 779-784.

[63] Killingsworth, CR; Wei, CC; Dell'Italia, LJ; Ardell, JL; Kingsley, MA; Smith, WM; Ideker, RE; Walcott, GP. Short-acting β-adrenergic antagonist esmolol given at reperfusion improves survival following prolonged VF. *Circulation* 2004, 109, 2469-2474.

[64] Wenzel, V; Krismer, AC; Arntz, HR; Sitter, H; Stadlbauer, KH; Lindner, KH. European Resuscitation Council Vasopressor during Cardiopulmonary Resuscitation Study Group, 2004. A comparison of vasopressin and epinephrine for out-of-hospital cardiopulmonary resuscitation. *N. Engl. J. Med.* 2004, 350, 105–113.

[65] Wenzel, V; Krismer, AC; Voelckel, WG; Mayr, VD; Raedler, C; Strohmenger, HU; Lindner, KH. The use of arginine vasopressin during cardiopulmonary resuscitation. An analysis of experimental and clinical experience and a view of the future. *Anaesthesist* 2002, 51, 191–202.

[66] Gibbs, CL; Papadoyannis, DE; Drake, AJ; Noble, MI. Oxygen consumption of the nonworking and potassium chloride-arrest dog heart. *Circ. Res.* 1980, 47, 408-417.

[67] Niemann, JT. Differences in cerebral and myocardial perfusion during closed-chest resuscitation. *Ann. Emerg. Med.* 1984, 13, 849-853.

[68] Paradis, NA; Martin, GB; Rivers, EP; Goetting, MG; Appleton, TJ; Feingold, M; Nowak, RM. Coronary perfusion pressure and the return of spontaneous circulation in human cardiopulmonary resuscitation. *JAMA* 1990, 263, 1106-1113.

[69] Brown, C; Wiklund, L; Bar-Joseph, G; Miller, B; Bircher, N; Paradis, N; Menegazzi, J; von Planta, M; Kramer, GC; Gisvold, SE. Future directions for resuscitation research. IV. Innovative advanced life support pharmacology. *Resuscitation* 1996, 33, 163-177.

[70] Ditchey, RV; Winkler, JV; Rhodes, CA. Relative lack of coronary blood flow during closed-chest resuscitation in dogs. *Circulation* 1982, 66, 297-302.

[71] Anonymous. Standards for cardiopulmonary resuscitation (CPR) and emergency cardiac care (ECC). 3. Advanced life support. *JAMA* 1974, 227, 852-860.

[72] Nolan, JP; Deakin, CD; Soar, J; Bottiger, BW; Smith, G. European Resuscitation Council guidelines for Resuscitation 2005. Section 4. Adult advanced life support. *Resuscitation* 2005, 67, S39-S86.

[73] Otto, CW; Yakaitis, RW. The role of epinephrine in CPR: a reappraisal. *Ann. Emerg. Med.* 1984, 13, 840–843.

[74] Ditchey, RV. The choice of vasopressor agents in cardiopulmonary resuscitation. *Curr. Opin. Crit. Care.* 1996, 2, 170-175.

[75] Otto, CW; Yakaitis, RW; Blitt, CD. Mechanism of action of epinephrine in resuscitation from asphyxial arrest. *Crit. Care Med.* 1981, 9, 364–365.

[76] Klouche, K; Weil, MH; Tang, W; Povoas, H; Kamohara, T; Bisera, J. A selective alpha(2)-adrenergic agonist for cardiac resuscitation. *J. Lab. Clin. Med.* 2002, 140, 27–34.

[77] Ditchey, RV; Lindenfeld, J. Failure of epinephrine to improve the balance between myocardial oxygen supply and demand during closed- chest resuscitation in dogs. *Circulation* 1988, 78, 382-389.

[78] Yakaitis, RW; Otto, CW; Blitt, CD. Relative importance of alpha and beta adrenergic receptors during resuscitation. *Crit. Care Med.* 1979, 7, 293–296.

[79] Kette, F. Increased survival despite a reduction in out-of hospital ventricular fibrillation in north-east Italy. *Resuscitation* 2007, 72, 52-58.

[80] Polentini, MS; Pirrallo, RG; McGill, W. The changing incidence of ventricular fibrillation in Milwaukee, Wisconsin (1992—2002). *Prehosp. Emerg. Care* 2006, 10, 52-60.

[81] Youngquist, ST; Kaji, AH; Niemann, JT. Beta-blocker use and the changing epidemiology of out-of-hospital cardiac arrest rhythms. *Resuscitation* 2008, 76, 376-380.

[82] Exner, DV; Reiffel, JA; Epstein, AE; Ledingham, R; Reiter, MJ; Yao, Q; Duff, HJ; Follmann, D; Schron, E; Greene, HL; Carlson, MD; Brodsky, MA; Akiyama, T; Baessler, C; Anderson, JL. Beta-blocker use and survival in patients with ventricular fibrillation or symptomatic ventricular tachycardia: the antiarrhythmics versus implantable defibrillators (AVID) trial. *J. Am. Coll. Cardiol.* 1999, 34, 325-333.

[83] Bassiakou, E; Xanthos, T; Koudouna, E; Goulas, S; Prapa, V; Papadimitriou, D; Rokas, G; Papadimitriou, L. Atenolol in combination with epinephrine improves the initial outcome of cardiopulmonary resuscitation in a swine model of ventricular fibrillation. *Am. J. Emerg. Med.* 2008, 26, 578-584.

[84] Cammarata, G; Weil, MH; Sun, S; Tang, W; Wang, J; Huang, L. Beta1-adrenergic blockade during cardiopulmonary resuscitation improves survival. *Crit. Care Med.* 2004, 32, S440-S443.

[85] Ditchey, RV; Rubio-Perez, A; Slinker, BK. Beta-adrenergic blockade reduces myocardial injury during experimental cardiopulmonary resuscitation. *J. Am. Coll. Cardiol.* 1994, 24, 804–812.

[86] Ditchey, R.V. and Slinker, B.K. (1994). Phenylephrine plus propranolol improves the balance between myocardial oxygen supply and demand during cardiopulmonary resuscitation from prolonged cardiac arrest in pigs: a prospective, randomized study. *Crit. Care Med. 22*, 282-290.

[87] Huang, L; Weil, M.X; Cammarata, G; Sun, S; Tang, W. Nonselective β-blocking agent improves the outcome of cardiopulmonary resuscitation in rat model. *Crit. Care Med.* 2004, 32, S378-S380.

[88] Tang, W; Weil, MH; Sun, S; Noc, M; Yang, L; Gazmuri, RJ. Epinephrine increases the severity of postresuscitation myocardial dysfunction. *Circulation* 1995, 92, 3089-3093.

[89] Anderson, JL; Rodier, HE; Green, LS. Comparative effects on beta-adrenergic blocking drugs on experimental ventricular fibrillation threshold. *Am. J. Cardiol.* 1983, 51, 1196-1202.

[90] Coram, WM; Olson, RW; Beil, ME; Cabot, CF; Weiss, GB. Effects on metoprolol, alone and in combination with lidocaine, on ventricular fibrillation threshold: comparison with atenolol, propranolol and pindolol. *J. Cardiovasc. Pharmacol.* 1987, 9, 611-621.

[91] Luketich, J; Friehling, TD; O'Connor, KM; Kowey, PR. The effect of beta-adrenergic blockade on vulnerability to ventricular fibrillation and inducibility of ventricular arrhythmia in short- and long-term feline infarction model. *Am. Heart J.* 1989, 118, 265-271.

[92] Srivatsa, UN; Ebrahimi, R; El-Bialy, A; Wachsner, RY. Electrical storm: case series and review of managment. *J. Cardiovasc. Pharmacol. Ther.* 2003, 8, 237-246.

[93] Tsagalou, EP; Kanakakis, J; Rokas, S; Anastasiou-Nana, MI. Supression by propranolol and amiodarone of an electrical storm referactory to metoprolol and amiodarone. *Int. J. Cardiol.* 2005, 99, 341-342.

[94] van Dantzig, JM; Koster, RW; Biervliet, JD. Treatment with esmolol of ventricular fobrillation unresponsive to lidocaine and procainamide. *J. Cardiothorac. Vasc. Anesth.* 1991, 5, 600-603.

[95] Dorian, P. and Wang, M.J. (1988). Defibrillation current and impedance Fare determinants of defibrillation energy requirements. *Pacing. Clin. Electrophysiol.* 11, 1996–2001.

[96] Huang, L. and Tang, W. (2004). Vasopressor agents: old and new components. *Curr. Opin. Crit. Care.* 10, 183–187.

[97] Elizur, A; Ben-Abraham, R; Manisterski, Y; Barak, A; Efrati, O; Lotan, D; Barzilay, Z; Paret, G. Tracheal epinephrine or norepinephrine preceded by beta blockade in a dog model. Can beta blockade bestow any benefits? *Resuscitation* 2003, 59, 271-276.

[98] Vaknin, Z; Manisterski, Y; Ben-Abraham, R; Efrati, O; Lotan, D; Barzilay, Z; Paret, G. Is endotracheal adrenaline deleterious because of the beta adrenergic effect? *Anesth. Analg.* 2001, 92, 1408-1412.

[99] Sloman, G; Robinson, JS; McLean, K. Propranolol (Inderal) in Persistent Ventricular Fibrillation. *Br. Med. J.* 1965, 1, 895-896.

[100] Ikram, H. Propranolol in persistent ventricular fibrillation complicating acute myocardial infarction. *Am. Heart J.* 1968, 75, 795-798.

[101] Mason, JR; Marek, JC; Loeb, HS; Scanlon, PJ. Intravenous propranolol in the treatment of repetitive ventricular tachyarrhythmias during resuscitation from sudden death. *Am. Heart J.* 1985, 110, 161-165.

[102] Rothfeld, EL; Lipowitz, M; Zucker, IR; Parsonnet, V; Bernstein, A. Management of persistently recurring ventricular fibrillation with propranolol hydrochloride. *JAMA* 1968, 204, 546-548.

[103] Besterman, E.M. and Friedlander, D.H. (1965). Clinical experiences with propranolol. *Postgrad. Med. J. 41*, 526-535

[104] Iwatsuki, K; Yusa, T; Hashimoto, Y; Watabe, Y. Effect of propranolol on paroxysmal ventricular fibrillation. *Tohoku J. Exp. Med.* 1966, 88, 257-262.

In: Drugs in Cardiopulmonary Resuscitation
Editor: Theodoros Xanthos

ISBN: 978-1-61122-512-9

Chapter 9

Nitroglycerin in the Emergency Setting

Vasiliki Kitsou
University of Athens, Medical School

Abstract

Nitroglycerin (glyceryl trinitrate, GTN) is a representative of the organic nitrates or nitrovasodilators. Its beneficial therapeutic effect is attributed to selective vasodilation of large arteries and large conductance veins with minimal effect on the arteriolar tone. Evidence indicates that GTN and other nitrates function as prodrugs that, when bioactivated, release nitric oxide (NO). It is hypothesised that the principal mechanism of GTN-induced vasorelaxation is the activation of the soluble guanylyl cyclase (sGC), an intracellular NO receptor, and the subsequent increase in tissue levels of the second messenger cyclic 3'5'-guanosine monophosphate (cGMP). cGMP, in turn, activates cGMP-dependent protein kinase C (PKC) which induces vasorelaxation. Recently, it has been demonstrated that the mitochondrial isoform of aldehyde dehydrogenase (mtALDH or ALDH2) is responsible for the bioactivation of GTN. Tolerance develops after continuous use of GTN, leading to reduced responsiveness of blood vessels to GTN and other organic nitrates or to the requirement of higher doses of these drugs. Tolerance is attributed to the formation of the strong oxidant peroxynitrite, a potent cellular oxidant. GTN has clear benefits for the treatment of angina pectoris, congestive heart failure, unstable angina, non-ST-segment myocardial infarction, acute myocardial infarction and variant angina. During cardiopulmonary resuscitation (CPR), the co-administration of a vasodilator, such as nitroglycerin, with one or even two vasopressors has been suggested, in animal models. Still, further investigation is necessary for the administration of GTN during CPR.

Introduction

GTN is the most prominent representative of the organic nitrates or nitrovasodilators. It has been used clinically since the late 19th century for the treatment of angina pectoris [1]. The beneficial therapeutic effect of GTN and other organic nitrates is attributed to selective vasodilation of large arteries and large conductance veins with minimal effect on the arteriolar tone [2].

Mechanism of Action of GTN

The mechanism by which GTN and other organic nitrates dilate blood vessels is still not fully understood. It is hypothesised that GTN exerts its effect through a, still unidentified, method of delivering NO via enzymatic transformation [3]. Evidence indicates that the principal mechanism of GTN-induced vasorelaxation is the activation of the sGC signalling pathway [4].

GTN and other nitrates function as prodrugs that, when bioactivated, release NO or S-nitrosothiol in vascular smooth muscle and endothelial cells. NO activates sGC, an intracellular NO receptor, subsequently increasing tissue levels of the second messenger cGMP. cGMP in turn activates cGMP-dependent PKC and cGMP-gated ion channels [5]. It has been shown that PKC mediates vasorelaxation through phosphorylation of proteins that regulate intracellular calcium (Ca^{2+}) levels. The mechanism of vasodilation includes a reduction in intracellular Ca^{2+} levels and desensitization of contractile proteins to Ca^{2+} in smooth muscle cells [6].

There is evidence that nitroglycerin, via its enzymatic transformation to NO, activates sensory nerve fibers to release calcitonin gene-related peptide (CGRP), a very potent vasodilator, in both central and periphery vascular tissues [7]. CGRP is a 37-amino acid residue vasoactive neuropeptide widely distributed in the nervous and cardiovascular systems. Most blood vessels are surrounded by a dense perivascular CGRP neural network, which plays an important role in modulating the tension of resistance vessels. Through interaction with its receptors, CGRP produces vasorelaxation. One study supports the conclusion that CGRP mediates, at least in part, the nitroglycerin-induced vascular relaxation [8].

Bioactivation of GTN

The pathway of GTN biotransformation yielding NO or a related bioactive species activating sGC is referred to as bioactivation. There has been an extensive search for the enzyme(s) catalysing GTN bioactivation and several candidates have been proposed in the past [9]. Recently, it has been demonstrated that ALDH2 is responsible for the bioactivation of GTN (Figure 1) [10,11].

ALDH2 is an important enzyme with two long-known enzyme activities. The dehydrogenase activity requires the cofactor nicotinamide adenine dinucleotide (NAD^+) and converts aldehydes to the respective carboxylic acid (e.g. acetaldehyde to acetic acid). The esterase activity does not require cofactors and converts carboxylic acid esters (probably also esters from other acids) to the free acid and the respective alcohol. The catalysis of these enzyme activities depends on thiols. The enzyme activities are inhibited by thiol-oxidizing compounds. In 2002, this enzyme was identified as an organic nitrate bioactivating enzyme. This so-called nitrate reductase activity denitrates organic nitrates and forms nitrite [10,12-14].

For the bioactivation of GTN, ALDH2 specifically catalyses the formation of 1,2-glycerol dinitrate (1,2 GDN) and nitrite from GTN. This activity differs from the others, since it reduces the nitrogen of the dissociated nitrite. The electrons for this reduction are not provided by NADH but by cysteine-thiols at the active site of the enzyme which are, thereby, converted to a disulfide.

Reductase activity of this oxidized ALDH2 can be restored by dithiol compounds such as dithiol dithiothreitol and dihydrolipoic acid. The mechanism of ALDH2 catalysed denitration is not fully understood. Currently, it is suggested that the initial step of the reaction resembles that of the classical ALDH2 activities. The reaction mediates the production of cGMP and the relaxation of vascular smooth muscle [8,10,15].

The effects of GTN are eliminated by ALDH2 inhibition or genetic deletion of ALDH2. Thus, it is demonstrated that ALDH2 is necessary and sufficient for vasoactivity derived from therapeutic levels of GTN. Nitrite generated within the mitochondria is metabolized further to generate NO-based bioactivity by reduction to NO and/or by conversion to S-nitrosothiol [16].

However, the exact reaction mechanism of this mitochondrial NO production, as well as the form in which NO bioactivity is conveyed from mitochondria to cytosolic sGC, remain unresolved [10,15,16]. Recently, the cytosolic isoform ALDH1, was also reported to metabolize GTN to a product that activates sGC in an NO-dependent fashion [17].

This nitrate-derived NO eventually supplements endothelial production of NO. In this sense, GTN and other nitrates are endothelium-independent vasodilators that are not reliant on functioning endothelium for their vasodilator activity.

Furthermore, the mechanism of reactivation of ALDH2, following GTN bioactivation, remains unknown. Oxidative inactivation of ALDH2 after one turnover implicates that a reducing cofactor is required for continuous recycling of the active enzyme.

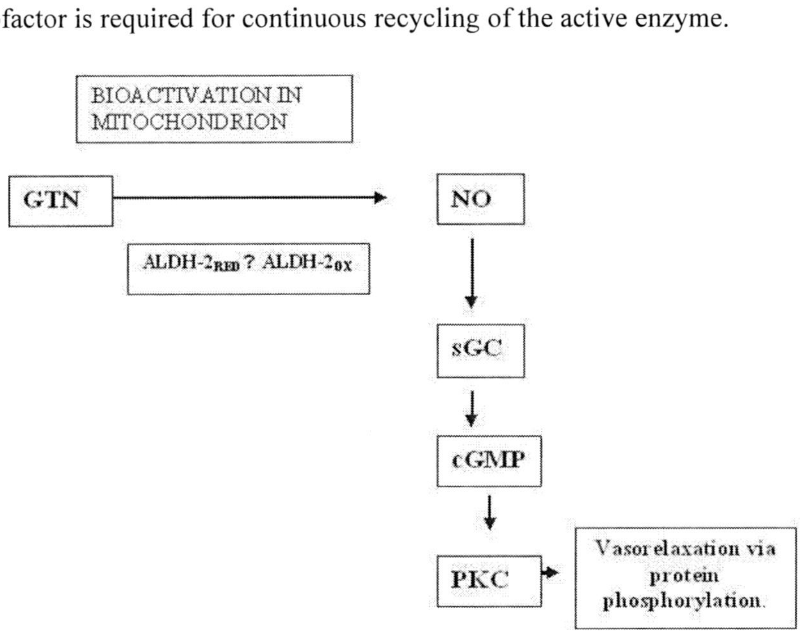

GTN: nitroglycerin; NO: nitric oxide; sGC: soluble guanylyl cyclase; cGMP: cyclic 3'5'-guanosine monophosphate; PKC: protein kinase C; ALDH2: mitochondrial isoform of aldehyde dehydrogenase

Figure 1. Bioactivation of GTN and mechanism of action.

Nitrate Tolerance

Nitrate tolerance is generally considered as a complex, presumably multifactorial, phenomenon, leading to reduced responsiveness of blood vessels to GTN and other organic nitrates or to the requirement of higher doses of these drugs.

Tolerance develops after their continuous use. Intermittent nitrate therapy allows a daily nitrate washout interval, preventing tolerance. Still, this regimen cannot provide a continuous and uninterrupted therapeutic effect [9,18].

Nitrate-induced tolerance to other endothelium dependent (e.g. acetylcholine) and endothelium-independent nitrovasodilators (e.g. nitroprusside) is termed cross-tolerance [5].

Experimental and clinical investigations suggest that nitrate tolerance is associated with the expression of potentially deleterious modifications such as increased oxidative stress, endothelial dysfunction, and sympathetic activation.

Therefore, nitrate tolerance cannot simply be viewed as a loss of the beneficial effects of nitrates but, also, as a condition, potentially, mediating extra harmful consequences [19-21].

Mechanism of Nitrate Tolerance

Despite extensive investigation, the underlying cause of nitrate tolerance has yet to be established. Recent studies indicate that stimulation of vascular production of reactive oxygen species (ROS) and inhibition of the GTN bioactivating mitochondrial enzyme ALDH2 can be considered as primary mechanisms [11].

Since 1995, it has been reported that sustained administration of GTN causes increased vascular formation of superoxide anion (O_2^-) catalysed by nicotinamide adenine dinucleotide phosphate (NADPH) oxidase [22]. Several other pathways may contribute to superoxide generation in GTN-exposed blood vessels [18].

The mitochondrial respiratory chain is the primary source of the nitrate-induced O_2^- overproduction in vessels. This overproduction overcomes the physiological scavenging mechanisms leading to a rapid reaction of the anion with NO (endothelium-produced and nitrate-derived) to form the strong oxidant peroxynitrite, a potent cellular oxidant. As a result, nitrate-derived NO bioavailability is reduced, sGC and PKC are inhibited and ALDH2 is inactivated impairing vasodilatory activity of GTN [16,23].

Interestingly, tolerance is prevented, or at least ameliorated, by co-administration of various antioxidants [5,16].

Endothelial dysfunction may be also aggravated by peroxynitrite leading to impaired endothelium-dependent vasodilation. Endothelial dysfunction may be an important deleterious complication of nitrate medication [24].

Furthermore, besides the early neuro-hormonal counter-regulatory mechanism mediated by the initial blood pressure drop, prolonged exposure to GTN has been shown to shift the physiological balance between the sympathetic and vagal nervous systems towards a prevalence of the sympathetic system, impairing baroreflex function. This autonomic dysfunction may be the result of oxidative stress [19].

Clinical Use

GTN has clear benefits for the treatment of angina pectoris, congestive heart failure, unstable angina, non-ST-segment myocardial infarction, acute myocardial infarction and variant angina due to its potent vasodilator capacities [25]. By dilation of the large coronary arteries, blood supply to the heart is improved and by venodilation, resulting in increased venous pooling, venous return and cardiac preload are reduced [26].

The reduction in preload is manifested by a decrease in cardiac chamber size, ventricular filling pressure, wall tension, and systemic blood pressure. Thus, it acutely relieves pulmonary congestion [27]. At high plasma nitrate concentrations, arteriolar vasodilation can occur, leading to increased arterial conductance and decreased peripheral vascular resistance with consequent reduction in left ventricular afterload. The effects of GTN on coronary circulation include improvement in the subendocardial/subepicardial blood flow ratio; prevention or reversal of coronary artery vasoconstriction (spontaneous or precipitated by exercise); dilatation of coronary collateral vessels [5,28].

The reduction in preload and afterload decreases cardiac work and lowers myocardial oxygen requirements. The combination of increased supply and decreased oxygen demand provides unique therapeutic benefit in cardiac ischaemia [2,26]. Though GTN and other nitrovasodilators are considered as being safe and free of serious side effects, their clinical use is limited by the phenomenon of nitrate tolerance, resulting in a complete loss of hemodynamic effects after 24–48 h of continuous application. In stable angina patients, nitrate tolerance is avoided by intermittent application of the drugs, for example, overnight removal of GTN patches [29]. However, nitrate tolerance seriously hampers continuous intravenous nitrate therapy of patients with acute heart failure, unstable angina or myocardial infarction [30, 31].

GTN in Cardiopulmonary Resuscitation

In order to enhance myocardial blood flow during CPR, the co-administration of a vasodilator, such as GTN, with one or even two vasopressors has been suggested, in animal models. The hypothesis that GTN can attenuate the untoward effects of the vasopressors without any observable harm was supported by the fact that coronary perfusion pressure (CPP), the only prognostic parameter to predict successful return of spontaneous circulation, remained significantly higher in groups of animals treated with combination regimens of vasopressor and nitroglycerin [32-36].

As a pharmacologic intervention, vasopressor agents aim to improve aortic diastolic pressure and, consequently, coronary and cerebral pressures. Epinephrine is the recommended drug for cardiac arrest. Furthermore, vasopressin seems to be a promising alternative vasopressor. The co-administration of vasopressin with epinephrine during CPR has resulted in a drastic improvement in the hemodynamic parameters necessary for the return of spontaneous circulation, in a porcine model of cardiac arrest [37].

In the doses given in CPR, epinephrine prevents arterial collapse thus increasing CPP; however, it increases myocardial oxygen consumption [38,39]. Although animal studies evaluating vital organ blood flow have indicated that vasopressin results in higher endocardial blood flow when compared with administration of epinephrine, endocardial perfusion during CPR remains suboptimal. Administration of either vasopressor agent during CPR may result in a critically decreased endocardial blood flow [40].

Vasodilator therapy with GTN may be particularly effective in a clinical setting of coronary artery disease and ischemia, which are usually present in patients suffering from cardiac arrest [35]. Still, further investigation is necessary for the administration of GTN during CPR.

Conclusion

Although clinical benefits of GTN are well established for over a century, further research is needed in order to clearly define the drug's bioactivation and mechanism of action. A major therapeutic limitation inherent to GTN is the development of tolerance which occurs during chronic treatment with this agent. The mechanisms underlying tolerance remain poorly defined, and are, likely, multifactorial. During CPR, the co-administration of a vasodilator, such as GTN, with one or even two vasopressors has been suggested. Coronary perfusion pressure in animal models of cardiac arrest remained significantly higher when they treated with a vasopressor combined with GTN. Extensive research is necessary to establish the administration of GTN during CPR.

References

[1] Murrel W. Nitro-glycerine as a remedy for angina pectoris. *Lancet* 1879;1:80-81.

[2] Harrison DG, Bates JN. The nitrovasodilators: new ideas about old drugs. *Circulation* 1993;87:1461-1467.

[3] Miller MR, Wadsworth RM. Understanding organic nitrates – a vein hope? *Br. J. Pharmacol.* 2009;157:565-567.

[4] Kleschyov AL, Oelze M, Daiber A. Does nitric oxide mediate the Vasodilator activity of nitroglycerin? *Circ. Res.* 2003;93:e104-112.

[5] Klemenska E, Beręsewicz A. Bioactivation of organic nitrates and the mechanism of nitrate tolerance. *Cardiol. J.* 2009;16:11-9.

[6] Munzel T, Feil R, Mulsch A, Lohmann SM, Hofmann F, Walter U. Physiology and pathophysiology of vascular signaling controlled by guanosine 3',5'-cyclic monophosphate-dependent protein kinase [corrected]. *Circulation* 2003;108:2172–2183.

[7] Booth BP, Tabrizi-Fard MA, Fung H. Calcitonin gene-related peptide-dependent vascular relaxation of rat aorta. An additional mechanism for nitroglycerin. *Biochem. Pharmacol.* 2000;59:1603-1609.

[8] Daiber A, Wenzel P, Oelze M, Munzel T. New insights into bioactivation of organic nitrates, nitrate tolerance and cross-tolerance. *Clin. Res. Cardiol.* 2008; 97:12–20.

[9] Fung HL. Biochemical mechanism of nitroglycerin action and tolerance: Is this old mystery solved? *Annu. Rev. Pharmacol. Toxicol.* 2004;44:67-85.

[10] Chen Z, Zhang J, Stamler JS. Identification of the enzymatic mechanism of nitroglycerin bioactivation. *Proc. Natl. Acad. Sci. USA* 2002;99:8306-8311.

[11] Daiber A, Wenzel P, Oelze M, Schuhmacher S, Jansen T, Munzel T. Mitochondrial aldehyde dehydrogenase (ALDH-2)-Maker of and marker for nitrate tolerance in response to nitroglycerin treatment. *Chem. Biol. Interact.* 2009;178:40-47.

[12] Racker E. Aldehyde dehydrogenase, a diphosphopyridine nucleotide-linked enzyme. *J. Biol. Chem.* 1949;177:883-892.

[13] Mann CJ, Weiner H. Differences in the roles of conserved glutamic acid residues in the active site of human class 3 and class 2 aldehyde dehydrogenases. *Prot. Sci.* 1999;8:1922-1929.

[14] Wymore T, Deerfield II DW, Hempel J. Mechanistic implications of the cysteine-nicotinamide adduct in aldehyde dehydrogenase based on quantum mechanical/molecular mechanical simulations. *Biochemistry* 2007;46:9495-9506.

[15] Chen Z, Foster MW, Zhang J et al. An essential role for mitochondrial aldehyde dehydrogenase in nitroglycerin bioactivation. *Proc. Natl. Acad. Sci. USA* 2005;102:12159-12164.

[16] Mayer B, Beretta M. The enigma of nitroglycerin bioactivation and nitrate tolerance: News, views and troubles. *Br. J. Pharmacol.* 2008;155:170-184.

[17] Beretta M, Gruber K, Kollau A et al. Bioactivation of nitroglycerin by purified mitochondrial and cytosolic aldehyde dehydrogenases. *J. Biol. Chem.* 2008; 283:17873-17880.

[18] Munzel T, Daiber A, Mulsch A. Explaining the phenomenon of nitrate tolerance. *Circ. Res.* 2005;97:618-628.

[19] Gori T, Floras JS, Parker JD. Effects of nitroglycerin treatment on baroreflex sensitivity and short-term heart rate variability in humans. *J. Am. Coll. Cardiol.* 2002;40:2000-2005.

[20] Gori T, Parker JD. The puzzle of nitrate tolerance: Pieces smaller than we thought? *Circulation* 2002;106:2404-2408.

[21] Gori T, Parker JD. Nitrate-induced toxicity and preconditioning: A rationale for reconsidering the use of these drugs. *J. Am. Coll. Cardiol.* 2008;52:251-254.

[22] Munzel T, Sayegh H, Freeman BA, Tarpey MM, Harrison DG. Evidence for enhanced vascular superoxide production in nitrate tolerance. A novel mechanism underlying tolerance and cross-tolerance. *J. Clin. Invest.* 1995;95: 187-194.

[23] Daiber A, Mulsch A, Hink U, et al. The oxidative stress concept of nitrate tolerance and the antioxidant properties of hydralazine. *Am. J. Cardiol.* 2005;96: 25I-36I.

[24] Schulz E, Jansen T, Wenzel P, Daiber A, Münzel T. Nitric oxide, tetrahydrobiopterin, oxidative stress, and endothelial dysfunction in hypertension. *Antiox. Redox. Signal.* 2008;10:1115-1126.

[25] Brunton LL, Lazo JS, Parker KL. Goodman and Gilman's *The Pharmacological Basis of Therapeutics*, 11th ed. New York: McGraw-Hill; 2006.

[26] Bode-Boger SM, Kojda G. Organic nitrates in cardiovascular disease. *Cell Mol. Biol. (Noisy-le-grand)* 2005;51:307-320.

[27] Steven M. Hollenberg Vasodilators in acute heart failure *Heart Fail Rev.* 2007; 12:143-147.

[28] Duncker DJ, Bache RJ. Regulation of coronary blood flow during exercise. *Physiol. Rev.* 2008;88:1009-1086.

[29] Abrams J. How to use nitrates. *Cardiovasc. Drugs Ther*. 2002;16:511-514.

[30] Thadani U. Nitrate tolerance, rebound, and their clinical relevance in stable angina pectoris, unstable angina, and heart failure. *Cardiovasc. Drugs Ther.* 1997;10:735-742.

[31] Elkayam U, Bitar F, Akhter MW, Khan S, Patrus S, Derakhshani M. Intravenous nitroglycerin in the treatment of decompensated heart failure: potential benefits and limitations. *J. Cardiovasc. Pharmacol. Ther.* 2004;9:227-241.

[32] Wenzel V, Lindner KH, Mayer H, Lurie KG, Prengel AW. Vasopressin combined with nitroglycerin increases endocardial perfusion during cardiopulmonary resuscitation in pigs. *Resuscitation* 1998;38:13-17.

[33] Kono S, Suzuki A, Obata Y, Igarashi H, Bito H, Sato S. Vasopressin with delayed combination of nitroglycerin increases survival rate in asphyxia rat model. *Resuscitation* 2002;54:297-301.

[34] Lurie KG, Voeckel WG, Iskos DN, McKnite SH, Zielinski TM, Sugiyama A. Combination drug therapy with vasopressin, adrenaline (epinephrine) and nitroglycerin improves vital organ blood flow in a porcine model of ventricular fibrillation. *Resuscitation* 2002;54:187-194.

[35] Kitsou V, Xanthos T, Stroumpoulis K, et al. Nitroglycerin and Epinephrine Improve Coronary Perfusion Pressure in a Porcine Model of Ventricular Fibrillation Arrest: A Pilot Study. *J. Emerg. Med.* 2009;37:369-375.

[36] Paradis NA, Martin GP, Rivers EP, et al. Coronary perfusion pressure and the return of spontaneous circulation in human cardiopulmonary resuscitation. *JAMA* 1990;263:1106-1113.

[37] Stroumpoulis K, Xanthos T, Rokas G, et al. Vasopressin and epinephrine in the treatment of cardiac arrest: an experimental study *Crit. Care*. 2008;12:R40.

[38] Grmec S, Mally S. Vasopressin improves outcome in out-ofhospital cardiopulmonary resuscitation of ventricular fibrillation and pulseless ventricular tachycardia: an observational cohort study. *Crit. Care.* 2006;10:R13.

[39] Varon J, Manik PE, Fronn RE Jr. Cardiopulmonary resuscitation: a review for clinicians. *Resuscitation* 1998;36:133-145.

[40] Lindner KH, Prengel AW, Pfenninger EG, et al. Vasopressin improves vital organ blood flow during closed-chest cardiopulmonary resuscitation in pigs. *Circulation* 1995;91:215-221.

In: Drugs in Cardiopulmonary Resuscitation
Editor: Theodoros Xanthos
ISBN: 978-1-61122-512-9

Chapter 10

Adenosine: Advanced Pharmacology, Basic Research and Clinical Aspects

Argyrios Krommidas, Evangelia Kouskouni and Theodoros Xanthos

Abstract

This chapter discusses the broad spectrum of clinical usage, diagnostic applications, experimental challenges and future perspectives of adenosine.

Adenosine, an adenylic nucleotide metabolite, widely distributed throughout the human body, exerts a wide range of regulatory effects.

From a cardiovascular perspective, data indicate that the adenosinergic system is important in mediating protection (e.g. via pre- and post-conditioning) and in determining myocardial resistance to insult or to reperfusion-ischemia injury.

Besides, adenosine exerts its effects through currently four known adenosine receptor (AR) subtypes namely A_1R, $A_{2A}R$, $A_{2B}R$ and A_3R. In general, $A_{2A}R$ is the predominant receptor subtype responsible for coronary blood flow regulation, which dilates coronary arteries. Interestingly, adenosine exerts its cardiac electrophysiologic effects via A_1R (e.g. anti-b-adrenergic action).

Regarding the supraventricular tissues, adenosine remains as a "first line" pharmacologic agent for the treatment of supraventricular arrhythmias, due to its effect on inhibiting rapidly the atrioventricular (AV) nodal conduction.

In addition to its clinical role as an antiarrhythmic agent, adenosine has been also administered under conditions of hypoxia, ischemia, and cardiac arrest. Thus, basic research has implicated adenosine as an endogenous distress molecule with essential impact on immune response, adaptation to limited oxygen availability, anti-inflammatory action.

Specific AR agonists or antagonists in conjunction with studies in genetic models for adenosine generation have identified a rapidly expanding field of biomedical roles and potential therapeutic applications of extracellular adenosine signaling.

Introduction

Adenosine is a natural compound in the human body, belonging to the molecular group of nucleosides. It is composed of a nitrogenous base of the purine class called adenine, which is attached to D-ribose - a pentose. This nucleobase is involved in many biological functions such as protein biosynthesis or cellular energy metabolism. It has also been shown to have a broad spectrum of physiological effects, which makes it effective as a cardioprotective agent.

1. Pharmacology

Extracellular adenosine functions as a signaling molecule through the activation of ARs on the extracellular surface of cell membranes. Especially during conditions of cellular distress (acute injury, hypoxia, inflammation), extracellular adenosine stems from phosphor-ester hydrolysis of its precursor molecules, adenosine-5'-triphosphate (ATP), 5'-adenosine diphosphate (ADP), or 5'-adenosine monophosphate (AMP) [1]. These nucleotides consist of adenosine, bound to a varying number of phosphor-esters attached to the 5'-designated atom of its ribose sugar ring [2]. Most cell types express enzymes on their cell surface that catalyze nucleotide-phospho-hydrolyzes via a three-step reaction. First, several cell types release intra-cellular stored nucleotides, mainly in the form of ATP and ADP [1,3,4]. This usually takes place during cellular damage or death (necrosis, lysis, apoptosis) or via specific gradient-driven channels [5,6]. An additional source of extracellular nucleotides comes from activated platelets that release ADP from stored intracellular vesicles through granular release [7]. Then extracellular ATP and ADP are rapidly converted to AMP by CD39, a surface-bound enzyme expressed on multiple cell types [8]. CD39 is responsible for extracellular adenosine production by generation of AMP and at the same time catalyzes the key step for extracellular breakdown of ATP and ADP, which are both important molecules, especially during thrombosis or inflammation [9,10]. The final step in extracellular adenosine generation is the rapid conversion of extracellular AMP to adenosine by CD73, a membrane-bound glycoprotein [2]. In conclusion, extracellular adenosine mainly stems from phosphor-hydrolysis of precursor nucleotides, a metabolic pathway which depends on the transcriptionally controlled enzymes (CD39 and CD73) [2].

1.1. Adenosine Receptors

There are four ARs: A_1R, $A_{2A}R$, $A_{2B}R$ and A_3R, two of which are involved in the cyclic AMP system. Thus, the A_1R inhibits the production of cyclic AMP, whereas the A_2R stimulates the formation of cyclic AMP [11].

1.1.a. A_1Rs

A_1 receptors have been located on neutrophils and myocytes. Their function is achieved by ATP sensitive potassium (K_{ATP}) channels activation through the inhibitory G-protein. As a result, the adenyl cyclase activity is reduced and the potassium outward conductance is stimulated. Moreover, the activation of K_{ATP} channels causes hyperpolarization and inhibits calcium (Ca^{2+}) conductance. At the level of physiology, the stimulation of the A_1R leads to negative chronotropy, dromotropy and antiadrenergic effects. On the other hand, neutrophil adherence and glycolysis are stimulated.

In addition, the A_1R activation offers myocardial protection by preserving ATP (improving nucleotide repletion on reperfusion) and by normalizing the `supply/demand ratio', mainly by limiting demand [12]. In fact, the A_1R is the most extensively adenosine receptor subtype studied within the context of cardiac protection. Specifically, exogenous or endogenous activation of myocardial A_1R protects the heart from injury during global ischemia [13] and ameliorates bio-energetic and mechanical recovery in reperfused myocardium [14-17]. Due to the fact that adenosine is actively produced from the degradation of ATP during ischemia, it is suggested that it plays a role in ischemic preconditioning.

Preconditioning, described for the first time by Murry *et al.* [18], is defined as an adaptation of the myocardium to the ischemic stress induced by short periods of ischemia, before a longer period of ischemia. This is the most powerful mechanism known to limit the infract size. This adaptation occurs in a biphasic pattern:

(a) early preconditioning (lasts for 2-3 h), and
(b) late preconditioning (starting at 24 h lasting until 72-96 h after initial ischemia) [19].

It is believed, that adenosine along with protein kinase C (PKC) and K_{ATP} channels, serve as important mediators of ischemic preconditioning in a range of species [20,21] Thus, a brief ischemic insult followed by reperfusion, generates endogenous adenosine, which in turn activates ARs. The activated ARs couple with G proteins and activate PKC, which opens the K_{ATP} channels [22]. Then, there is an efflux of potassium from cells during repolarization [23,24], which decreases the duration of the myocardial action potential and the time available for voltage-dependent Ca^{2+} influx [24].

Therefore, increases of intracellular Ca^{2+} are prevented, myocardial ATP concentrations are preserved and the myocytes are better protected during a subsequent ischemic insult. In addition, there are data indicating that, pentazocine, a non selective δ-opiod receptor agonist, improves postresuscitation myocardial dysfunction along with the duration of survival via opening K_{ATP} channels [25]. Although there is evidence supporting that more than one of the four ARs subtypes promote myocardial protection, it seems that the A_1R is of main importance concerning ischemic preconditioning [26].

However, there is conflicting evidence regarding A_1R involvement in ischemic preconditioning (IPC) in some species. For example, studies in rat myocardium acquired evidence against an essential role for adenosine in preconditioning in rats [27,28]. Also, Auchampach [29] suggested that A_1R blockade does not modify protection with multiple cycle IPC in canine hearts, although the author had previously indicated a role for A_1R with single cycle IPC in dogs [30].

Finally, de Jong *et al.* revealed the involvement of the A_1R [31] and the previous notions, which had supported that adenosine was not involved in preconditioning of rat myocardium, have generally been disregarded. This is further accentuated, as shown from recent studies, which demonstrate inhibition of remote preconditioning in A_1R knockout mice [32,33].

Taken together, adenosine and A_1Rs are essential in mediating cardiac protection with both intrinsic and remote preconditioning in multiple species [34]. Furthermore, adenosine can also induce late or delayed preconditioning (the so-called second window of protection) [35,36], where ischemia in another organ (e.g. brain) leads to cardioprotection [37]. Late preconditioning is triggered by a similar sequence of events, attenuates myocardial stunning, but in addition, depends also on newly synthesized proteins, which include inducible nitric oxide synthase (iNOS), cyclooxygenase-2 (COX-2), manganese superoxide dismutase, and possibly heat shock proteins [19].

There is also controversy regarding the involvement of iNOS in adenosine-dependent delayed preconditioning [35,36], at least between different animal models (mouse vs. rat). Several data claim that iNOS acts as a powerful, cardioprotective mediator required for the response of the heart to stress [38], while others report that iNOS has no role in mediating adenosine A_1 receptor delayed preconditioning in rat myocardium [39].

Currently, the effects of IPC are generally well recognized, and as result, the infarct-reducing effect is observed irrespective of animal species - rats [40,41], rabbits [42,43], dogs [44,45], pigs [46,47] -. Nonetheless, resistance to ischemia has been also proved in isolated human myocardium [48]. It has also been demonstrated that drug-induced delayed cardiac protection operates in rabbits with hypercholesterolaemia and atherosclerosis [49], and thus, it is effective even under pathological conditions.

Another interesting finding is that phosphodiesterase-5 (PDE-5) inhibitors such as sildenafil and vardenafil, which have been used to treat erectile dysfunction [50] and pulmonary artery hypertension [51], have provided cardioprotection against ischemia-reperfusion injury to the rabbit [52]. It is suggested, that sildenafil can result in increased release of adenosine, via generation of nitric oxide (NO), which activates the A_1R and leads to a subsequent protection from ischemia-reperfusion injury 24 hours later [53].

The A_1R activation contributes to the protection of other tissues from ischemic injury [54,55]. There are some models which link A_1R agonism to several kinase systems such as PKC, MAPKs (mitogen-activated protein kinases), P13-kinase, Akt [56,57]. These paths may be involved in parallel with mitochondrial targets, such as the mitochondrial permeability transition pore (mPTP) [58] and the mitochondrial K_{ATP} channel [59]. However, specific kinase involvement remains controversial [34]. In this respect, prior studies point K_{ATP} channels and PKC as mediators to acute AR protection [60], consistent with parallel signaling paths.

Undoubtedly, the work of Germack in isolated cardiomyocytes shows, that although A_1Rs stimulate both Akt and Erk1/2 (extracellular signal-regulated kinase), yet only Erk1/2 is involved in cardiac protection [61]. In addition, there is evidence concerning MAPK involvement in A_1R protection. A p38 MAPK pathway has also been found as a potential mediator of acute A_1R mediated protection in the *in vivo* porcine myocardium [62].

There are also numerous studies indicating that ischemia can cause major shifts in localization and activity of MAPKs and these stimuli can generate different response profiles [63,64]. In parallel, research showed that the protective actions of adenosine are partly mediated via sarcolemmal, as opposed to mitochondrial channels [65].

Finally, regarding the functional effects of myocardial A_1Rs overexpression, it probably leads to a reduction in heart rate, whereas contractile function and coronary resistance remain unchanged [66]. A possible explanation about the existence of several studies with conflicting data regarding the ability of exogenous adenosinergic therapy to reduce injury during ischemia-reperfusion, is that the lack of such response to an exogenous adenosine receptor agonist may reflect maximal endogenous activity [67].

In conclusion, the activation of endogenous adenosine ameliorates contractile recovery mainly through amelioration of post-ischemic diastolic dysfunction [66]. Post-ischemic elevation in diastolic tension possibly reflects altered Ca^{2+} with enhanced diastolic Ca^{2+} [68]. Thus, increased expression of cardiac A_1Rs appears beneficial during ischemia [66]. On the other hand, chronically increased receptors may be counterproductive in states which require maximal cardiac output such as shock [66].

1.1.b. A_{2A}Rs

There is lots of evidence suggesting that A_{2A}Rs play a pivotal role regarding adenosine-mediated inhibition of tissue ischemia reperfusion injury [69]. A_{2A}Rs are found on platelets, vascular smooth muscle, endothelial cells, and neutrophils [70]. Thus, the A_{2A}-mediated inhibition of tissue ischemia-reperfusion injury has also been documented in several organs, including the liver, lung, kidney and heart [71-75]. In addition, A_{2A}Rs regulate the inflammatory/immune processes in a variety of organs and cells [76].

Inflammation has a profound role in both the early and late aspects of injury and remodeling with ischemia-reperfusion. Therefore, it seems possible that the activation of the A_{2A}Rs is protective in this setting. The mechanisms involved in A_{2A}-dependent cardioprotection include inhibition of leukocyte-dependent inflammatory process [77], vasodilatation [78], effects on organ parenchymal cells [79] and likely a direct inotropic action [80], which seems selective for post-ischemic tissue [75]. Several experimental studies [81] show enhanced vasodilatation with A_{2A} agonism during reperfusion. Nevertheless, due to species differences, this usually takes place in guinea-pig, pig and murine hearts [82].

Taken together, an A_{2A} dependent reduction in ischemia-reperfusion injury has been confirmed *in vivo* [72], in agreement with data that A_{2A}Rs can attenuate the injurious effects of neutrophil activation and proapoptotic signaling [83]. However, there is evidence indicating that this subtype does not have "direct" protection *in vitro* in the absence of circulating blood cells [17]. The beneficial effect on A_{2A} activation against myocardial ischemia-reperfusion injury has also been documented in intact animal models [72] and in several *ex vivo* experiments [79].

In addition, there is evidence that A_{2A} activation can modify myocardial contractile outcomes [81]. For example, immediately after a large myocardial infarction (MI), regional contractile dysfunction develops, not only at the infarct site, but also in non ischemic regions of the left ventricle (LV) remote from the infracted area. This remote LV dysfunction has been documented in patients shortly after reperfused MI [84] and also in canines [85], sheep [86] and rodents [87].

Therefore, specific stimulation of A_{2A}Rs significantly improved global LV function after a large transmural MI, by preventing contractile dysfunction that normally afflicts non-infarcted regions of myocardium [88]. The protective effects of A_{2A} stimulation were also associated with an inhibition of myocardial NF-κB (nuclear factor kappa-light-chain enhancer of activated B cells) and of myocardial iNOS, which contribute to myocardial injury and dysfunction in a variety of clinical settings [89].

On the other hand, Linden and colleagues found that the infarct-sparing actions of A_{2A}Rs agonism are mediated solely through regulation of bone marrow-derived cells [90] identified as CD4+ T lymphocytes [91]. Thus, agonism of A_{2A}Rs on CD4+ T lymphocytes lowers the accumulation of such cells and of neutrophils in ischemic tissue, hinders interferon-gamma (IFNγ) release and as a result, reduces infarct development [91]. Therefore, the A_{2A}-dependent inhibition of vascular-neutrophils interactions and apoptotic signaling modifies CD4+ T lymphocyte functionality [83]. This is of vital importance, due to the fact, that leukocytes are the main effector cells of reperfusion injury, according to data obtained from both animals and clinical studies [92].

Reperfusion causes a vigorous inflammatory response and a dramatic augmentation in neutrophil adherence to the reperfused endothelium leading to edema, capillary plugging and to a limitation in coronary blood flow [92]. Another crucial finding is that the administration of a specific A_{2A}R agonist dramatically attenuated inflammatory responses [93] and appeared to be an elegant therapeutic approach in ventilator-induced lung injury (VILI) [94]. Vinten-Johansen and colleagues have also found a protective part for the A_{2A}R in post-conditioning [95], both in the presence and absence of blood cells [90].

Post-conditioning is a term first used by Vinten-Johansen and colleagues describing a form of graded reperfusion which has similarities with IPC [96]. Thus, ischemic post-conditioning involves brief episodes of ischemia-reperfusion immediately following an index ischemia, which leads to reductions in MI, stunning, and apoptosis [34]. It is shown, that mitochondrial K_{ATP} channels and PKC are also involved in post-conditioning cardioprotection [97]. In addition, post-conditioning protects against infarct size extension without significantly increasing or reducing the developed post-ischemic ventricular pressure in rabbits [98].

Additionally, evidence suggests that A_{2A} and/or A_{2B}Rs are essential for expression of cardioprotection with pre-ischemic A_1 agonism [99]. The exact finding was that A_{2A} /A_{2B} antagonism blocks cardioprotection triggered by an A_1 agonist in the *in situ* rat heart, despite the absence of protective effects of A_{2A} agonism alone, suggesting that A_1R protection is partly dependent on A_2Rs. Another interesting finding is that the A_{2A}Rs have also been implicated in promotion of angiogenesis, which may have salutary effects on post-ischemia remodeling and possibly facilitate recovery [100].

1.1.c. A_{2B}Rs

The A_{2b}R is even less well studied than A_{2A}Rs at least in the field of myocardial ischemia-reperfusion. In particular, there is no "direct" evidence of ventricular myocyte A_{2B} expression [34]. Although the A_{2B}R is known to activate angiogenic factors [101] and enhance coronary endothelial growth [102], it also impairs neovascularization in non cardiac tissues [103]. Thus, it has an essential role in modulating vascular growth and tissue remodeling [34].

Moreover, the expression of A_{2B}Rs in cardiac fibroblasts results in anti-fibrotic and anti-proliferative actions [104], dictating the progression of post-ischemic alterations in myocardial phenotype, promoting angiogenic growth, reducing fibrosis and modulating post-ischemic remodeling [105]. In addition, the A_{2B}R contributes to the infarct-sparing effects of post-conditioning in the rabbit myocardium [106]. There is also data showing a beneficial effect of $A_{2B}R$ in preconditioning [107] and in cardioprotection via A_1R agonism [99].

However, there is low sensitivity between adenosine and $A_{2B}R$, a fact which limits the activation of $A_{2B}R$ only to periods of excessive extracellular adenosine accumulation [34]. Finally, a new role for the $A_{2B}R$ has recently been published. It has been found that the A_{2B} modulates platelet function beyond mediating the immediate effect of adenosine on aggregation [108]. It has also been demonstrated that the platelet $A_{2B}R$ is up-regulated *in vivo* under stress, and, thus, controls ADP receptor expression and inhibits agonist-induced platelet aggregation [108].

1.1.d. A_3Rs

The A_3R is the only adenosine subtype which has been cloned, before its pharmacological identification [109]. It has been mapped on the human chromosome 1p21-p13 [110] and consists of 318 amino-acid residues. The A_3R is a G-protein-coupled receptor (GPCR) characterized by a C-terminal region and 7 trans-membrane domains. This C-terminal region is important for the rapid receptor desensitization upon agonist application [111].

The A_3R is widely expressed in various organs such as kidneys, placenta, brain, heart, testis, lung, spleen, bladder, liver and uterus [112-114]. In cardiomyocytes, there was no direct evidence of the presence of A_3R [34], but, according to many studies, A_3R is cardioprotective in a variety of species included isolated human cardiomyocytes [115-117].

The main pathways associated with A_3R activation are the inhibition of the adenyl cyclase activity via the coupling with Gi proteins and the stimulation of phospholipase C (PLC), inositol triphosphate (IP3) and intracellular Ca^{2+}, through Gq proteins [118]. Moreover, additional intracellular pathways have been described explaining the cardioprotective effects of A_3Rs through K_{ATP} channel activation [109].

In addition, a subsequent stimulation of phospholipase D (PLD) mediates protection of cardiac myocytes from ischemia [119]. Therefore, the protection through this subtype shares some similarities with the A_1R such as the involvement of PKC, Akt/p13-kinase, ERK, and MAPK. All these molecular signals contribute to the cardioprotection induced by ischemic preconditioning [59]. Specifically, the activation of the A_3R not only offers acute protection, but more sustained preconditioning effects [34].

Thus, the first selective adenosine A_3 receptor agonist, IB-MECA, induces cardioprotection against myocardial ischemia/reperfusion injury, when given before onset of ischemia, by triggering pharmacological preconditioning [116]. Moreover, IB-MECA improves cardiac contractile function, reduces apoptosis [120] and protects the heart by minimizing either stunning or necrosis, both *in vitro* and *in vivo* [116].

These data suggest that IB-MECA given at reperfusion (or re-oxygenation) prevented stunning in guinea pig myocardium by reducing reperfusion injury, infarct size and maintaining the heart in a sustained defensive state [121]. Other beneficial effects of IB-MECA in the heart include the protection against other types of stress-induced cardiac damage, angiotensin II apoptosis, doxorubicin-induced cardiotoxicity and the blockade of phenylephrine-induced hypertrophy [122].

On the other hand, the activation of A_3R induces hypotension in rats by promoting degranulation of mast cells [123], whereas cardiac-specific over-expression of the A_3R leads to decreased basal heart rate and contractility, short-term ischemic ATP preservation and protection from post-ischemic contractile and energetic dysfunction [124].

Considerable interest has also been shown concerning the involvement of A_3R in normal and pathological conditions of the central nervous system (CNS), despite its low expression in the brain. One of the main factors contributing to the overall neuroprotective profile of chronic treatment with A_3R agonists is believed to be the reduction in post-ischemic expression of NO synthase, the enzyme involved in NO generation [125].

Different evidences reported that a part of neuroprotection induced by A_3R is due to its modulation of the brain immune system [126]. Data suggest that functional A_3R are expressed in mouse microglia cells and that their activation produces a biphasic effect on ERK1/2 phosphorylation [127] and in murine astrocytes, where A_3R stimulation prompts the release of the neuroprotective chemokine CCL2 [128]. In conclusion, extracellular adenosine serves as a signaling molecule which can activate any of four G-protein coupled receptors [129]. A_1 and A_3 are primarily coupled to Gi family G proteins and A_{2A} and A_{2B} are mostly coupled to Gs like G proteins [129].

It seems that higher adenosine concentrations are required for the activation of the $A_{2B}R$, compared with the other three receptors, and that are mainly achieved under pathophysiological conditions (inflammation, hypoxia, ischemia) [94,129].

As biologic functions caused by adenosine signaling, depend on the adenosine concentrations at the cell surface, various other factors, such as the functionality of the intracellular signaling pathways, coupled to adenosine receptors, and the density of the receptors are important determinants of signaling effects [130]. AR signaling occurs via the alterations in adenylyl cyclase activity, resulting in subsequent changes of intracellular cAMP levels as second messenger [129].

Examples of typical physiologic responses associated with the activation of individual ARs include adenosine-mediated bradycardia through stimulation of the A_1R [131], arterial vasodilatation or inhibition of platelet aggregation through activation of the $A_{2A}R$ [132], ischemic preconditioning of different organs via stimulation of the $A_{2B}Rs$ [133], or rodent mast cell degranulation via A_3R-dependent attenuation of intracellular cAMP concentrations [134].

2. Demand/Supply Oxygen Ratio Mediated by Adenosine

2.1. Vascular Reactivity

Adenosine is believed to be an important mediator of the adaptation blood flow to metabolic demand. Vasodilatation is the common response to adenosine with the exception of the afferent arterioles of the kidney, which respond with contraction to adenosine coming from the interstitium [132], via A_1Rs. Besides, there are data supporting that A_{2A} and A_{2B} receptors also regulate vascular reactivity. For example, $A_{2A}Rs$ regulate local blood flow by reducing platelet aggregation [135].

2.2. Cell Work

Adenosine can both indirectly and directly reduce cellular workload. More specifically, tubular transport work is decreased via an A_1R-mediated reduction in renal blood flow [129]. Respectively, adenosine acts directly on the nervous system through A_1Rs, by hindering the release of excitatory neurotransmitters and by hyperpolarizing the nerves, resulting in decreased rates of firing [136]. Furthermore, adenosine, via A_1Rs, limits epileptic seizures and seizure-dependent cell death [137].

2.3. Temperature Regulation

There is interesting evidence suggesting that central temperature control plays a profound role on the organism expected life span [138]. It is possible that adenosine A_1R activation is one of the most efficient means of lowering the body temperature [139] and that mice lacking A_1Rs have elevated body temperatures and reduced survival [140].

2.4. Adaptation to Hypoxia

Adenosine is also essential in the adaptive changes in circulation and respiration triggered, by hypoxia sensing cells in the carotid body; for example $A_{2A}Rs$ are found in type I cells of the carotid body. During acute hypoxia, respiratory stimulation is mediated by these receptors which also appear to interact with dopamine D_2 receptors [141]. Therefore, the increased firing in the afferent nerves from the carotid body stimulates respiration, and increases blood pressure [129].

2.5. Angiogenesis

There are many studies demonstrating that adenosine also serves by enhancing vascular growth in areas with reduced oxygen tension [142]. In addition, adenosine may stimulate the expression of the vascular endothelial growth factor (VEGF) in many cell types [142], mainly via A_{2A} and A_{2B} receptors. Besides, angiogenesis contributes to brain repair after stroke and, therefore, angiogenic factors such as adenosine and VEGF [143] may be useful in therapy. Thus, adenosine in physiologically relevant concentrations can stimulate migration and proliferation of endothelial cells [129].

2.6. Immune System

It is known, that many of the cells of the immune system, have lots of adenosine receptors and that endogenous adenosine influences their function [76]. Adenosine and the precursor ATP control neutrophil function which plays a major role as the first line defense against pathogens. All four ARs are expressed. More specifically, A_1Rs have been shown to enhance adhesion, $A_{2A}Rs$ regulate some of the surface molecules on neutrophils, $A_{2B}Rs$

maintain a barrier to leukocyte migration and A_3Rs also mediate the migration of the neutrophil leukocytes [5]. Thus, during hypoxia, adenosine provides an essential signal to limit excessive infiltration of neutrophils and subsequent tissue damage [144].

Additionally, there is strong evidence involving adenosine in monocyte-macrophage-microglial cell function [129]. Although some reports have often conflicting data due to differences among species, it is clear that the migration of monocytes into tissues is decreased via A_{2A}Rs [145]. For example, in mice lacking CD73, and thus having low adenosine levels, macrophage levels in tissues are increased after any inflammatory insult [146].

Furthermore, ARs are found also in T lymphocytes and thus adenosine can regulate several lymphocyte functions, despite the fact that A_1Rs' expression is low [145]. On the other hand, A_{2A}Rs significantly decrease the T cell-mediated inflammatory response in a variety of tissues [147] and A_{2B}Rs also contribute to that.

Finally, both adenosine and ATP seem to influence dendritic cells [145]. There is recent data suggesting, that a novel type of dendritic cell, the interferon-producing killer dendritic cell, is of major importance regarding tumor immuno-surveillance, but so far, little is known about the role of ARs in regulating the processing of antigen and its presentation [129].

3. Adenosine Metabolism

The biotransformation of adenosine is very rapid and is done by circulating enzymes in vascular endothelial cells and in erythrocytes [148], with two means; firstly, by deamination, primarily to inactive inosine (which is further degraded to hypoxanthine and then to uric acid) [149] and, secondly, by phosphorylation to AMP [148]. Thus, the half life of adenosine is less than 10 seconds [148].

3.1.a. Extracellular Adenosine Uptake

The main mechanism for the fast decline of vascular adenosine levels after intravenous injection is adenosine uptake from the extracellular to the intracellular compartment [150], followed by fast intracellular metabolism through the adenosine deaminase (conversion to inosine) or adenosine kinase (conversion to AMP) [151]. Adenosine can cross the cell membrane via equilibrative nucleotide transporters such as ENT_1 and ENT_2 [150]. These transporters represent diffusion-limited channels that allow adenosine to freely traverse the cell membrane after a concentration gradient [150].

Under normal circumstances, the net flow through ENTs is very small [150], due to the fact that there are only minimal differences between intra- and extracellular adenosine concentrations. On the other hand, extracellular adenosine concentrations augment substantially after intravenous bolus application of adenosine and the flow via ENTs is directed from the extracellular to the intracellular space, resulting in rapid adenosine uptake [2]. ENTs are widely expressed, including erythrocytes, epithelial, vascular endothelial or inflammatory cells [2].

Under injurious conditions, such as ischemia, inflammation, hypoxia, in which adenosine levels rise, there are similar transport phenomena, which direct adenosine transport via ENTs, towards the intracellular space [2]. This is the reason for the prolonged actions of extracellular adenosine after pharmacological inhibition of adenosine transporters (e.g. with dipyridamole) [150].

3.1.b. Intracellular Adenosine Metabolism

There are two alternative pathways resulting in the rapid metabolization of adenosine in the intracellular compartment. The first is the conversion of adenosine to inosine via the enzymatic activity of the adenosine deaminase [152] and the second the conversion of adenosine to AMP by adenosine kinase [151]. Therefore, inhibition of adenosine kinase increases extracellular adenosine signaling, leading to attenuation of the detrimental effects of hypoxia or ischemia [151]. Similarly genetic deletion of the adenosine deaminase in mice results in dramatic high extracellular adenosine levels leading to pulmonary adenosine toxicity [152].

3.2. Adenosine and the Aged Heart

Advancing age is associated with decreased myocardial resistance to ischemic insult, in humans and animals models [153]. Besides, aging is linked with a loss in preconditioning "potential" [153], whereas the adenosine-mediated protection is also decreased or lost with age [154]. The mechanism explaining the loss of the protective responses may involve changes or defects in receptor-coupled signaling cascades [155,156].

Further abnormalities in post-receptor signaling lead to the loss of adenosine-mediated protection with senescence, whereas the functionality of ARs does not seem to contribute to that [156]. Several studies report the maintenance of A_1Rs functionality with age, implying a malfunction in downstream protective signaling with age [154], such as the loss of adenosine-mediated NO release in the aged heart, where NO is involved in acute and delayed preconditioning responses [157]. Thus, the protective function of adenosine in aged hearts remains controversial [34].

4. Electrophysiology

4.1. Negative Chronotropic Action

Adenosine suppresses the activity of cardiac pacemakers including the sinus node (SN), AV junction and the His-Purkinje system. This action is mediated via A_1Rs and with the activation of a potassium outward current (IK^+Ado). In addition, the inward Ca^{2+} current (ICa^{2+}) and the hyper-polarization-activated current (If) are suppressed. It is also known, that nor-epinephrine shifts the activation curve of If to the right and enhances ICa^{2+} [158]. Thus, this anti-adrenergic role of adenosine contributes to its negative chronotropic effects. Moreover, the over-expression of A_1R results in a 20-fold rise in the potency of 2-chloroadenosine in slowing heart rate and in a 35% decrease in maximal heart rate induced by d-adrenoceptor stimulation [159]. It is also associated with reduced positive chronotropic response to exercise with minimal effect on the resting heart rate [160].

On the other hand, over-expression of A_3Rs leads to decreased heart rate, mainly at rest [161]. Therefore, the prime mechanism for the negative chronotropic action of adenosine and its anti-b-adrenergic effects is mediated by A_1Rs.

4.2. Negative Dromotropic Action

Adenosine prolongs the PR and AH intervals without affecting HV interval and can cause complete AV nodal conduction block. It has been demonstrated, that adenosine mediates hypoxia-ischemia-induced AV nodal conduction block, hyperpolarizes cell membrane potential, shortens action potential duration, slows the recovery of ICa^{2+} and prolongs post-repolarization refractoriness in isolated single AV nodal cells. Thus, the main dromotropic effects of adenosine involve the AV node and are mediated by A_1Rs.

4.3. Atrial and Ventricular Myocardium

The activation of IK^+Ado in atrial myocytes via the A_1Rs explains the direct and indirect anti-b-adrenergic effects of adenosine. Hove-Madsen *et al.* [162] have shown that $A_{2A}R$ is expressed in the human right atrium and distributed in a banded pattern along the Z lines, overlapping with the ryanodine receptor, suggesting that the activation of $A_{2A}R$ stimulates the ryanodine receptor itself [162].

On the contrary, adenosine does not directly affect ventricular myocytes, although it exerts pronounced anti-b-adrenergic effects in the ventricular myocardium. This is mediated via A_1Rs and by the subsequent decrease of intracellular levels of cAMP. Adenosine lessens the catecholamine-dependent rise in inward L-type Ca^{2+} current ($ICa^{2+}L$), the delayed rectifier potassium current and chloride current (ICl), and attenuates the transient inward current (Iti)-dependent after-depolarizations and triggered activity [163].

Moreover, adenosine terminated episodes of ventricular tachycardia (VT) and abolished the delayed after-depolarizations (DAD) associated with digoxin toxicity in the guinea-pig and canine heart [164]. Thus, according to several reports adenosine, by its anti-b-adrenergic action [164]. can exert an antiarrhythmic effect in the setting of catecholamine/cAMP dependent VTs.

5. Clinical Indications

5.1.a. Supraventricular Tachycardias

Adenosine was introduced into the American clinical setting in 1989 as an antiarrhythmic drug for the immediate termination of reentrant paroxysmal supra-ventricular tachycardia (PSVT) involving the AV node - AV reentrant tachycardia (AVRT), AV nodal re-entrant tachycardia (AVNRT) -. Adenosine, by binding to its receptor in the AV node, can sufficiently slow conduction to break the circuit which causes the tachycardia. In about 10% of supra-ventricular tachycardia (SVT) not involving AV nodal reentry, adenosine will slow AV nodal conduction, reduce the ventricular rate and unmask P waves (e.g. atrial flutter) [165].

Adenosine has an indirect effect on atrial tissue by shortening the refractory period. When administered through a central lumen catheter, adenosine has been shown to initiate atrial fibrillation because of its effect on atrial tissue. In individuals with accessory pathways, the onset of atrial fibrillation can lead to a life-threatening ventricular fibrillation (VF). Interestingly, a second generation of adenosine receptor-related drug candidates (e.g. tecadenoson - a novel selective A_1R agonist) have been developed for the acute suppression of PSVT [166].

Verapamil, diltiazem and adenosine compounds exert their maximum effect on the AV node by lengthening intranodal conduction time significantly. In 1971, it was demonstrated that intravenous diltiazem can also terminate narrow complex PSVT. There are many clinical trials which compare adenosine and verapamil in the treatment of SVT and these have shown that the arrhythmia was terminated in more than 90% of cases with both drugs [167]. There was an 8.6% recurrence of SVT vs 3.4% rate in the adenosine and in the verapamil-treated group respectively, but this difference was not statistically significant. Moreover, premature ventricular beats were noted after the termination of the SVT in 33% of the patients having taken adenosine and in 27% of the patients who received verapamil [167]. In addition, three out of the 77 patients in the adenosine group developed atrial fibrillation, with two of them spontaneously reverting to normal sinus rhythm within two minutes, whereas none of the patients receiving verapamil developed atrial fibrillation.

Adenosine is frequently accompanied by transient side effects (facial flushing, chest discomfort, breathlessness in up to 75% of subjects), and a recurrence rate for SVT varying from 9 to 57%. On the other hand, verapamil can cause a fall in blood pressure which is usually transient.

Several reports have established the efficacy and safety of adenosine in patients with PSVTs presenting in an emergency department (ED). A current study took into account the patients` characteristics (age, sex, past PSVT occurrences, symptoms, heart rate, dose, blood pressure and a response to adenosine), and proposed a prognostic index that would allow the emergency physician to have a useful and reliable method with sufficient sensitivity and specificity to guide treatment planning [168]. The formula, (age/heart rate at admission) + number of past PSVT episodes, yields a sensitivity of 96.2% and a specificity of 71.2% and becomes a simple and attractive tool in the ED [168]. For example, when a patient presents in an ED with a result lower than the cutoff value of 1.18 according to the preceding index, then is more possible to respond to adenosine after failure of vagal maneuvers [168].

5.1.b. Ventricular Tachycardia/Fibrillation

Idiopathic left VT has been classified into three subgroups according to mechanism: verapamil-sensitive, adenosine-sensitive, and propranolol-sensitive. The mechanism of LF outflow tract VT is most likely adenosine-sensitive triggered activity. Only 10% of patients with adenosine-sensitive VT have a LV site of origin. Yeh *et al.* [169] reported cases with adenosine-sensitive LV outflow tract VT, which were successfully ablated from the anterior aspect of the LV, just below the mitral annulus.

In a recent study, adenosine terminated sustained, exercise-triggered VT in four patients with structurally normal hearts, due to its aforementioned anti-b-adrenergic effects [170]. This action of adenosine is mediated by A_1Rs. Also, Lerman *et al.* [171] observed that adenosine can terminate frequent ectopic beats and salvos of VT which occur typically at rest.

Besides, among the adenosine-sensitive VTs, are the idiopathic VT, the right outflow tract VT, which is the most common form and presents as repetitive monomorphic VT or exercise-induced VT, and the left outflow tract VT. The proposed mechanism for the responsiveness to adenosine of such tachycardias is cAMP-mediated triggered activity.

VF is a dynamic pulseless cardiac dysrhythmia that is recognizable on the surface electrocardiogram (ECG), by its distinctive chaotic pattern. The natural course of prolonged VF is a gradual deterioration over time which is shown in the ECG waveform as a transition from a coarse pattern at onset to a fine tracing as asystole is approached.

In a swine model of prolonged VF, a selective A_1R antagonist accelerated the deterioration in the VF waveform suggesting that endogenous adenosine exerts cardioprotective effects during sudden cardiac arrest associated with VF (see below) [172]. Nonetheless, reports in human subjects show conflicting evidence regarding the use of an A_1R antagonist in this setting, due to the fact that endogenous adenosine may perpetuate asystole [173].

Thus, in this setting of cardiac arrest, the use of aminophylline, a non selective AR antagonist, has been proposed to ameliorate resuscitation outcome [173]. However, other studies raised doubts regarding the use of aminophylline in this situation [174].

5.1.c. Adenosine for Wide-Complex Tachycardia

The use of adenosine for wide-complex tachycardias has raised safety concerns, including paradoxic enhancement of accessory tract conduction, and acceleration of the ventricular response, when the underlying rhythm is atrial fibrillation with a bypass tract or atrial flutter.

If there is a history of Wolff Parkinson White Syndrome or the wide-complex tachycardia is irregularly irregular, and thus consistent with atrial fibrillation, then adenosine should not be administered.

Most accessory pathways are not adenosine sensitive. Exceptions occur mainly in pathways with long refractory periods. On the other hand, the absence or presence of a change in heart rhythm after intravenous adenosine infusion remains a useful and safe way to distinguish between supraventricular and ventricular origin in patients with stable sustained regular wide-complex tachycardia.

More specifically, in narrow or wide-complex tachycardia termination means that the AV node is part of the circuit, whereas development of AV block without termination of the tachycardia excludes AV reentry and is in favor of atrial tachycardia. In wide-complex tachyarrhythmia, absence of adenosine responsiveness, yields strong evidence to a ventricular origin, and, precipitating VA block, confirms VT. Likewise, in a typical left-bundle branch morphology of the tachycardia, termination also suggests a supraventricular origin and usually an orthodromic tachycardia with a left lateral accessory pathway.

5.1.D. Adenosine and Bradyarrhythmias

Adenosine has been associated as mediator of late bradyarrhythmias during an inferior wall MI (48 hours after). These arrhythmias are often atropine-resistant, suggesting, that they result from another mechanism, besides increased vagal tone.

5.2. Detection of Coronary Artery Disease

Adenosine has been used as an agent in conjunction with radio nucleotide myocardial perfusion imaging (MPI) in patients who were unable to perform adequate exercise stress. Dipyridamole, an adenosine uptake blocker, was also used earlier for this reason, due to its effect on blocking the metabolism of adenosine and increasing its extracellular concentration.

Adenosine dilates coronary arteries, and through a steal phenomenon, ischemic regions in the heart may be diagnosed with MPI. On the other hand, adenosine-induced vasodilatation of coronary arteries, is mediated, primarily, by A_{2A}Rs leading to the discovery of more selective agonists for the A_{2A} subtype, such as CGS-21680. Yet, a nonselective analog, NECA resulted in greater relaxation, implicating the A_{2B} subtype for the additional relaxation that was produced [175].

6. Adenosine as a Diagnostic Tool

6.1.a. QT Interval

Many diagnostic applications of adenosine including the aforementioned diagnosis of wide-complex tachycardia are used in clinical practice. Adenosine challenge induces changes in QT interval distinguishing patients with long QT syndrome (LQTS) from healthy subjects [176]. These observations explain the several cases of adenosine-induced Torsades-de-Pointes [177].

6.1.b. Sick Sinus Syndrome (SSS)

Another application of adenosine is associated with the identification of patients with sick sinus syndrome (SSS). Fragakis *et al.* found that, when a cutoff value of 535 ms for sinus recovery time (i.e. the time elapsed from sinus arrest until the appearance of the first sinus beat) was used to identify sinus node dysfunction, it had 74% sensitivity and 100% specificity, whereas the recovery time following adenosine administration had 94% sensitivity and 84% specificity [178].

6.1.d. PCI

Several studies have tested the safety and benefits of either intracoronary or intravenous infusion of adenosine during percutaneous interventions in the catheterization-laboratory setting. They were based on the fact that adenosine reduces the severity of ischemia during subsequent balloon inflations, via ischemic preconditioning (i.e. the initial balloon inflation).

Regarding the injury occurring during the balloon inflation itself, Strauer and associates observed that intracoronary administration of dypiridamole, before balloon inflation, reduced ventricular systolic and diastolic dysfunction by increasing adenosine levels in the myocardium [179].

Furthermore, similar reports suggest the attenuation of ST-segment elevation and angina, when adenosine was administered intracoronary as a pretreatment, before repetitive balloon inflations [180].

In addition, the AMISTAD (Acute Myocardial Infarction Study of Adenosine) trial, demonstrated the cardioprotective effects of intravenous adenosine, before thrombolytic therapy was initiated in 236 patients [181]. The results reported a 33% decrease in relative infarct size with adenosine treatment compared with control patients who were treated with thrombolytic therapy alone.

6.1.d. Coronary Artery Bypass Graft (CABG)

Nevertheless, there was a trend toward increased deaths and heart failure in adenosine-treated patients, which was without statistical significance. Lee *et al.* first reported benefits with pretreatment of adenosine preoperatively to patients with poor LV function and three-vessel disease undergoing CABG surgery [182].

Other studies also noted that when adenosine was infused before the initiation of cardiopulmonary bypass, the cardiac index was improved postoperatively and the creatine-kinase-MB fraction release was less.

Finally, it is has been observed, that adenosine was cardioprotective either when it was administered alone or as an adjunct to hyperkalemic crystalloid cardioplegia.

6.2. Fractional Flow Reserve (FFR)

Adenosine is also the most commonly used agent in clinical practice, both intracoronary and intravenously, for the measurement of FFR. FFR is defined as the ratio of the maximal blood flow achievable in a stenotic vessel to the theoretical maximal flow in the same vessel, if no stenosis was present. In a normal coronary artery there should be no pressure gradient between the aorta and the distal artery resulting in a FFR value of 1.

Several studies have shown that a FFR < 0.75 reliably identifies a stenosis with the potential to induce reversible myocardial ischemia. This is achieved because adenosine induces maximal hyperemia.

6.3. Adenosine in Pregnancy and in Pediatrics

Atrial premature beats are frequently diagnosed during pregnancy, whereas SVT is diagnosed less frequently. For short-term management, when vagal maneuvers fail, intravenous adenosine is the "first choice" drug and may safely terminate the arrhythmia in stable patients [183]. The reported human clinical experience with adenosine during pregnancy, indicates no teratogenicity or other adverse effects to the fetus, and it is as effective in terminating SVT (efficacy rates >90%) in pregnant women, as it is in patients who are not pregnant [183]. Paroxysmal supraventricular reentrant tachycardia is the most frequent symptomatic dysrhythmia in infants, children and adolescents [184]. In the newborn period, or during the first year of life, administration of verapamil is contradicted due to its potential harmful side effects. On the contrary, adenosine is well recognized as the first line pharmacological agent to terminate PSVTs in children and adults. The dosage of adenosine in children is as follows: After a rapid bolus of 0.05 mg/kg as initial dose, the dosage is increased in 0.05-0.10 mg/kg and rises to a maximum dose of 0.25-0.30 mg/kg or until the tachycardia is terminated [185]. The efficacy is comparable to that observed in adults [184].

7. Hemodynamic Effects

The hemodynamic response to adenosine is associated with the mode of administration. An increase of 10-15 mmHg initially in systolic and diastolic blood pressure may be observed after intravenous bolus infusion at the time of prolongation of AV conduction, followed by a decrease of blood pressure during subsequent tachycardia. In the setting of continuous administration to conscious patients, the pulmonary vascular resistance is decreased.

In addition, at high doses, the heart rate, stroke volume and cardiac index are increased. Because of its short half life, adenosine has short-lasting hemodynamic effects.

7.1. Dosage

As an antiarrhythmic, adenosine is given rapidly (over 1 to 3 seconds) intravenously with a dose of 6 mg followed by a 20 ml saline flush. If the first dose is not effective within one to two minutes, a 12 mg rapid intravenous push may be given and repeated 1-2 minutes later, if necessary. The total cumulative dose should not exceed 30 mg. As a diagnostic tool adjunct, the dose is 0.14 mg/kg/min intravenously, given for six minutes.

7.2. Drug Interactions

Carbamazepine may increase heart block caused by adenosine, while dipyridamole potentiates the effects of adenosine by inhibiting cellular uptake; thus, dose reduction is recommended. On the other hand, xanthines and, especially, caffeine and theophylline antagonize the effects of adenosine. Therefore, larger doses of adenosine may be required.

7.3. Medical Considerations/Contradictions

Adenosine should not be used, except under special circumstances, when there is second or third degree AV block, without pacemaker, because of the risk of complete heart block.

Furthermore, adenosine is contraindicated for toxin-induced tachycardias and for atrial fibrillation and atrial flutter. The risk-benefit should be considered when there is angina pectoris and unstable angina, because of the fact that adenosine may increase the risk of developing fatal cardiac arrest, life threatening ventricular arrhythmias and MI.

Additionally, inhaled adenosine has been reported to cause bronchoconstriction in asthmatic patients. Also patients with autonomic dysfunction, stenotic valvular heart disease, pericarditis or pericardial effusions, stenotic carotid artery disease with cerebrovascular insufficiency, are at greater risk of developing hypotensive complications.

7.4. Side/Adverse Effects

Side effects after intravenous bolus injection may be seen in up to 30% of adult patients and are usually short-lasting. The most frequent are facial flushing due to vasodilatation, dyspnea in up to 12%, but without significant changes seen in measured airway resistance, chest pain, headache, gastrointestinal discomfort, such as abdominal or stomach pain, diarrhea, nausea, or vomiting.

Others, are arrhythmias, including sinus tachycardia, atrial fibrillation, non-sustained VT, torsades-de-pointes requiring cardioversion, sinus bradycardia, prolonged sinus arrest and AV block [186]. Thus, cardiac monitoring is essential when this drug is administered. Less frequently, cough and lightheadedness are observed.

Occasionally, severe bronchospasm has been reported [185], but the adverse pulmonary effects of adenosine remain unclear. It is believed that adenosine activates purinoreceptors via indirect inflammatory mediators, causing bronchospam.

Finally, increased intracranial pressure after adenosine infusion has been observed to an adult patient, and therefore, it is recommended that the agent should be used with caution in patients with already elevated intracranial pressure.

8. Adenosine and Resuscitation

8.1.a. Neuroprotection

Cardiac arrest and resuscitation produce global ischemia and reperfusion damage to the brain, which result in high mortality and delayed neuronal death. Protein synthesis is very sensitive to blood flow and may be equally sensitive to depressed tissue ATP post-ischemia. More specifically, there is an increased synthesis of heat shock and stress-induced proteins, in parallel with a significant reduction in the proteins needed to maintain cellular structure and function [187].

Adenosine has been suggested as an endogenous neuroprotective molecule and has been proposed as a possible post-ischemic treatment approach, due to its multiple interactions with the pathophysiological mechanisms activated during ischemia and reperfusion. 2-Chloroadenosine, is an adenosine A_1 receptor agonist, which has showed a protective role against ischemic cell loss in the rat hippocampus. In another study, propentofylline, an adenosine uptake blocker, protected hippocampal CA1 pyramidal cells from ischemia-induced delayed hippocampal neuronal death [188].

Taken together, it is suggested that the enhanced extracellular concentrations of adenosine protect the brain from the ischemic and reperfusion insult. More specifically, adenosine reduces the release of excitotoxic neurotransmitters, such as N-methyl-D-asparate (NMDA), decreases metabolism, acts as a scavenger for free radicals, has anti-inflammatory effects, leads to vasorelaxation and produces moderate reduction of brain temperature [125]. More recent data suggest that adenosine crosses the blood brain barrier (BBB) and has a central effect on the brain [189].

Moreover, Kui Xu *et al.* suggested that post-resuscitation treatment with adenosine, following a 12-min cardiac arrest improved the overall survival and the preservation of hippocampal neurons in rats [189]. Another beneficial effect of adenosine is that it depresses brain temperature; thus, part of the neuroprotective impact of adenosine is the result of its hypothermia-inducing properties. Studies report that hypothermic neuroprotection involves mechanisms such as reduction of excitotoxic amino acid release, decrease of cerebral metabolic rate, attenuation of depletion of ATP, reduction of post-ischemic radical activity, and, thus, leads to less consumption of endogenous antioxidants and to reduced lipid peroxidation [190]. Therefore, post-resuscitation administration of adenosine of 7.2 mg/kg, depressed brain temperature after resuscitation through the 6h monitoring period, whereas prevention of adenosine-induced hypothermia lowered survival rates and increased hippocampal neuronal death [189]. On the other hand, reperfusion after global ischemia is frequently characterized by an initial hyperemia, followed by a period of hypoperfusion, which results in a significant decrease of cerebral blood flow (CBF) below pre-ischemic baseline [192]. However, adenosine may increase CBF via local vasodilatation and inhibition of clot formation, whereas the increasing interstitial levels of adenosine, secondary to adenosine transport blockade, significantly lessens the magnitude of perfusion deficit in the setting of global cerebral ischemia [192]. In addition, another determinant of postresuscitation survival is the extent of brain edema. This is due to the fact that brain edema increases intracranial pressure producing further tissue damage via secondary ischemia, especially in regions such as brainstem, which contains respiratory and cardiovascular centers. High mortality because of brain edema peaks at 1, 6 and 24 hours after resuscitation in the cortex and hippocampus, and 24 hours in the brainstem [189]. Nevertheless, mild hypothermia has been proposed to decrease brain edema. Taken together, it is suggested that adenosine protects the brain from reperfusion injury induced by cardiac arrest and resuscitation, mainly through adenosine-induced hypothermia and via improvement of postresuscitation blood flow. Finally, ATL-146e, a novel adenosine A_{2A} receptor agonist, that has anti-inflammatory, neuroprotective and coronary vasodilator properties, combined with 1L Hextend (HEX), a colloid solution approved for volume expansion during surgery, safely and effectively counteracted a reduction in cardiac performance noted after traumatic brain injury and hemorrhage, without causing hypotension or bradycardia [192].

8.1.b. Adenosine and the VF Waveform

It has been proposed, that there is a three-distinct-phase model of VF: (1) an electrical phase, in which defibrillation is the most effective therapy lasting 4-5 min (2) a circulatory phase, in which cardiopulmonary resuscitation (CPR) and other therapies may be useful prior to defibrillation, involving approximately 5-10 min after the patient collapses and (3) a metabolic phase, in which the prolonged period of tissue ischemia results in release into circulation of tumor necrosis factor, endotoxins, and cytokines, all of which suppress myocardial contractility, and for which therapeutic interventions have yet to be defined [193].

Although there is total interruption of coronary blood flow, the myocardium continues in an energy consuming state [194]. The VF Scaling Exponent (ScE) curve, a non-linear geometric measure of the ECG waveform that estimates the fractal dimension of the ECG waveform during VF, has been noted to go three phases as well; an initial gradual increase during the first 4 min, followed by a 3-4min plateau and then a steep rise after 8min. T

The ScE has been demonstrated to bc directly proportional to the duration of untreated cardiac arrest [195]. The progression of ScE from low (1.1) to high (1.8) is associated with a reduction in cardiac susceptibility to defibrillation shocks, as demonstrated by the decrease observed in probability of the return of spontaneous circulation (ROSC), as ScE was increasing, both in animal and human studies [196].

It is suggested, that during untreated VF, accumulating endogenous adenosine modulates the degeneration of VF waveform over time, during the period which corresponds to the circulatory phase of VF cardiac arrest. Additionally, treatment with a selective A_1 adenosine antagonist changed the ScE significantly during the plateau phase, by enhancing the deterioration in the VF waveform [172]. A_1R antagonism resulted in a profoundly earlier fall in the frequency during VF. As lower ScE and higher frequencies are associated with a greater possibility of successful defibrillation, it is suggested that the adenosine receptor produces an essential protective response to the ischemia of VF [172].

Furthermore, several studies report, that prehospital intra-arrest cooling improves the ScE compared to normothermic controls with equal arrest duration [197]. There are also data supporting a relationship between myocardial energy stores and the VF ScE [198].

Therefore, the fact that the decaying electrical activity of the VF ECG corresponds to the depletion of ATP stores, suggests that disarrangement of the energy metabolism apparatus of myocardium is a mediator of defibrillation susceptibility [198].

Interestingly, there are gender differences regarding the VF waveform. More specifically, female gender may be associated with a slower natural decay in ECG VF waveform morphology over time, and may have statistically significant greater rate of ROSC and short-term survival than males [199]. It is also possible that due to the fact that gender differences are more pronounced during the early phases of cardiac arrest, they are of no consequences in prolonged VF [199].

Taken together, the restoration of ATP concentrations in the myocardium is believed to be a key concept regarding the therapeutic interventions for cardiac arrest [198]. Besides, the ischemic decaying of energy stores hinders the reestablishment of a productive cardiac rhythm, and thus, the administration of energy substrates to the myocardium during cardiac arrest has been proposed, as one means of reversing or preventing ATP depletion.

8.1.C. Adenosine and Asystolic Cardiac Arrest

Cardiac asystole remains to be an ominous rhythm with survival rates below 3%. As noted above, adenosine acts as an extracellular messenger to regulate myocardial oxygen supply and demand. Despite its well demonstrated cardioprotective response, adenosine can have detrimental effect by inducing a state of refractory atropine-resistant asystole [200].

It has been demonstrated that adenosine attenuates the stimulatory action of catecholamines on cardiac myocytes, and hinders the release of nor-epinephrine from presynaptic adrenergic nerve terminals. Moreover, one of the factors for the development of bradyasystole, despite the large amounts of endogenous catecholamines, which are released during cardiac arrest, is the local accumulation of adenosine.

However, the use of a potent and selective antagonist of the A_1 subtype of adenosine receptor (BG9719) that mediates the negative chronotropic, dromotropic and inotropic actions of endogenous adenosine on the heart had no effect on either the rate of ROSC or short-term survival in a porcine model of prolonged VF cardiac arrest [201].

Furthermore, the use of aminophylline, a nonspecific adenosine receptor antagonist capable of reversing ischemia-induced bradyasystole [200], failed to obtain statistically significant improvement in ROSC, when given during the early phase of asystolic cardiac arrest resuscitation in the out-of-hospital setting [202].

8.1.d. Adenosine and Defibrillation Threshold (DFT)

Although a metabolic mechanism has been suggested, hypoxia, metabolic acidosis or alkalosis does not affect DFT during VF cardiac arrest [203]. On the other hand, there are data supporting that adenosine markedly elevates trans-thoracic and trans-myocardial DFT [203]. These adverse effects on the threshold are mediated by the A_1R, since they are reversed by CPT, a specific A_1 receptor antagonist [203]. Moreover, catecholamines that are released during hypoxia have been shown to reduce DFT, whereas b-blockers increase it.

To reveal the mechanism of action of adenosine on DFT, its effects were determined in the same dog during both the innervated and denervated states [203]. Its lack of effect during the denervated condition, in contrast to its adverse effect on DFT in the innervated state, indicates a anti-adrenergic or cAMP-dependent effect of adenosine on DFT.

On the contrary, adenosine by functioning as a negative feedback inhibitor of b-adrenergic stimulation protects the myocardium against excessive O_2 demand [203]. Besides, catecholamines cause coronary spam, put myocardial metabolism into hyper-metabolic overdrive to support the “fight or flight” reflex, and enhance the depletion of ATP needed for cardiac and mechanical recovery. In addition, although the value of epinephrine to resuscitation has never been demonstrated, its potential damage has been largely ignored. Thus, the deleterious effects of adenosine on DFT are a “paradoxical” consequence of its otherwise protective role, consistent with its anti-adrenergic mechanism of action and suggesting that the spectrum of adenosine`s effects are more complex than previously believed [203].

8.2. Adenosine and Apoptosis

Data support, that the induction of cardiomyocyte`s apoptosis, is an essential part of the ischemia-reperfusion injury [204]. More specifically, apoptosis is defined as a morphologically distinct type of cell death, which is characterized by shrinkage of the cell and fragmentation into apoptotic bodies, which are rapidly phagocytosed by neighboring cells [205]. In addition, the apoptosis of cardiomyocytes is associated with the ischemia-reperfusion injury during an open heart surgery [205]. Nonetheless, the apoptosis can be prevented during experimental ischemia-reperfusion injury. Adenosine is shown to decrease cardiac tumor necrosis factor (TNF) production, which is significantly raised during ischemia [206]. Furthermore, high circulating TNF levels contribute to myocardial dysfunction and cardiomyocyte death, in ischemia-reperfusion injury [206]. Although adenosine showed some signs of positive outcome against ischemia-reperfusion injury, yet no statistical significance was reached [205].

8.3. Adenosine and Myocardial Protection during Resuscitation

An electrically stable and mechanically competent cardiac activity is essential for the successful treatment of cardiac arrest. Abnormalities in this setting, such as refractory VF, ischemic contracture, post-resuscitation ectopic activity (with recurrent episodes of VF), and post-resuscitation myocardial dysfunction (with hemodynamic dysfunction), compromise the resuscitation effort.

Ischemic contracture is a result of severe ischemia and is associated with a decrease in ATP levels to less than 10% of normal. It is also characterized by progressive thickening of the LV wall with reductions in ventricular cavity size [207]. Thus, ventricular preload is compromised and the amount of blood ejected by chest compressions is decreased.

Moreover, the severity of ischemic contracture is proportional to the interval of untreated VF in a porcine model of VF [207]. In humans, ischemic contracture has been observed during open-chest resuscitation and has been suggested to compromise resuscitation [208]. Furthermore, ischemic contracture increases coronary vascular resistance, suggesting that interventions that could decrease ischemic contracture may improve resuscitation outcome.

However, coronary artery perfusion pressure has been shown to be an important hemodynamic determinant of successful experimental and human CPR. Although, after adenosine infusion, coronary artery perfusion was reduced below the threshold necessary for rodent survival, the mobilization of coronary flow reserve by adenosine may explain why survival after CPR was not compromised.

Consequently, the reduction of coronary vascular resistance by adenosine, decreases myocardial oxygen demands, improves recovery of cardiac function after prolonged cardioplegic arrest, increases coronary microvasular flow and attenuate myocardial reperfusion injury.

Delivery of electrical shocks immediately upon recognition of VF is highly effective if the preceding interval of untreated VF is brief (i.e. below 3 min). Nevertheless, electrical shocks delivered after longer intervals may fail to reverse VF or even precipitate asystole or pulseless electrical activity (PEA).

Electrical instability with recurrent episodes of VF occurs frequently after resuscitation from cardiac arrest. They are partly related to opening of the sarcolemmal potassium ATP channels.

Global systolic and diastolic myocardial dysfunction develops after resuscitation from cardiac arrest. This kind of myocardial stunning usually resolves within hours or days, but it may hinder ROSC [209]. Systolic dysfunction represents decreases in contractility and in ejection fraction, whereas diastolic dysfunction is characterized by reductions in end-diastolic volume and by myocardial wall thickening.

It is suggested that the adenosine pathway may represent an agent that could minimize these myocardial abnormalities which take place during cardiac arrest.

Conclusion

Adenosine is an endogenous nucleoside, which has been extensively studied and has been shown to have an essential cardioprotective role. It has been used for the treatment of SVT for many decades. Recent data have highlighted important aspects of adenosine receptors, particularly during conditions of limited oxygen availability, regarding tolerance to ischemia, treatment of hypoxia-induced vascular leakage, excessive inflammation, ischemia-reperfusion injury, preconditioning (early and delayed) and post-conditioning.

Specific AR agonists, in conjunction with studies in genetic models, have identified a rapidly expanding field of biochemical roles and therapeutic applications of extracellular adenosine signaling. Despite the wealth of background data, many controversies remain to be resolved and further basic research is needed to elucidate the whole spectrum of adenosinergic protection.

References

[1] Eltzschig, HK, Ibla, JC, et al. Coordinated adenine nucleotide phospho-hydrolysis and nucleoside signaling in posthypoxic endothelium: Role of ectonucleotidases and adenosine A2B receptors. *J. Exp. Med,* 2003; 198:783-96.

[2] Eltzschig, HK. Adenosine: an old drug newly discovered. *Anesthesiology,* 2009; 111(4):904-15.

[3] Eltzschig, HK, Weissmüller, T, Mager, A, Eckle, T. Nucleotide metabolism and cell-cell interactions. *Methods Mol. Biol,* 2006; 341:73-87.

[4] Faigle, M, Seesle, J, Zug, S, El Kasmi, KC, Eltzschig, HK. ATP release from vascular endothelia occurs across Cx43 hemichannels and is attenuated during hypoxia. *PLos One,* 2008; 3:e2801.

[5] Chen, Y, Corriden, R, et al. ATP release guides neutrophil chemotaxis via P2Y2 and A3 receptors. *Science,* 2006; 314:1792-5.

[6] Eltzschig, HK, Eckle, T, et al. ATP release from activated neutrophils occurs via connexin 43 and modulates adenosine-dependent endothelial cell function. *Circ. Res,* 2006;99:1100-8.

[7] Weissmüller, T, Cambell, EL et al. PMNs fascilitate translocation of platelets across human and mouse epithelium and together alter fluid homeostasis via epithelial cell-expressed ecto-NTPDases. *J. Clin. Invest,* 2008; 118:3682-92.

[8] Robson, SC, Wu, Y, et al. Ectonucleotidases of CD39 family modulate vascular inflammation and thrombosis in transplantation. *Semin. Thromb Hemost,* 2005; 31:217-33.

[9] Enjyoji, K, Sévigny, J, et al. Targeted disruption of cd39/ATP diphospho-hydrolase results in disordered hemostasis and thromboregulation. *Nat. Med,* 1999; 5:1010-7.
[10] Pinsky, DJ, Broekman, MJ et al. Elucidation of the thromboregulatory role of CD39/ectoapyrase in the ischemic brain. *J. Clin. Invest,* 2002; 109:1031-44.
[11] Van Calker, D, Muller, M, Hamprecht, B. Adenosine regulates via two different types of receptors. The accumulation of cyclec AMP in cultured brain cells. *J. Neurochem,* 1979; 33:995-1005.
[12] Ely, S.W. and Berne, R.M. (1992). Protective effects of adenosine in myocardial ischemia. *Circulation* 85, 893-904.
[13] Lasley, R.D., Rhee, J.W., Van Wylen, D.G.L., and Mentzer, R.M., Jr.(1992) Adenosine A1 receptor mediated protection of the globally ischemic isolated rat heart. *J. Mol. Cell. Cardiol. 22*, 39-47.
[14] Angello, D.A., Headrick, S.P., Coddington, N.M., and Berne, R.M., (1991). Adenosine antagonism decreases metabolic but not functional recovery from ischemia. *Am. J. Physiol. 260*, H193-H200.
[15] Lasley, R.D., and Mentzer, R.M., Jr. (1992). Adenosine improves recovery of postischemic myocardial function via an adenosine A1 receptor mechanism. *Am. J. Physiol. 263*, H1460-H1465.
[16] Zhao, Z.Q., McGee, D.S., et al and Vinten-Johansen, J. (1993). Receptor-mediated cardioprotective effects of endogenous adenosine are exerted primarily during reperfusion after coronary occlusion in the rabbit. *Circulation. 88,* 709-719.
[17] Finegan, B.A, Lopaschuk, G.D., Gandhi, M., and Clanachan, A.S., (1996). Inhibition of glycolysis and enhanced mechanical function of working rat hearts as a result of adenosine A1 receptor stimulation during reperfusion following ischaemia. *Br. J. Pharmacol.* 118, 355-363.
[18] Murry, C.E., Jennings, R.B., Reimer, K.A., (1986). Preconditioning with ischemia, a delay of lethal cell injury in ischemic myocardium. *Circulation. 74*, 1124-1136.
[19] Das, M, Das, DK. Molecular mechanism of preconditioning. *IUBMB Life,* 2008;60(4):199-203.
[20] Parratt, J.R., (1994). Protection of the heart by ischaemic preconditioning: mechanisms and possibilities for pharmacological exploitation. *Trends Pharmacol. 118*, 355-363.
[21] Headrick, J.P., (1996) Ischemic preconditioning: bioenergetic and metabolic changes and the role of endogenous adenosine. *J. Mol. Cell. Cardiol. 28*, 1227-1240.
[22] Tang, W, Weil, MH, Sun, S, Pernat, A, Mason, E. K(ATP) channel activation reduces the severity of post resuscitation myocardial dysfunction. *Am. J. Physiol. Heart Circ. Physiol*, 2000; 279(4):H1609-15.
[23] Hu, K, Duan, D, Li, GR, Nattel, S. Protein kinase C activates ATP-sensitive K^+ current in human and rabbit ventricular myocytes. *Circ. Res*, 1996; 78:492-498.
[24] Shigematsu, S, Sato, T, et al. Pharmacological evidence for the persistent activation of ATP-sensitive K^+ channels in early phase of reperfusion and its protective role against myocardial stunning. *Circulation*, 1992; 92:2266-2275.
[25] Fang, X, Tang, W, et al. Mechanism by which activation of delta-opioid receptor reduces the severity of postresuscitation myocardial dysfunction. *Care Med,* 2006; 34(10):2607-12.

[26] Mizimura, T., Auchampach, J.A., Linden, J., Bruns, R.F., and Gross, G.J., (1996) PD81,723, an allosteric enhancer of the A1 adenosine receptor, lowers the threshold for ischemic preconditioning in dogs. *Circ. Res. 79*, 415-423.

[27] Cave, A.C., et al. (1993) Improved functional recovery by ischaemic preconditioning is not mediated by adenosine in the globally ischaemic isolated rat heart. *Cardiovasc. Res. 27*, 663−668.

[28] Headrick, J. P. (1996a). Ischemic preconditioning: bioenergetic and metabolic changes and the role of endogenous adenosine. *J. Mol. Cell. Cardiol 28*, 1227- 1240.

[29] Auchampach, J. A., Jin, X., et al. (2004). Comparison of three different A1 adenosine receptor antagonists on infarct size and multiple cycle ischemic preconditioning in anesthetized dogs. *J. Pharmacol. Exp. Ther. 308*, 846−856.

[30] Auchampach, J. A., Ge, Z. D., (2003) .A3 adenosine receptor agonist IB-MECA reduces myocardial ischemia–reperfusion injury in dogs. *Am. J. Physiol. Heart. Circ. Physiol. 285*, H607−H613.

[31] de Jong, J. W., de Jonge, R., Keijzer, E., and Bradamante, S., (2000). The role of adenosine in preconditioning. *Pharmacol. Ther. 87*, 141−149.

[32] Schulte, G., Sommerschild, H., et al (2004) Adenosine A1 receptors are nece-ssary for protection of the murine heart by remote, delayed adaptation to isch-aemia. *Acta. Physiol. Scand. 182*, 133−143.

[33] Lankford, A. R., Yang, J. N., et al. (2006). Effect of modulating cardiac A1 adenosine receptor expression on protection with ischemic preconditioning. *Am. J. Physiol. Heart. Circ. Physiol. 290,* H1469−H1473.

[34] Peart, JN, Headrick, JP. Adenosinergic cardioprotection: multiple receptors, multiple pathways. *Pharmacol. Ther*, 2007; 114(2): 208-21.

[35] Baxter, G. F., and Yellon, D. M. (1997). Time course of delayed myocardial protection after transient adenosine A1-receptor activation in the rabbit. *J. Cardiovasc. Pharmacol .29*, 631−638.

[36] Kristo, G., Yoshimura, Y., et al. (2004) Adenosine A1/A2a receptor agonist AMP-579 induces acute and delayed preconditioning against in vivo myocar-dial stunning. *Am. J. Physiol. Heart. Circ. Physiol. 287*, H2746−H2753.

[37] Schulte, G, Sommerschild, H, et al. Adenosine A receptors are necessary for protection of the murine heart by remote, delayed adaptation to ischaemia. *Acta Physiol. Scand*, 2004; 182: 133–143.

[38] Bolli, R. Cardioprotective function of inducible nitric oxide synthase and role of nitric oxide in myocardial ischemia and preconditioning: an overview of a decade of research. *J. Mol. Cell Cardiol,* 2001*;* 33:1897–1918.

[39] Lasley, RD, Keith, BJ, Kristo, G, Yoshimura, Y, Mentzer, RM Jr. Delayed adenosine A1 receptor preconditioning in rat myocardium is MAPK depen-dent but iNOS independent. *Am. J. Physiol. Heart Circ. Physiol*, 2005; 289(2):H785-91.

[40] Li, Y, Kloner, RA. The cardioprotective effects of ischemic preconditioning are not mediated by adenosine receptors in rat hearts. *Circulation,* 1993; 87: 1642–7.

[41] Speechly-Dick, ME, Mocanu, MM, Yellon, DM. Protein kinase C: its role in ischemic preconditioning in the rat. *Circ. Res,* 1994; 75: 586–90.

[42] Iwamoto, T, Miura, T, Adachi, T, et al. Myocardial infarct size-limiting effect of preconditioning was not attenuated by oxygen free-radical scavengers in the rabbit. *Circulation,* 1991; 83: 1015–22.

[43] Sakamoto, J, Miura, T, Goto, M, et al. Limitation of myocardial infarct size by adenosine A1-receptor activation is abolished by protein kinase C inhibitors in the rabbit. *Cardiovasc. Res,* 1995; 29: 682–8.

[44] Murry, CE, Jennings, RB, Recmer, KA. Preconditioning with ischemia: a delay of lethal cell injury in myocardium. *Circulation* ,1986; 74: 1124–36.

[45] Armstrong, S, Ganote, CE. Adenosine receptor specificity in preconditioning of isolated rabbit cardiomyocytes: evidence of A3-receptor involvement. *Cardiovasc. Res,* 1994; 28: 1049–56.

[46] Schott ,RJ, Rohmann, S, Braun, ER, Schaper, W. Ischemic preconditioning reduces infarct size in swine myocardium. *Circ. Res,* 1990; 66: 1133–42.

[47] Toombs, CF, Wiltse, AL, Shebuki, RJ. Ischemic preconditioning fails to limit infarct size in reserpineized rabbit myocardium: implication of norepinephrine release in the preconditioning effect. *Circulation,* 1993; 88: 2351–8.

[48] Yellon, DM, Alkhulaifi, AM, Pugsley, WB. Preconditioning the human myo-cardium. *Lancet,* 1993; 342: 276–7.

[49] Szekeres, L., Szilva´ssy, Z., et al. (1997). Delayed cardiac protection against h-armful consequences of stress can be induced in experimental atherosclerosis in rabbits. *J. Mol. Cell. Cardiol,. 29,* 1977– 1983.

[50] Kukreja, RC, Salloum , FN, Xi, L. Nonurologic applications of phosphodie-sterase type 5 inhibitors. *Curr. Sex Health Rep*, 2007;4:64–70.

[51] Galiè, N, Ghofrani, HA, et al. Sildenafil citrate therapy for pulmonary arterial hypertension. *N. Engl. J. Med.* 2005; 353(20):2148–57.

[52] Ockaili ,R, Salloum ,F, Hawkins, J. Sildenafil (Viagra) induces powerful cardioprotective effect via opening of mitochondrial K(ATP) channels in rabbits. *Am. J. Physiol: Heart Circ. Physiol,* 2002; 283:H1263–9.

[53] Salloum ,FN, Das, A, et al. Adenosine A1 receptor mediates delayed cardio-protective effect of sildenafil in mouse. *J. Mol. Cell Cardio,* 2007; 43: 545–551.

[54] Von Lubitz, D.K., Beenhakker, M., et al. (1996). Reduction of postischemic brain damage and memory deficits following treatment with the selective adenosine A1 receptor agonist. *Eur. J. Pharmacol. 302*, 43-48.

[55] Heurteaux, C., Lauritzen, I., et al. (1995). Essential role of adenosine, adenosine A1 receptors, and ATP-sensitive K^+ channels in cerebral ischemic preconditioning. *Proc. Natl. Acad. Sci. U.S.A*. 92, 4666-70.

[56] Dana, A., Skarli, M., Papakrivopoulou, J., and Yellon, D.M. (2000). Adenosine A1 receptor induced delayed preconditioning in rabbits: induction of p38 mi-togen-activated protein kinase activation and Hsp27 phosphorylation via a tyrosine inase- and protein kinase C-dependent mechanism. *Circ. Res. 86*, 989−997.

[57] Headrick, J. P., Hack, B., and Ashton, K. J. (2003a). Acute adenosinergic cardioprotection in ischemic-reperfused hearts. *Am. J. Physiol. Heart. Circ. Physiol. 285*, H1797−H1818.

[58] Pepe, S. (2000). Mitochondrial function in ischaemia and reperfusion of the ageing heart. *Clin. Exp. Pharmacol. Physiol. 27*, 745−750.

[59] Cohen, M. V., Baines, C. P., and Downey, J.M. (2000). Ischemic preconditio-ning: from adenosine receptor to KATP channel. *Annu. Rev. Physiol. 62*, 79−109.

[60] Peart, J., Willems, L., and Headrick, J. P. (2003). Receptor and non-receptor-dependent mechanisms of cardioprotection with adenosine. *Am. J. Physiol. Heart. Circ. Physiol. 284*, H519–H527.
[61] Germack, R., and Dickenson, J. M. (2005). Adenosine triggers preconditioning through MEK/ERK1/2 signalling pathway during hypoxia/reoxygenation in neonatal rat cardiomyocytes. *J. Mol. Cell. Cardiol. 39*, 429–442.
[62] Yoshimura, Y., Kristo, G., et al. and Lasley, R. D. (2004). The p38 MAPK inhibitor SB203580 blocks adenosine A1 receptor-induced attenuation of in vivo myocardial stunning. *Cardiovasc. Drugs. Ther. 18*, 433–440.
[63] Liu, Q., and Hofmann, P. A. (2003). Modulation of protein phosphatase 2a by adenosine A1 receptors in cardiomyocytes: role for p38 MAPK. *Am. J. Physiol. Heart. Circ. Physiol. 285*, H97–H103.
[64] Ballard-Croft, C., Kristo, G., et al. (2005). Acute adenosine preconditioning is mediated by p38 MAPK activation in discrete subcellular compartments. *Am. J. Physiol. Heart. Circ. Physiol. 288*, H1359–H1366.
[65] Light, P. E., Kanji, H. D., et al. (2001). Distinct myoprotective roles of cardiac sarcolemmal and mitochondrial KATP channels during metabolic inhibition and recovery. *FASEB. J. 15*, 2586–2594.
[66] Matherne, GP, Linden, J et al. (1997). Transgenic A1adenosine receptor over-expression increases myocardial resistance to ischemia. *Proc. Natl. Acad. Sci. U.S.A. 94*, 6541-6.
[67] Vander Heide, R.S., Reimer, K.A. (1996). Effect of adenosine therapy at reperfusion on myocardial infarct size. *Cardiovasc. Res. 31*, 711-8.
[68] Meissner, A, Morgan, J.P. (1995). Contractile dysfunction and abnormal Ca^{2+} modulation during postischemic reperfusion in rat heart. *Am. J. Physiol. 268,* H100-11.
[69] Yang, Z., Day, YJ., et al. (2005). Infarct-Sparing Effect of A2A-Adenosine Receptor Activation Is Due Primarily to Its Action on Lymphocytes. *Circulation. 111,* 2190-7.
[70] Vinten-Johansen, J., Thourani, V.H., et al. (1999). Broad-spectrum cardio-protection with adenosine. *Ann. Thorac. Surg. 68*, 1942-8.
[71] Harada N, Okajima K, et al. Adenosine and selective A(2A) receptor agonists reduce ischemia/reperfusion injury of rat liver mainly by inhibiting leukocyte activation. *J. Pharmacol. Exp. Ther*, 2000; 294:1034 –1042.
[72] Jordan JE, Zhao ZQ, et al. Adenosine A2 receptor activation attenuates reperfusion injury by inhibiting neutrophil accumulation, superoxide generation and coronary endothelial adherence. *J. Pharmacol. Exp. Ther*, 1997;280:301–309.
[73] Okusa MD, Linden J, et al. Selective A2A adenosine receptor activation reduces ischemia-reperfusion injury in rat kidney. *Am. J. Physiol*, 1999;277:F404 –F412.
[74] Ross SD, Tribble CG, et al. Selective adenosine-A2A activation reduces lung reperfusion injury following transplantation. *J. Heart Lung Transplant*,1999;18: 994–1002.
[75] Lasley RD, Jahania MS, Mentzer RM Jr. Beneficial effects of adenosine A(2a) agonist CGS-21680 in infarcted and stunned porcine myocardium. *Am. J. Physiol. Heart Circ. Physiol*, 2001;280:H1660–H1666.
[76] Cronstein, B. N. (1994). Adenosine, an endogenous anti-inflammatory agent. *J. Appl. Physiol. 76*, 5–13.

[77] Visser, S. S., Theron, A. J., et al. and Anderson, R. (2000). Apparent involve-ment of the A2A subtype adenosine receptor in the anti-inflammatory inter-actions of CGS 21680, cyclopentyladenosine, and IB-MECA with human neutrophils. *Biochem. Pharmacol. 60*, 993–999.

[78] Shryock JC, Snowdy S, et al. A2A-adenosine receptor reserve for coronary vasodilation. *Circulation*, 1998; 98:711–718.

[79] Lozza G, Conti A, Ongini E, Monopoli A. Cardioprotective effects of adenosine A1 and A2A receptor agonists in the isolated rat heart. *Pharmacol. Res*, 1997; 35:57– 64.

[80] Dobson, J. G., Jr., and Fenton, R. A. (1997). Adenosine A2 receptor function in rat ventricular myocytes. *Cardiovasc. Res. 34*, 337–347.

[81] Maddock, H. L., Broadley, K. J., et al. (2001). Role of endothelium in ischa-emia-induced myocardial dysfunction of isolated working hearts: cardioprotec-tion by activation of adenosine A2A receptors. *J. Auton. Pharmacol. 21*, 263–271.

[82] Lew, M. J., and Kao, S. W. (1999). Examination of adenosine receptor-media-ted relaxation of the pig coronary artery. *Clin. Exp. Pharmacol. Physio.l 26*, 438–443.

[83] Zhao, Z. Q., Budde, J. M., et al. (2001). Adenosine attenuates reperfusion-induced apoptotic cell death by modulating expression of Bcl-2 and Bax proteins. *J. Mol. Cell. Cardiol .33*, 57–68.

[84] Bogaert, J, Bosmans, H, et al. Remote myocardial dysfunction after acute anterior myocardial infarction: impact of left ventricular shape on regional function. *J. Am. Coll. Cardiol,* 2000;35: 1525–1534.

[85] Weiss CR, Aletras AH, et al. Stunned, infarcted, and normal myocardium in dogs: simultaneous differentiation by using gadolinium-enhanced cine MR imaging with magnetization transfer contrast. *Radiology* ,226: 723–730, 2003.

[86] Kramer CM, Lima JA, et al. Regional differences in function within non-infarcted myocardium during left ventricular remodeling. *Circulation,* 1993; 88:1279–1288.

[87] Epstein FH, Yang Z, et al. MR tagging early after myocardial infarction in mice demonstrates contractile dysfunction in adjacent and remote regions. *Magn. Reson Med.* 48: 399–402, 2002.

[88] Toufektsian, MC, Yang, Z et al. Stimulation of A2A-adenosine receptors after myocardial infarction suppresses inflammatory activation and attenuates contractile dysfunction in the remote left ventricle. *Am. J. Physiol. Heart,* 2006; 290: H1410-8.

[89] Kelly, RA, Balligand, JL, Smith, TW. Nitric oxide and cardiac function. *Circ. Res.* 1996; 79: 363–380.

[90] Yang, X. M., Philipp, S., Downey, J. M., and Cohen, M. V. (2005a). Postconditioning's protection is not dependent on circulating blood factors or cells but involves adenosine receptors and requires PI3-kinase and guanylyl cyclase activation. *Basic. Res. Cardiol. 100*, 57–63.

[91] Yang, Z., Day Y.-J., et al. (2006). Myocardial infarct-sparing effect of adenosine A2A receptor activation is due to its action on CD4+ T-lympho-cytes. *Circulation, 114*, 2056–2064.

[92] Engler, RL, Schmid-Schonbein, GW, Pavelec, RS. Leukocyte capillary plugging in myocardial ischemia and reperfusion in the dog. *Am. J. Pathol*, 1983;111:98 –111.

[93] Chen, CM, Penuelas, O, et al. Protective effects of adenosine A2A receptor agonist in ventilator-induced lung injury in rats. *Crit. Care Med,* 2009; 37:2235-41.

[94] Eckle, T, Grenz, A, et al. A2B adenosine receptor signaling attenuates acute lung injury by enhancing alveolar fluid clearance in mice. *J. Clin. Invest,* 2008; 118: 3301–3315.

[95] Kin, H., Zatta, A. J., et al. (2005). Postconditioning reduces infarct size via adenosine receptor activation by endogenous adenosine. *Cardiovasc. Res. 67*, 124−133.

[96] Zhao, Z. Q., Corvera, J. S., et al. (2003). Inhibition of myocardial injury by ischemic postconditioning during reperfusion: comparison with ischemic preconditioning. *Am. J. Physiol. Heart. Circ. Physiol. 285*, H579−H588.

[97] Penna, C, Rastaldo, R, et al. Post-conditioning induced cardioprotection requires signaling through a redox-sensitive mechanism, mitochondrial ATP-sensitive K^+ channel and protein kinase C activation. *Basic Res. Cardio,* 2006; 101:180-9.

[98] Gelpi ,R,J,, Morales, C,, et al. (2002). Xanthine oxidase contributes to pre-conditioning`s preservation of left ventricular developed pressure in isolated rat heart: developed pressure may not be an appropriate end-point for studies of preconditioning. *Basic. Res. Cardio.l 97*, 40–46.

[99] Lasley, R. D., Kristo, G., Keith, B. J., and Mentzer, R. M., Jr. (2006). The A2a/A2b receptor antagonist ZM241385 blocks the cardioprotective effect of adenosine receptor agonist pretreatment in in vivo rat myocardium. *Am. J. Physiol. Heart. Circ. Physiol., 292,* H426-31.

[100] Montesinos, M. C., Desai, A., et al. (2002). Adenosine promotes wound he-aling and mediates angiogenesis in response to tissue injury via occupancy of A2A receptors. *Am. J. Pathol., 160*, 2009−2018.

[101] Feoktistov, I., Goldstein, A. E., et al. (2002). Differential expression of ade- sine receptors in human endothelial cells: role of A2B receptors in angiogenic factor regulation. *Circ. Res. 90*, 531−538.

[102] Dubey, R. K., Gillespie, D. G., and Jackson, E. K. (2002). A2B adenosine receptors stimulate growth of porcine and rat arterial endothelial cells. *Hypertension. 39*, 530−535.

[103] Afzal, A., Shaw, L. C., et al. (2003). Reduction in preretinal neovascula-rization by ribozymes that cleave the A2B adenosine receptor mRNA. *Circ. Res. 93*, 500−506.

[104] Chen, Y., Epperson, S., et al. (2004). Functional effects of enhancing or silencing adenosine A2b receptors in cardiac fibroblasts. *Am. J. Physiol. Heart. Circ. Physiol. 287*, H2478−H2486.

[105] Wakeno, M., Minamino, T., et al. (2006). Long-term stimulation of adenosine A2b receptors begun after myocardial infarction prevents cardiac remodeling in rats. *Circulation.,114*; 1923-32

[106] Philipp, S., Yang, X. M., et al. (2006). Postconditioning protects rabbit hearts through a protein kinase C-adenosine A2b receptor cascade. *Cardiovasc. Res. 70*, 308−314.

[107] Solenkova, N. V., Solodushko, V., et al. (2006). Endogenous adenosine protects preconditioned heart during early minutes of reperfusion by activating Akt. *Am. J. Physiol. Heart. Circ. Physiol. 290*, H441−H449.

[108] Yang, D, Chen, H et al. A new role for the A2b adenosine receptor in regu-lating platelet function. *J. Thromb. Haemost* , 2010; [Epub ahead of print].

[109] Gessi, S, Merighi, S et al. The A3 adenosine receptor: An enigmatic player in cell biology. *Pharmaco. Ther,* 2008; 117:123-40.

[110] Atkinson, M. R., Townsend-Nicholson, A., et al.(1997). Cloning, characteri-sation and chromosomal assignment of the human adenosine A3 receptor (ADORA3) gene. *Neurosci. Res. 29*, 73–79.
[111] Palmer, T. M., and Stiles, G. L. (2000). Identification of threonine residues controlling the agonist-dependent phosphorylation and desensitization of the rat A3 adenosine receptor. *Mol. Pharmacol. 57*, 539–545.
[112] Zhou, Q. -Y., Li, C., Olah, M. E., et al. (1992). Molecular cloning and characterization of an adenosine receptor: the A3 adenosine receptor. *Proc. Natl .Acad. Sci. U. S. A. 89,* 7432–7436.
[113] Salvatore, C. A., Jacobson, et al. (1993). Molecular cloning and character-rization of the human A3 adenosine receptor. *Proc. Natl. Acad. Sci. U. S. A. 90*, 10365–10369.
[114] Dixon, A. K., Gubitz, A. K., et al.(1996). Tissue distribution of adenosine receptor mRNAs in the rat. *Br. J. Pharmacol.118*, 1461–1468.
[115] Tracey, W. R., Magee, W., et al. (1997). Selective Adenosine A3 receptor stimulation reduces ischemic myocardial injury in the rabbit heart. *Cardiovasc. Res. 33,* 410–415.
[116] Xu, Z., Jang, Y., Mueller, R. A., and Norfleet, E. A. (2006). IB-MECA and cardioprotection. *Cardiovasc. Drug. Rev. 24,* 227–238.
[117] Harrison, G. J., Cerniway, R. J., et al. (2002). Effects of A3 adenosine receptor activation and gene knock-out in ischemic-reperfused mouse heart. *Cardiovasc. Res. 53,* 147–155.
[118] Abbracchio, M. P., Brambilla, R., et al. (1995). G protein-dependent activation of phospho-lipase C by adenosine A3 receptors in rat brain. *Mol. Pharmacol. 48,* 1038–1045.
[119] Mozzicato, S., Joshi, B. V., Jacobson, K. A., and Liang, B. T. (2004). Role of direct RhoA-phospholipase D1 interaction in mediating adenosine-induced protection from cardiac ischemia. *FASEB. J.* 18, 406–408.
[120] De Jonge, R, Out, M, Maas, WJ, De Jong, JW. Preconditioning of rat hearts by adenosine A1 or A3 receptor activation. *Eur. J. Pharmacol,* 2002;441:165–172.
[121] Maddock, HL, Gardner, NM, Khandoudi, N, Bril, A, Broadley, KJ. Protection from myocardial stunning by ischaemia and hypoxia with the adenosine A3 receptor agonist, IB-MECA. *Eur. J. Pharmacol,* 2003;477: 235–245.
[122] Goldenberg, I, Shainberg, A, et al. Adenosine protects against angiotensin II-induced apoptosis in rat cardiocyte cultures. *Mol. Cell Biochem,* 2003;252:133–139.
[123] . Hannon, JP, Pfannkuche, HJ, Fozard, JR. A role for mast cells in adenosine A3 receptor-mediated hypotension in the rat. *Br. J. Pharmacol,* 1995;115:945–952.
[124] .Cross, HR, Murphy, RG, et al. Overexpression of A3 adenosine receptors decreases heart rate, preserves energetics, and protects ischemic hearts. *Am. J. Physiol. Heart Circ. Physiol,* 2002;283:H1562-8.
[125] Von Lubitz, D. K. J. E. (1999). Adenosine and cerebral ischemia: therapeutic future or death of a brave concept? *Eur. J. Pharmacol. 371*, 85–102.
[126] Haskó, G., Pacher, P., Vizi, E. S., and Illes, P. (2005). Adenosine receptor signaling in the brain immune system. *Trends. Pharmacol. Sci. 26*, 511–516.
[127] Hammarberg, C., Schulte, G., and Fredholm, B. B. (2003). Evidence for functional adenosine A3 receptors in microglia cells. *J. Neurochem .86*, 1051–1054.
[128] 128. Wittendorp, M. C., Boddeke, H. W. G. M., and Biber, K. (2004). Adenosine A3 receptor-induced CCl2 synthesis in cultured mouse astrocytes. *Glia 46*, 410–418.

[129] . Fredholm ,BB. Adenosine, an endogenous distress signal, modulates tissue damage and repair. *Cell Death Differ,* 2007; 14:1315–23.

[130] Haskó, G, Linden, J, et al. Adenosine receptors: Therapeutic aspects for inflammatory and immune diseases. *Nat. Rev. Drug Discov,* 2008; 7:759–70.

[131] .Prystowsky, EN, Niazi, I, et al. Termination of paroxysmal supraventricular tachycardia by tecadenoson (CVT-510), a novel A1-adenosine receptor agonist. *J. Am. Coll. Cardiol, 2003*; 42:1098–102.

[132] Hansen, PB, Schnermann, J. Vasoconstrictor and vasodilator effects of adenosine in the kidney. *Am. J. Physiol. Renal. Physiol,* 2003; 285:F590–9.

[133] Eckle, T, Köhler, D, Lehmann, R, El Kasmi, K, Eltzschig, HK. Hypoxia-inducible factor-1 is central to cardioprotection: A new paradigm for ischemic preconditioning. *Circulation,* 2008; 118:166–75.

[134] Jin, X, Shepherd, RK, Duling, BR, Linden, J. Inosine binds to A3 adenosine receptors and stimulates mast cell degranulation. *J. Clin. Invest,* 1997; 100:2849–57.

[135] Ledent, C, Vaugeois, JM, et al. Aggressiveness, hypoalgesia and high blood pressure in mice lacking the adenosine A2A receptor. *Nature,* 1997; 388: 674–678

[136] . Fredholm , BB, Chen, JF, Masino, SA, Vaugeois, JM. Actions of adenosine at its receptors in the CNS: insights from knockouts and drugs. *Annu. Rev. Pharmacol. Toxicol,* 2005; 45: 385–412.

[137] . Boison, D. Adenosine kinase, epilepsy and stroke: mechanisms and therapies. *Trends Pharmacol. Sci,* 2006; 27: 652–658.

[138] Conti, B, Sanchez-Alavez ,M, et al. Transgenic mice with a reduced core body temperature have an increased life span. *Science,* 2006; 314: 825–828.

[139] Johansson, B, Halldne,r L, Dunwiddie, TV, L et al. Hyperalgesia, anxiety, and decreased hypoxic neuroprotection in mice lacking the adenosine A1 receptor. *Proc. Natl. Acad. Sci. USA,* 2001; 98: 9407–9412.

[140] . Giménez-Llort, L, Fernández-Teruel, A, et al. Mice lacking the adenosine A1 receptor are anxious and aggressive, but are normal learners with reduced muscle strength and survival rate. *Eur. J. Neurosci*, 2002; 16: 547–550.

[141] . Fredholm ,BB, Bättig, K, et al. Actions of caffeine in the brain with special reference to factors that contribute to its widespread use. *Pharmacol. Rev,* 1999; 51: 83–133.

[142] Adair, TH. Growth regulation of the vascular system: an emerging role for adenosine. *Am. J. Physiol. Regul. Integr. Comp. Physiol*, 2005; 289: R283–R296.

[143] . Greenberg, DA, Jin, K. From angiogenesis to neuropathology. *Nature,* 2005; 438: 954–959.

[144] Eltzschig, HK, Thompson, LF, et al. Endogenous adenosine produced during hypoxia attenuates neutrophil accumulation: coordination by extracellular nucleotide metabolism. *Blood,* 2004; 104: 3986–3992.

[145] Bours , MJ, Swennen, EL, et al. Adenosine 5'- triphosphate and adenosine as endogenous signaling molecules in immunity and inflammation. *Pharmacol. Ther,* 2006; 112: 358–404.

[146] Zernecke, A, Bidzhekov, K, et al. CD73/ecto-50-nucleotidase protects against vascular inflammation and neointima formation. *Circulation,* 2006; 113: 2120–2127.

[147] Akkari, R, Burbiel, JC, et al. Recent progress in the development of adenosine receptor ligands as antiinflammatory drugs. *Curr. Top Med. Chem.* 2006; 6: 1375–1399.

[148] Parker, RB, McCollam, PL. Adenosine in the episodic treatment of paroxysmal supraventricular tachycardia. *Clin. Pharm,* 1990; 9: 261-71.

[149] Pelleg, A, Porter, RS. The pharmacology of adenosine. *Pharmacotherapy,* 1990; 10(3): 157-74.

[150] Löffler, M, Morote-Garcia, JC, et al. Physiological roles of vascular nucleoside transporters. *Arterioscler. Thromb. Vasc. Biol,* 2007; 27:1004–13.

[151] Morote-Garcia, JC, Rosenberger, et al. HIF-1-dependent repression of adenosine kinase attenuates hypoxia-induced vascular leak. *Blood,* 2008; 111:5571–80.

[152] Blackburn, MR, Volmer, JB, et al. Metabolic consequences of adenosine deaminase deficiency in mice are associated with defects in alveogenesis, pul-monary inflammation, and airway obstruction. *J. Exp. Med,* 2000; 192:159–70.

[153] Taylor, R. P., and Starnes, J. W. (2003). Age, cell signalling and cardioprotection. *Acta. Physiol. Scand.178*, 107−116.

[154] Gao, F., Christopher, T. A., et al. (2000). Mechanism of decreased adenosine protection in reperfusion injury of aging rats. *Am. J. Physiol. Heart. Circ. Physiol. 279,* H329−H338.

[155] Schulman, D., Latchman, D. S., and Yellon, D. M. (2001). Effect of aging on the ability of preconditioning to protect rat hearts from ischemia–reperfusion injury. *Am. J. Physiol. Heart. Circ. Physiol. 281,* H1630−H1636.

[156] 156. Headrick, J. P.,Willems, L., (2003b). Ischaemic tolerance in aged mouse myocardium: the role of adenosine and effects of A1 adenosine receptor overexpression. *J. Physiol. 549*, 823−833.

[157] Jones, S. P., and Bolli, R. (2006). The ubiquitous role of nitric oxide in cardioprotection. *J. Mol. Cell. Cardiol. 40,* 16−23.

[158] DiFrancesco, D., Borer, J.S., (2007). The funny current: cellular basis for the control of heart rate. *Drugs 67*, 15–24.

[159] Headrick, J.P., Gauthier, N.S., et al. (2000). Chronotropic and vasodilatory responses to adenosine and isoproterenol in mouse heart: effects of adenosine A1 receptor overexpression. *Clin. Exp. Pharmacol. Physiol. 27,* 185–190.

[160] Kirchhof, P., Fabritz, L., (2003). Altered sinus nodal and atrioventricular nodal function in freely moving mice overexpressing the A1 adenosine receptor. *Am. J. Physiol. Heart. Circ. Physiol. 285,* H145–H153.

[161] Fabritz, L., Kirchhof, P., (2004). Gene dose-dependent atrial arrhythmias, heart block, and brady-cardiomyopathy in mice overexpressing A(3) adenosine receptors. *Cardiovasc. Res. 62,* 500–508.

[162] Hove-Madsen, L., Prat-Vidal, C., (2006). Adenosine A_{2A} receptors are expressed in human atrial myocytes and modulate spontaneous sarcoplasmic reticulum calcium release. *Cardiovasc. Res. 72,* 292–302.

[163] Song, Y., Thedford, S., et al (1992). Adenosine-sensitive afterdepolarizations and triggered activity in guinea pig ventricular myocytes. *Circ. Res. 70,* 743–753.

[164] Xu , J., Hurt, C.M., Pelleg, A. (1995). Digoxin-induced ventricular arrhyth-mias in the guinea pig heart in vivo: evidence for a role of endogenous cate-cholamines in the genesis of delayed afterdepolarizations and triggered activity. *Heart. Vessels. 10,* 119–127.

[165] DiMarco ,J, Seller, TD, et al. Diagnostic and therapeutic use of adenosine in patients with supraventricular tachyarrhythmias. *J. Am. Coll. Cardiol.* 1985;6:417-25.

[166] Cheung, J.W., Lerman, B.B., (2003). CVT-510: a selective A1 adenosine receptor agonist. *Cardiovasc. Drug. Rev. 21,* 277–292.

[167] DiMarco, J., Miles, W., et al. (1990). Adenosine for paroxysmal supra-ventricular tachycardia-dose ranging and comparison with verapamil. *Ann. Intern. Med. 113*, 104-10.

[168] Xanthos, T, Ekmektzoglou, K.A, et al. A prognostic index for the successful use of adenosine in patients with paroxysmal supraventricular tachycardia in emergency settings: a retrospective study. *Am. J. Emerg. Med,* 2008;26:304-9.

[169] Yeh, SJ, Wen, MS, et al. Adenosine sensitive ventricular tachycardia from the anterobasal left ventricle. *J. Am. Coll. Cardiol,* 1997;30:1339–1345.

[170] 170. Lerman, B.B,, Belardinelli, L., et al. (1986) . Adenosine-sensitive ventricular tachycardia: evidence suggesting cyclic AMP-mediated triggered activity. *Circulation. 74,* 270–280.

[171] Lerman, B.B., Stein, K., (1995). Mechanism of repetitive monomorphic ventricular tachycardia. *Circulation. 92,* 421–429.

[172] Mader, T.J., Menegazzi, J.J., et al. (2006). Adenosine A1 receptor antagonism hastens the decay in ventricular fibrillation waveform morphology during porcine cardiac arrest. *Resuscitation. 71,* 254–259.

[173] Viskin, S., Belhassen, B., (1993). Aminophylline for bradyasystolic cardiac arrest refractory to atropine and epinephrine. *Ann. Intern. Med. 118,* 279–281.

[174] Hayward, E., Showler, L., Soar, J., (2007). Aminophylline in bradyasystolic cardiac arrest. *Emerg. Med. J. 24*, 582–583.

[175] . Makujina, S.R., Sabouni, M.H., et al. (1992). Vasodilatory effects of adenosine A2 receptor agonists CGS 21680 and CGS 22492 in human vasculature. *Eur. J. Pharmacol. 221,* 243–247.

[176] Viskin, S., Ross, R., et al. (2006). Provocation of sudden heart rate oscillation with adenosine exposes abnormal QT responses in patients with long QT syndrome: a bedside test for diagnosing long QT syndrome. *Eur. Heart. J. 27,* 469–475.

[177] Pelleg, A., Pennock, R.S., Kutalek, S.P., (2002). Proarrhythmic effects of adenosine: one decade of clinical data. *Am. J. Ther . 9,* 141–147.

[178] Fragakis, N., Iliadis, I., et al. (2007) ,The value of adenosine test in the diagnosis of sick sinus syndrome: susceptibility of sinus and atrioventricular node to adenosine in patients with sick sinus syndrome and unexplained syncope. *Europace. 9,* 559–562

[179] Strauer, B.E., Heidland, U.E., et al. (1996). Pharmacologic myocardial pro-tection during percutaneous transluminal coronary angioplasty by intracoro-nary application of dipyridamole: impact on hemodynamic function and left ventricular performance. *J. Am. Coll. Cardiol. 1996*, 28: 1119–26.

[180] Leesar, MA, Stoddard, M, et al. Preconditioning of human myocardium with adenosine during coronary angioplasty. *Circulation* ,1997;95:2500–7.

[181] Mahaffey, KW, Puma, JA, et al. Adenosine as an adjunct to thrombolytic therapy for acute myocardial infarction: results of a multicenter, randomized, placebo-controlled trial: the Acute Myocardial Infarction Study of Adenosine (AMISTAD) trial. *J. Am. Coll. Cardiol,* 1999;34:1711–20

[182] Lee, HT, LaFaro, RJ, Reed, GE. Pretreatment of human myocardium with adenosine during open heart surgery. *J. Cardiac. Surg,* 1995;10:665–76.

[183] Trappe, HJ. Acute therapy of maternal and fetal arrhythmias during pregnancy. *J. Intensive Care Med,* 2006;21:305-15.

[184] Paul, T, Pfammatter JP. Adenosine: an effective and safe drug in pediatrics. *Pediatr. Cardiol,* 1997;18:118-26.

[185] . Till, J.A., (1992). The use of adenosine in children. *Res. Clin. For. 14:*45–55

[186] Harrington, GR, Froelich ,EG. Adenosine-induced torsades de pointes. *Chest* 1993;103:1299–301.

[187] Paskitti, M, Reid, KH. Use of an adenosine triphosphate-based 'cocktail' early in reperfusion substantially improves brain protein synthesis after global ischemia in rats. *Neurosci. Lett,* 2002;331:147-50.

[188] Andine, P., Rudolphi, K.A., et al. (1990). Effect of propentofylline (HWA 285) on extracellular purines and excitatory amino acids in CA1 of rat hippocampus during transient ischaemia. *Br. J. Pharmacol. 100,* 814–818.

[189] Xu, K, Puchowicz, MA, et al. Adenosine treatment delays postischemic hippocampal CA1loss after cardiac arrest and resuscitation in rats. *Brain Res,* 2006;

[190] Karibe, H., Chen, S.F., (1994). Mild intraischemic hypothermia suppresses consumption of endogenous antioxidants after temporary focal ischemia in rats. *Brain Res. 649,* 12–18.

[191] .Gidday, J.M., Kim, Y.B., et al. (1996). Adenosine transport inhibition ameliorates postischemic hypoperfusion in pigs. *Brain Res. 734*, 261–268.

[192] Crookes, BA, Cohn, SM, et al. Building a Better Fluid for Emergency Resuscitation of Traumatic Brain Injury. *J. Trauma,* 2004;57:547-54.

[193] Weisfeldt, ML, Becker ,LB. Resuscitation after cardiac arrest: a 3-phase time-sensitive model. *JAMA,* 2002;288:3035-8.

[194] Kern, KB, Garewal, HS, et al. Depletion of myocardial adenosine triphos-phate during prolonged untreated ventricular fibrillation: effect on defibrillation success. *Resuscitation*, 1990;20:221-9.

[195] Callaway, CW, Sherman, LD, et al. Scaling structure of electrocardiographic waveform during prolonged ventricular fibrillation in swine. *Pacing and Clinical Electrophysiology*, 2000;23:180–91.

[196] Sherman, LD, Rea, TD, et al. Logarithm of the absolute correlations of the ECG waveform estimates duration of ventricular fibrillation and predicts successful defibrillation. *Resuscitation, 2008;*78:346–54.

[197] Menegazzi, JJ, Rittenberger, JC, et al. Effects of pre-arrest and intraarrest hypothermia on ventricular fibrillation and resuscitation. *Resuscitation,* 2009;80:126–32.

[198] Salcido, DD, Menegazzi, JJ, et al. Association of intramyocardial high energy phosphate concentrations with quantitative measures of the ventricular fibrillation electrocardiogram waveform. *Resuscitation,* 2009;80:946-50.

[199] Sherman LD, Mader TJ, et al. Sex differences exist in porcine ventricular fibrillation morphology [abstract]*Circulation,* 2006;114(suppl II):100.

[200] Mader, TJ, Gibson, P. Adenosine receptor antagonism in refractory asystolic cardiac arrest: results of a human pilot study. *Resuscitation,* 1997;35:3-7.

[201] Mader, TJ, Menegazzi, JJ, et al. The effect of adenosine A1 receptor antagonism on return of spontaneous circulation and short-term survival in prolonged ventricular fibrillation. *Prehosp. Emerg. Care*, 2008;12:352-8.

[202] Mader, TJ, Smithline, HA, et al. A Randomized Controlled Trial of Intravenous Aminophylline for Atropine-resistant Out-of-hospital Asystolic Cardiac Arrest. *Acad. Emerg. Med,* 2003;10:192-7.

[203] Lerman, BB, Engelstein, ED. Metabolic determinants of defibrillation. Role of adenosine. *Circulation,* 1995;91:838-44.

[204] Saraste, A, Pulkki, K, Kallajoki ,M, et al. Apoptosis in human acute myocar-dial infarction. *Circulation,* 1997; 95: 320–323.

[205] Vähäsilita, T, Virtanen, J, et al. Adenosine in myocardial protection given through three windows of opportunity. An experimental study with pigs. *Scand. Cardiovasc. J,* 2001;35:409-14

[206] Cain, BS, Meldrun, DR, Adenosine reduces cardiac TNF production and human myocardial injury following ischemia-reperfusion. *J. Surg. Res,* 1998; 76: 117–123.

[207] Klouche, K, Weil, MH, Sun, S, et al. Evolution of the stone heart after prolonged cardiac arrest. *Chest,* 2002, 122:1006–1011.

[208] Takino, M, Okada, Y. Firm myocardium in cardiopulmonary resuscitation. *Resuscitation,* 1996, 33:101–106.

[209] Deantonio , HJ, Kaul, S, Lerman, BB. Reversible myocardial depression in survivors of cardiac arrest. *Pacing Clin. Electrophysiol,* 1990; 13:982–985.

In: Drugs in Cardiopulmonary Resuscitation
Editor: Theodoros Xanthos

ISBN: 978-1-61122-512-9

Chapter 11

Inotropes and Vasopressors in Post-Resuscitation Care

Sotirios Kakavas and Theodoros Xanthos
University of Athens, Medical School

Abstract

The post-resuscitation period should comprise a second, more complex phase of interventions which are likely to influence, significantly, the final outcome. As a critical component of post-resuscitation care, prompt optimisation of hemodynamic status by means of targeted interventions is vital in order to maximize the likelihood of a good outcome. In this setting, prompt administration of fluids and potentially vasopressors and inotropes are common treatment modalities of circulatory support after cardiac arrest. Furthermore, vasoactive agents may be required in the setting of underlying conditions complicating the post-resuscitation condition of the patient. The clinical efficacy of inotropes and vasopressors has been largely investigated through examination of their impact on hemodynamic end points, and clinical practice has been driven in part by expert opinion, extrapolation from animal studies, and physician preference. Careful and frequent monitoring of hemodynamic parameters and other measures, as required, is crucial to ensure optimal outcomes with the use of vasoactive agents. Clearly these agents are all supportive measures to stabilise the patient prior to some form of definitive therapy, and it is important to emphasise that all these pharmacological agents are associated with potentially significant side effects.

Introduction

Return of spontaneous circulation (ROSC) is just the first step toward the goal of complete recovery from cardiac arrest [1,2]. Unfortunately, data shows that only a small percentage of patients with ROSC survive to hospital discharge [3] although there is considerable variation in post-cardiac arrest treatment and patient outcome between institutions [4,5]. Care of the post-cardiac arrest patient is time-sensitive, as most post-resuscitation deaths occur during the first 24 hours [6]. Data from clinical research on sepsis [7] suggest that outcomes are optimized when interventions are both goal-directed and initiated as early as possible [8-10].

Hemodynamic instability, possibly multifactorial in origin, is common after cardiac arrest with abnormalities of cardiac rate, rhythm, systemic blood pressure (BP), and organ perfusion [2]. This circulatory deregulation is often related to a transient myocardial dysfunction that has been described by several case series [6,11] and is manifested by tachycardia and elevated left ventricular end-diastolic pressure, hypotension and low cardiac output (CO) [6,12]. Moreover, a systemic ischemic-reperfusion response may develop after ROSC, which is associated with inadequate tissue oxygen delivery, microcirculatory failure and subsequent generalized activation of immunologic and coagulation pathways [13,14]. This systemic response shares many common features with sepsis [15,16] and clinical manifestations include intravascular volume depletion, impaired vasoregulation, impaired oxygen delivery and utilization, and increased susceptibility to multiple organ failure and infection [15-17]. In addition, the pathophysiology of post-resuscitation hemodynamic instability is commonly complicated by persisting acute pathology that caused or contributed to the cardiac arrest itself, such as acute coronary syndrome (ACS), heart failure (HF) and dysrhythmias.

A significant body of knowledge suggests that the pathologies responsible for hemodynamic instability are potentially treatable [18,19]. Initial treatment with supplemental high flow oxygen will go some way to reducing tissue hypoxia and early recourse to mechanical ventilation will help by reducing the work of breathing as well as the preload and afterload. Adequate fluid resuscitation and treatment of associated arrhythmia, myocardial ischemia and electrolyte abnormalities is essential. During post-resuscitation care, it may be necessary to augment BP and CO by one of three ways: (1) pharmacological inotropic or/and vasopressor support, (2) intra-aortic balloon counterpulsation and (3) revascularisation with thrombolysis, percutaneous intervention or coronary artery bypass surgery [2]. Inotropic and vasopressor agents have increasingly become a therapeutic cornerstone for the management of critically ill patients in the setting of several important cardiovascular syndromes. The principal aim of these drugs is to restore inadequate systemic and regional perfusion to physiological levels by the enhancement of CO or modulation of vascular tone that have been severely compromised during the post-resuscitation period. The hemodynamic effects of vasoactive agents vary from drug to drug, but may also vary in a dose-dependent manner in a single agent. This variation results from differing pharmacological actions on receptors.

Receptors and Drugs

Inotropes, such as dobutamine and milrinone, are defined as drugs that increase the force of cardiac contraction and thus may result in increased CO and BP [20,21]. Vasopressors, such as norepinephrine and phenylephrine, exert a predominantly vasoconstrictive action on the peripheral vasculature and are used primarily to increase mean arterial pressure (MAP). The distinction between these two groups of drugs is often confusing. Some agents, such as dopamine and epinephrine, possess combined inotrope/vasopressor properties, while others have variable effects on the peripheral vasculature. Given the overlap of pharmacodynamic effects of these drugs, the term 'vasoactive agents' seems as a more appropriate description.

Vasopressors and inotropes can be subdivided in three major subgroups, namely, catecholamines, phosphodiesterase-III inhibitors (PDIs) and, more recently, calcium (Ca^{2+}) sensitizers (levosimendan). Vasopressin can also be regarded as a potent vasopressor. The following table summarizes the clinical indications, standard dosing and major side effects of significant inotropic and vasopressors drugs.

Table 1. Inotropes and Vasopressors, Clinical Indications, Standard Dose Range and Major Clinical Side Effects

Drug	Clinical Indication	Dose Range	Major Side Effects
Catecholamines			
Dopamine	Shock (cardiogenic, vasodilatory), HF symptomatic bradycardia unresponsive to atropine or pacing	2.0 to 20 μg/kg/min (max. 50 μg/kg/min)	Severe hypertension (especially in patients taking nonselective *β*-blockers), ventricular arrhythmias, cardiac ischemia, tissue ischemia/gangrene (high doses or due to tissue extravasation)
Dobutamine	Low CO (decompensated HF, cardiogenic shock, sepsis-induced myocardial dysfunction), symptomatic bradycardia unresponsive to atropine or pacing	2.0 to 20 μg/kg/min (max. 40 μg/kg/min)	Tachycardia, increased ventricular response rate in patients with AF, ventricular arrhythmias, cardiac ischemia, hypertension (especially nonselective *β*-blocker patients), hypotension
Norepinephrine	Shock (vasodilatory, cardiogenic)	0.01-3 μg/kg/min	Arrhythmias, bradycardia, peripheral (digital) ischemia, hypertension (especially nonselective *β*-blocker patients)
Epinephrine	Shock (cardiogenic, vasodilatory, CA, bronchospasm/anaphylaxis, symptomatic bradycardia or heart block unresponsive to atropine or pacing	Infusion: 0.01-0.10 μg/kg/min Bolus: 1 mg IV every 3-5 min IM: (1:1000): 0.1 to 0.5 mg (max 1 mg)	Ventricular arrhythmias, severe hypertension resulting in cerebrovascular hemorrhage, cardiac ischemia, sudden cardiac death
Isoproterenol	Bradyarrhythmias unresponsive to atropine or pacing	2-10 μg/min	Ventricular arrhythmias,cardiac ischemia, hypertension, hypotension
Phenylephrine	Hypotension (vagally mediated, medication-induced)	Bolus: 0.1-0.5 mg IV every 10-15 min Infusion: 0.4-9.1 μg/kg/min	Reflex bradycardia,h ypertension (especially with nonselective *β*-blockers), severe peripheral and visceral vasoconstriction, tissue necrosis with extravasation

Table 1. (continued)

Drug	Clinical Indication	Dose Range	Major Side Effects
PDIs			
Milrinone	Low CO (decompensated HF, after cardiotomy)	Bolus: 50 μg/kg bolus over 10 to 30 min Infusion: 0.375 to 0.75 μg/kg/min (dose adjustment necessary for renal impairment)	Ventricular arrhythmias, hypotension, cardiac ischemia, torsade des pointes
Amrinone	Low CO (refractory HF)	Bolus: 0.75 mg/kg over 2 to 3 min Infusion: 5 to 10 μg/kg/min	Arrhythmias, enhanced AV conduction (increased ventricular response rate in AF), hypotension, thrombocytopenia, hepatotoxicity
Vasopressin	Shock (vasodilatory, cardiogenic), CA	Infusion: 0.01 to 0.1 U/min (common fixed dose 0.04 U/min) Bolus: 40-U IV bolus	Arrhythmias, hypertension, decreased CO (at doses >0.4 U/min), cardiac ischemia, severe peripheral vasoconstriction causing ischemia (especially skin), splanchnic vasoconstriction
Ca^{2+} sensitizers			
Levosimendan	Decompensated HF	Loading dose: 12 to 24 μg/kg over 10 min Infusion: 0.05 to 0.2 μg/kg/min	Tachycardia, enhanced AV conduction, hypotension

HF: heart failure; CO: cardiac output; AF: atrial fibrillation; CA: cardiac arrest; IV: intravenous; IM: intramuscular; AV: atrioventricular; Ca^{2+}: calcium

The ideal vasoactive agent should increase contractility, MAP and CO, and enhance tissue perfusion without increasing myocardial oxygen consumption. Furthermore, its use should not be associated with an increased possibility for tachycardia, arrhythmias or toxicity. Ideally, such an agent should be cost effective, compatible with other drugs and, finally, easily titratable. Therefore, its action should be characterized by rapid onset and termination, and the lack of tolerance. Unfortunately, no agent possesses all the prementioned features. Apparently, inotropes and vasopressors display considerable differences in their pharmacokinetics and pharmacodynamics, because of their differential abilities to stimulate individual receptors or modulate distinct cellular processes. Accordingly, each agent must be considered separately.

Catecholamines (Sympathomimetic Amines)

Sympathomimetic amines (catecholamines) are the most frequently used vasoactive agents in the intensive care unit (ICU) [20,21]. These include the naturally occurring catecholamines dopamine, norepinephrine (noradrenaline) and epinephrine (adrenaline), as well as synthetic substances such as dobutamine, isoprenaline and dopexamine. The latter carry out their pharmacological effects mainly by mimicking the physiological responses of endogenous catecholamines, which mediate the action of sympathetic nervous system (SNS) upon individual tissues. The postganglionic receptors of SNS are termed adrenergic receptors and noradrenaline is the major endogenous neurotransmitter. Natural occurring and synthetic catecholamines bind to populations of adrenergic receptors, largely divided into alpha (α) and beta (β) subgroups, and dopaminergic receptors (DA). Further subgroups of α- (α_{1A}, α_{1B}, α_{1D}, α_{2A}, α_{2B}, α_{2C}), β- (β_1, β_2, β_3) and DA receptors (DA_1 and DA_2) have been identified [22,23].

Catecholamines consist of an aromatic ring attached to a terminal amine by a carbon chain. Epinephrine (adrenaline), a natural catecholamine extracted from the adrenal gland, was the principal active substance to be discovered [24]. Since then, various endogenous and synthetic catecholamines or "sympathomimetics" have been characterized [25]. Norepinephrine is the predominant peripheral sympathetic neurotransmitter. It is formed through the hydroxylation of dopamine in a synthetic pathway shared by all catecholamines, including L-dopa, dopamine, norepinephrine and epinephrine. The release of norepinephrine from sympathetic terminals is augmented by epinephrine released from the adrenal gland at times of stress. Norepinephrine is converted to form epinephrine that is subsequently metabolized in liver and lung.

The cardiovascular actions of individual catecholamines depends on their relative binding affinities to adrenergic receptors, predominantly α_1, β_1, β_2, and dopaminergic receptors [20,21,26]. Direct acting drugs act by stimulating the SNS receptors, whereas indirect acting agents cause the release of endogenous catecholamines which subsequently produce the effect. Some agents are characterized by mixed properties. Post synaptic α_1- and α_2-adrenergic receptors stimulation, mainly in smooth muscle and splachnic vessels, results in vasonstriction and an increase in systemic vascular resistance (SVR). Presynaptic α_2 receptors in heart and vasculature appear to mediate negative feedback inhibition of further norepinephrine release. β_1 Receptors are predominant postsynaptic adrenergic receptors in the heart, and their activation leads to enhanced myocardial contractility and enhanced chronotropy. Stimulation of postsynaptic β_2-adrenergic receptors, predominantly in skeletal muscle blood vessels, results in vasodilation. Finally, peripheral DA_1 dopaminergic receptors mediate renal, coronary and mesenteric arterial vasodilatation and a natriuretic response, while DA_2 dopaminergic receptors act as presynaptic receptors on sympathetic nerve endings and inhibit norepinephrine release.

The physiological actions of adrenergic receptors are mediated through the activation of distinct second-messenger systems [22,23,26]. Subsequent phosphorylation of substrate proteins via protein kinases act as third messengers to trigger a cascade of events which lead to specific cardiovascular effects. The β receptor is linked with a stimulatory Gs-guanidine triphosphate unit (Gs-GTP), which activates the adenyl cyclase system resulting in increased concentrations of cyclic AMP (cAMP). In cardiac myocytes, β_1-mediated increase of cAMP concentration activates Ca^{2+} channels and increases cytosolic Ca^{2+}, which leads to Ca^{2+}-

mediated enhanced chronotropic responses and enhanced myocardial contractility (positive inotropy) through Ca^{2+}-mediated facilitation of the actin-myosin complex binding with troponin C. In vascular smooth muscle, β_2-mediated increase of cAMP results in stimulation of a cAMP-dependent protein kinase, phosphorylation of phospholamban, and augmented Ca^{2+} uptake by the sarcoplasmic reticulum (SR), which leads to vasodilation. The α_1 receptor, on the other hand, activates a different regulatory G protein (Gq), which acts through the phospholipase C system and the production of 1,2-diacylglycerol (DAG) and, via phosphatidyl-inositol-4,5-biphosphate (PiP2), of inositol 1,4,5-triphosphate (IP3). IP3 activates the release of Ca^{2+} from the SR, which by itself and through the Ca^{2+}-calmodulin dependent protein kinases influences cellular processes, which in vascular smooth muscle leads to vasoconstriction. DAG, simultaneously, activates protein kinase C, which leads to the phosphorylation of other proteins within the cell.

The configuration of each drug is important for determining affinity to respective receptors [20,21]. Naturally occurring catecholamines (epinephrine, norepinephrine and dopamine) are all predominantly β-agonists at low doses, with increasing α-effects becoming evident as the dose is increased. Synthetic catecholamines derived from dopamine are characterised by increased length of the carbon chain, which confers affinity for β-receptors. These agents are all predominantly β-agonists and have relatively little affinity for α-receptors due to the configuration of the terminal amine, which differs from the endogenous catecholamines. Epinephrine, norepinephrine and isoprenaline are associated with 100-fold greater potency than dopamine or dobutamine due to the presence of hydroxyl groups on the β-carbon atom of the side chain. Table 2 summarizes the differing potency and efficacy of various catecholamines at specific receptor types.

A continuum exists between the effects of the predominantly α_1-stimulation of phenylephrine (intense vasoconstriction) to the β-stimulation of isoproterenol (marked increase in contractility and heart rate - HR -) [20,21].

Specific cardiovascular responses are further modified by reflexive autonomic changes after acute BP alterations, which impact HR, SVR, and other hemodynamic parameters. In addition to adrenergic regulation, vasomotor tone is also modulated by neurohumoral pathways. These are mediated through the renin-aldosterone-angiotensin axis and local mediators such as vasopressin, corticosteroids, nitric oxide (NO), endothelin and the eicosanoids [27].

Table 2. Catecholamines and receptor binding

Drug	Receptor Binding			
	α_1	β_1	β_2	DA
Dopamine	+++	++++	++	+++++
Dobutamine	+	+++++	+++	N/A
Norepinephrine	+++++	+++	++	N/A
Epinephrine	+++++	++++	+++	N/A
Isoproterenol	0	+++++	+++++	N/A
Phenylephrine	+++++	0	0	N/A

α_1 indicates α_1 receptor; β_1, β_1 receptor; β_2, β_2 receptor; DA: dopamine receptors; 0: zero significant receptor affinity; + through +++++: minimal to maximal relative receptor affinity; N/A: not applicable

Therefore, the final hemodynamic effect depends upon a multitude of factors. Moreover, the systemic effects of these agents may vary greatly between patients and within individuals at different times. Table 3 summarizes the cardiovascular effects of the catecholamines under physiological conditions [20].

Table 3. Cardiovascular effects of catecholamines

	Effect on hemodynamic parameters			
	HR	CI	SVR	MAP
Epinephrine				
≤0.2 mcg/kg/min (β_1, β_2)	Increase	Increase	Decrease	Variable
>0.2 mcg/kg/min (α)	None	None or decrease	Increase	Increase
Norepinephrine (α > β)	Variable	None or decrease	Increase	Increase
Phenyleprine (α)	Decrease	None or decrease	Increase	Increase
Dopamine				
0.5-2 mcg/kg/min (DA)	None	None	None but renal and mesenteric vasodilation	None or decrease
2–5 mcg/kg/min (β_1)	Increase	Increase	None	None or slight increase
>10 mcg/kg/min (α)	None	None or decrease	Increase	Increase
Dobutamine (β_1, β_2 > α)	Increase	Increase	Decrease	Variable
Isoproterenol (β_1, β_2)	Increase	Increase	Decrease	Variable

HR: heart rate; CI: cardiac index; MAP: mean arterial pressure; SVR: systemic vascular resistance

Theoretically, in cases of prominent peripheral vasodilatation (for example in septic shock) it seems entirely reasonable to administer agents that antagonise this vasodilatation by causing vasoconstriction due to activation of α-receptors. Where there is evidence of impaired heart performance, addition of an agent that augments such performance by acting on β-receptors, seems wise. However, adequacy of response is often unpredictable and depends on the aetiology of circulatory failure and systemic comorbidities. In some patients, dramatic responses to small doses may occur, whilst in others, large doses of inotropes may be required to support the failing circulation. Thus, the selection of the most appropriate agent for each patient should be based not only on the pharmacology of the drug but also on careful consideration of the clinical status of the patient.

All catecholamines have very short biological half-lives (1-2 minutes) and are generally very short acting [20,21,26]. These agents should be administered via a central line via an infusion controller. A steady state plasma concentration is achieved within 5-10 minutes after the start of a constant infusion. This allows rapid titration of drug to a clinical end-point such as the MAP. α_1-Mediated responses have slower onset and longer duration than β_1 receptor mediated responses. In the failing myocardium, β-adrenergic receptors may be desensitized and downregulated [28]. In these situations, α_1 and α_2 receptors have an important role in maintaining peripheral vasoresponsiveness and inotropy. This may render catecholamines, particularly β-agonists such as dobutamine, ineffective; this is termed 'tolerance' or tachyphylaxis. This phenomenon may explain the requirement for high doses of catecholamines in refractory shock states. Furthermore, the relative binding affinities of individual catecholamines to adrenergic receptors and subsequently their clinical effect can be diminished under hypoxia [29] or acidosis [30].

The administration of catecholamines requires close monitoring, as side effects may occur including tachycardia, arrhythmias, and hyper- or hypotension [20,21]. Furthermore, catecholamines may precipitate or deteriorate myocardial ischaemia by increasing myocardial oxygen consumption and, due to activation of proteolytic enzymes, proapoptotic signal cascades, mitochondrial damage, and eventual membrane disruption and necrosis [31]. All catecholamines are equally effective in increasing splanchnic perfusion and renal blood flow primarily because of increased CO and MAP. However the resultant natriuresis is not accompanied by alterations in glomerular filtration rate (GFR). In addition, concerns exist about agents that induce α-mediated splanchnic vasoconstriction and may lead to mesenteric and hepatic ischaemia. Similarly, the possibility for development of digital ischemia or gangrene has been attributed to catecholamine-induced vasoconstriction. Under physiological conditions, catecholamines do not normally cross the blood-brain barrier. However, if the blood-brain barrier is disrupted, for example following traumatic brain injury, exogenous catecholamines may directly enter the cerebral circulation. The resultant outcome remains undetermined, but there is some evidence suggesting that dopamine has a direct effect causing increased cerebral blood flow and intracranial pressure [32]. Catecholamine-mediated β-stimulation may result in hyperglycaemia, hypokalaemia and hypophosphataemia, which may need monitoring and correcting. Finally, adrenaline is associated with the development of adverse metabolic effects including hyperlactataemia and acidaemia [33]. Therefore, the lowest possible doses of inotropic and pressor agents should be used to adequately support vital tissue perfusion while limiting adverse consequences.

Epinephrine

Epinephrine (adrenaline), mainly secreted by the adrenal medulla, is an endogenous catecholamine which acts as a neurotransmitter in the SNS [24,25]. It is synthesized from norepinephrine and binds to both α- and β-receptor subgroups [20,21]. β-Effects are prominent at low doses, and α-effects predominate at high doses. Its primary efficacy is due to its α-adrenergic, vasoconstrictive effects, while β_1-adrenergic actions of epinephrine result in increased HR and force of contraction. Therefore, epinephrine is a powerful vasoconstrictor, a positive inotrope, and a positive chronotrope. Increased HR and force of contraction produce an increase in CO. Systolic BP rises, but with low doses diastolic BP may fall due to vasodilation and increased blood flow through skeletal muscle beds resulting from ß2-adrenoceptor effects. At higher doses, the vasoconstrictive effects of α_1 stimulation become more apparent causing an increase in SVR and in both systolic and diastolic BP.

Arterial and venous pulmonary pressures are increased through direct pulmonary vasoconstriction and increased pulmonary blood flow. Bronchial smooth muscle is relaxed due to β_2 action resulting in bronchodilation. Coronary blood flow is enhanced through an increased relative duration of diastole at higher HR and through stimulation of myocytes to release local vasodilators, which largely counterbalance direct α_1-mediated coronary vasoconstriction [34].

However, concomitant increases in myocardial oxygen consumption and transient hypoxaemia due to pulmonary arteriovenous shunting may offset these benefits. Moreover, high and prolonged doses can cause direct cardiac toxicity through damage to arterial walls, which causes focal regions of myocardial contraction band necrosis, and, through direct stimulation of myocyte, apoptosis [35]. Epinephrine increases the irritability of automatic conducting system and may predispose to ectopic ventricular dysrhythmias (particularly when the myocardium is acidotic). Administration of this agent is associated with a decrease in the splanchnic blood flow and an increase in blood glucose and systemic lactate concentrations [33].

Commercial solutions of epinephrine are available in concentrations of 1:1000 (i.e. 1 mg in 1 ml) and 1:10,000 (i.e. 1 mg in 10ml). Epinephrine is the first drug used in cardiac arrest of any aetiology [36]. It is included in the advanced cardiac life support (ACLS) algorithm for use every 3-5 min of cardiopulmonary resuscitation (CPR) (1 mg intravenous - IV - bolus).

Furthermore, epinephrine is preferred in the treatment of anaphylaxis (0.1 to 0.5 mg intramuscular - IM - , max. 1 mg) and is a second-line inotrope for cardiogenic and vasodilatory shock (IV infusion at rate 0.01-0.20 μg/kg/min) in patients who are unresponsive to first-line agents [20,21,26]. Major undesirable effects include an increase in lactate levels, a potential to produce myocardial ischemia or arrhythmias, and a reduction in splanchnic flow. Care should be taken with halothane anaesthesia as arrhythmias may frequently occur.

Norepinephrine

Norepinephrine is a major endogenous neurotransmitter liberated by postganglionic adrenergic nerves. It is a potent α_1-adrenergic receptor agonist with modest β_1 effects and no clinically significant β_2 effects [20,21,26]. Therefore, it is a powerful vasoconstrictor and acts primarily as a vasopressor increasing SVR and MAP. Norepinephrine has a minimal impact on CO resulting in no change or slight decrease in CO due to increased afterload.

Due to its minimal chronotropic effects, norepinephrine is less likely to cause tachycardia than epinephrine. On the contrary, unopposed vasoconstriction may induce reflex bradycardia. Coronary flow is increased due to elevated diastolic BP and indirect stimulation of cardiomyocytes, which release local vasodilators [37].

However, prolonged norepinephrine infusion can have a direct toxic effect on cardiac myocytes by inducing apoptosis via protein kinase A activation and increased cytosolic Ca^{2+} influx [38]. Despite its vasoconstrictive properties, norepinephrine may increase renal blood flow and urine output in hypotensive patients by increasing perfusion pressure.

It is indicated for the treatment of refractory hypotension [20,21,26]. As a vasopressor, it can successfully increase BP in shock (vasodilatory, cardiogenic), especially in the case of septic shock, where peripheral vasodilation is prominent. Nevertheless, norepineprhine, as others vasopressors, is not recommended as first-line agent in cardiogenic shock and is only indicated in patients who remain hypotensive when the combination of an inotropic agent and fluid challenge fails to restore systolic BP, despite an improvement in CO.

The rate of norepinephrine infusion may vary from 0.01 to 1.5 mcg/kg/min. Large doses, as high as 3.0 mcg/kg/min, may be required because of the α-receptor down-regulation in persons with sepsis. Major side effects include arrhythmias, bradycardia and hypertension (especially in patients under medication with a non-selective β-blocker).

Isoproterenol (Isoprenaline)

Isoproterenol is a powerful, nonselective, synthetic β-adrenergic agonist with virtually no affinity for α-adrenergic receptors [20,21,26]. This agent causes potent β_1-mediated chronotropy and inotropy and β_2-mediated bronchodilation. β_2-Mediated potent systemic vasodilatory effects lead to a drop in SVR and diastolic BP. However, with usual doses this is counterbalanced by an increase in CO that is usually enough to maintain or even raise MAP in some cases. The main indication of isoproterenol is bradyarrhythmias including complete heart block, overdose of beta blockers, severe bradycardia unresponsive to atropine or bradycardia-induced torsade des pointes. It is administered by IV infusion usually at a rate of 2-10 μg/min. Isoproterenol can also be used to treat asthma, but is considered less suitable than drugs that act only on b_2 receptors e.g. salbutamol. Side effects include ventricular arrhythmias, cardiac ischemia and hyper- or hypotension.

Phenylephrine

Phenylephrine is potent synthetic α-adrenergic agonist with virtually no affinity for β-adrenergic receptors [20,21,26]. Its vasoconstrictive properties are similar to those of norepinephrine, but phenylephrine is even shorter acting. Thus, phenylephrine increases systolic and diastolic BP in a dose-dependent manner, but because of its minimal β-effects, HR and contractility are generally not affected. However, rapid alterations in MAP by the use of phenylephrine may induce significant reflex bradycardia. Phenylephrine is used primarily for immediate correction of sudden severe vagally mediated hypotension or hypotension induced by medication or anesthesia. It can also be administered to raise MAP in patients with severe refractory hypotension resulting from shock although it has been largely replaced by other catecholamines (norepinphrine, dopamine). An initial IV bolus of 0.1-0.5 mg over 1 min may be given in urgent situations. If required, infusion at an initial rate of 20–50 mcg/min may follow. Possible side-effects include the induction of hypertension (especially in patients under medication with non-selective β-blockers) and severe peripheral and visceral vasoconstriction.

Ephedrine

Ephedrine is naturally occurring amine with both direct and indirect sympathomimetic effects [20,21,26]. It acts directly on β-receptors, and, primarily, indirectly on α-receptors by causing norepinephrine release from postganglionic sympathetic nerve endings. The haemodynamic effects are similar to epinephrine but ephedrine has a longer duration of action and is active when administered orally. The produced increased cardiac contractility and HR lead to increased CO. α-Mediated peripheral vasoconstriction is balanced by simultaneous vasodilation with little overall change in SVR. Collectively, ephedrine raises MAP by causing a greater increase in systolic than diastolic BP. Moreover, it relaxes bronchial and other smooth muscle, but less effectively compared to epinephrine. Ephedrine is not catabolized by monoamine oxidase (MAO) and, thus, it is excreted unchanged by kidney. The primary indication of IV ephedrine is to treat hypotension due to vasodilation e.g. following spinal or epidural anaesthesia. It may also be used to treat hypotension resulting from sympathectomy or overdose of antihypertensive drugs. It is considered as the best vasopressor to use in pregnancy as it does not reduce placental blood flow. Ephedrine is administered in IV boluses of 3-10 mg repeated as necessary within a short time (maximum dose is 60 mg). Its length of action is 5-15 minutes, but repeated doses may be less effective due to the induction of tachyphylaxis. Side effects include tachycardia and hypertension. The possibility of arrhythmias is greater if ephedrine is used with halothane.

Methoxamine

Methoxamine produces direct and indirect effects acting both as an α-agonist and a β-blocker [20,21,26]. The primary effect is peripheral vasoconstriction resulting in rise in systolic and diastolic BP. Bradycardia may occur due to β-blocking action and a reflex decrease in HR. This combined effect renders methoxamine useful in the case of hypotension with tachycardia. Methoxamine is indicated in hypotensive states due to spinal or epidural block. It is administered IV in bolus doses of 2-10 mg repeated as necessary within 2 mins. Hypertension, bradycardia and precipitation myocardial ischaemia are possible side effects.

Metaraminol

Metaraminol acts on adrenoreceptors both, directly, as a selective α_1-agonist and, indirectly, by causing the release of endogenous norepinephrine [20,21,26]. Its haemodynamic effects are similar to ephedrine except that overall peripheral resistance is increased. Increased SVR and CO due to prominent vasoconstriction and β-mediated positive inotropy lead to a greater increase in BP, especially diastolic BP. Reflex bradycardia can result from vasoconstriction but less likely than methoxamine or phenylephrine. Metaraminol is indicated for the prevention and treatment of acute hypotension during spinal anesthesia and as an adjunct in the treatment of hypotension due to various aetiologies. It can be administered as IV boluses of 1 mg or by infusion at 1-20 mg/hr. The dose for subcutaneous (SC) or IM administration is 2-10 mg.

Dopamine

Dopamine is an endogenous neurotransmitter found in both the central and peripheral nervous systems. It is the immediate precursor to norepinephrine in the catecholamine synthetic pathway. Dopamine directly stimulates dopaminergic and adrenergic receptors, and it, indirectly, causes the release of endogenous norepinephrine to elicit a multitude of clinical effects [20,21,26]. The action of dopamine is complex and dose dependent. At low doses (0.5 to 2 μg/kg/min) dopamine directly stimulates DA_1 postsynaptic receptors concentrated in the coronary, renal, mesenteric, and cerebral beds and DA_2 presynaptic receptors present in the vasculature and renal tissues and promotes vasodilation and increased blood flow to these tissues. Dopamine also has direct natriuretic effects through its action on renal tubules [39]. Such doses are still used by some for renal protection ('renal dose') since urine output may increase, while BP and HR are usually not affected. However, the clinical efficacy of "renal-dose" dopamine seems contradictory, as it does not increase GFR and it has not been demonstrated to prevent renal failure [40,41]. Intermediate doses (3 to 10 μg/kg/min) are commonly used for inotropy due to a modest activation of β-receptors, as well as the promotion of release and the inhibition of reuptake of norepinephrine in sympathetic nerve terminals. These actions result in positive inotropic and chronotropic effects, while increased myocardial contractility and HR lead to enhanced CO. At higher infusion rates (10 to 20 μg/kg/min), an additional α_1-adrenergic action becomes prominent. Extensive vasoconstriction causes SVR and MAP to increase. At doses greater than 20 μg/kg/min, the effects of dopamine are similar to those of norepinephrine.

Dopamine is primarily used for haemodynamic support in cases of shock (cardiogenic, vasodilatory) as well as acute or decompensated chronic HF [20,21,26]. It is usually initiated at a rate of 5-10 mcg/kg/min IV, and the infusion rate is adjusted according to MAP and other hemodynamic parameters. If the patient remains hypotensive despite dopamine administration, a direct vasoconstrictor (e.g. norepinephrine) should be added and titrated to maintain an MAP of 60 mm Hg. Dopamine may also be administered in symptomatic bradycardia unresponsive to atropine or pacing at a dose of 1 μg/kg/min. Available data do not support administration of low doses of dopamine solely to maintain renal function [38,39]. Undesirable effects include the induction of tachycardia or ventricular arrhythmias and the potential to decrease splanchnic perfusion and increase pulmonary shunting. Although dopamine increases myocardial contractility, at the same time it may increase myocardial oxygen demand and deteriorate cardiac ischemia. Severe hypertension may occur, especially in patients taking nonselective β-blockers.

Dopexamine

Dopexamine is a synthetic catecholamine structurally related to dopamine. It exerts a marked direct agonist activity on β_2-receptors and to a lesser degree on β_1- and DA receptors [20,21,26]. Moreover, it acts indirectly on adrenoreceptors by inhibiting the uptake of endogenous catecholamines. As a result, HR and CO are enhanced, while afterload is reduced due to pronounced arterial vasodilatation. Renal perfusion is increased by selective renal vasodilatation and mild direct and indirect positive inotropy. Dopexamine is not as effective as dopamine at increasing renal blood flow, but causes a substantially greater increase in cardiac index (CI). This agent can be used for haemodynamic support in the setting of acute HF or following cardiac surgery. IV infusion is initiated at 0.5 mcg/kg/min and titrated upwards in increments of 1 mcg/kg/min to a maximum of 6 mcg/kg/min. Tachycardia may occur as an adverse effect and precipitate a pre-existing ischaemic heart disease. Although dopexamine is considered not to be arrhythmogenic, its use is associated with ventricular ectopies. Finally, it may cause reversible reductions in neutrophil and platelet counts.

Dobutamine

Dobutamine is a synthetic catecholamine derived from isoprenaline. It shares the same basic structure with dopamine but has a bulky ring substitution on the terminal amino group. Although dobutamine is undoubtedly an inotrope, some authors consider it also a vasopressor, whereas others consider it a vasodilator. The reason for this disparity is because the pharmacology of dopamine is quite complex [42]. Generally, it possesses a strong affinity for both β_1- and β_2-receptors, which it binds to at a 3:1 ratio, with little affinity for α-receptors because of the configuration of the terminal amine. However, this agent is actually a racemic mixture of 2 isomers. Both enantiomers are β-adrenoceptor agonists, but one enantiomer is a potent α_1-agonist and can act as a vasopressor, while the second enantiomer is a potent α_1-antagonist. Overall, dobutamine induces significant β_1-mediated positive inotropic effects with mild chronotropic effects leading to enhanced CO [20,21,26]. Due to the β_2-mediated vasodilation and the mixed pharmacological action of α-agonism balanced by some α-blockade, SVR may remain unchanged or moderately decrease. MAP may thus rise, fall slightly or remain unchanged. Mild peripheral vasodilation (decrease in afterload) is more likely particularly at lower doses, whereas vasoconstriction progressively dominates at infusion rates higher than 5 μg/kg/min. Nevertheless, these effects are weak compared to the myocardial effects of dobutamine.

Dobutamine is considered by many a reasonable choice for short-term inotropic support in the presence of low CO (decompensated HF, cardiogenic shock, sepsis-induced myocardial dysfunction) with normal MAP or mild hypotension [20,21,26]. It is usually initiated with a 2-5 μg/kg/min infusion rate without a loading dose. The infusion rate may then be progressively increased according to symptoms, diuretic response and clinical status until the desired effect on CI or venous saturation or a maximum of 20 mcg/kg/min has been reached. In general, dobutamine should be avoided in patients with moderate or severe hypotension because of its vasodilative properties. Symptomatic bradycardia, unresponsive to atropine or pacing, is also an indication for dobutamine. Despite its mild chronotropic effects at low to medium doses, dobutamine significantly increases myocardial oxygen consumption and this may limit its utility in clinical conditions in which induction of ischemia is potentially harmful. However, it has the advantage of not affecting myocardial oxygen demand as much as dopamine. Moreover, the resulting tachycardia may preclude the use of this inotropic agent in some patients, and malignant ventricular arrhythmias can be observed at any dose. Tolerance can develop after just a few days of therapy [43]. Dobutamine, like dopamine is rapidly inactivated under alkaline solutions.

Vasopressin

Vasopressin is a naturally occurring antidiuretic hormone which is stored primarily in granules in the posterior pituitary gland [20]. The release of endogenous vasopressin is promoted by increased plasma osmolality or hypotension, as well as pain, nausea, and hypoxia. Secondary sites of vasopressin synthesis to a lesser degree include the heart, in response to elevated cardiac wall stress, [44] and the adrenal gland, in response to increased catecholamine secretion [45]. There are 3 vasopressin receptors (V_1,V_2,V_3) [20]. V_1 receptors cause vasoconstriction of systemic, splanchnic, renal, and coronary arteries via activation of voltage-gated Ca^{2+} channels resulting in an increase in intracellular Ca^{2+}. Stimulation of V_2 receptors mediates the antidiuretic effect of vasopressin by enhancing renal collecting duct permeability and water reabsorption. Finally, V_3 receptors are located in the anterior pituitary gland and cause secretion of adrenocorticotropin hormone. As an antidiuretic hormone, vasopressin is indicated to inhibit diuresis in patients with diabetes insipidus. At the same time, it is also a distinctive vasopressor because its vasoconstrictive effects do not result from its interaction with adrenoceptors.

In high doses, vasopressin acts as a powerful vasopressor and may raise BP by increasing SVR [20,21,26]. Its pressor effects are further enhanced by a vasopressin-modulated increase in vascular sensitivity to norepinephrine. This agent may also directly influence mechanisms involved in the pathogenesis of vasodilation, through inhibition of ATP-activated potassium channels [46], attenuation of interleukin-induced generation of NO [47], and reversal of adrenergic receptor downregulation [48].

Vasopressin exerts a neutral or inhibitory impact on CO, depending on its dose-dependent increase in SVR and the reflexive increase in vagal tone. However, it may have a modest inotropic effect on the myocardium via V_1-mediated increases in intracellular Ca^{2+} [49]. Vasopressin promotes splanchnic vasoconstriction, but causes less direct coronary and cerebral vasoconstriction than catecholamines.

Interestingly, the pressor effects of vasopressin are relatively preserved during hypoxic and acidotic conditions, which, commonly, develop during cardiac arrest or shock of any origin. Thus, the American Heart Association (AHA) recommends that vasopressin (40 IU bolus IV) could be administered as an alternative to epinephrine for the treatment of adult cardiac arrest [36].

Vasodilatory or cardiogenic shock represents another possible indication for the administration of vasopressin [20,21,26]. The use of vasopressin at low to moderate doses (IV infusion 0.0-0.1 IU/min) may be particularly useful in settings of catecholamine hyposensitivity such as norepinephrine-resistant vasodilatory shock [50].

Apart from improving MAP and CI, vasopressin therapy may also reduce the need for catecholamines, resulting in improved coronary blood flow and decreased cardiotoxicity and malignant arrhythmias due to catecholamine sparing [49]. However, the use of high doses (>0.4 U/min) can be associated with the appearance of arrhythmias, hypertension, decreased CO or cardiac ischemia.

Phosphodiesterase Inhibitors (PDIs)

Although natural and synthetic catecholamines are considered more potent inotropic and chronotropic agents, serious drawbacks have been associated with their clinical use. Furthermore, the downregulation and desensitization of adrenoreceptors may render these agents ineffective. This has led to interest in the use of inotropes which exert their action by a different mechanism such as PDIs and, more recently, the Ca^{2+} sensitizer levosimendan [20,21,26].

Phosphodiesterase III is an intracellular enzyme associated with the SR in myocytes that inactivates cAMP. Inhibition of this enzyme by PDEIs results in an increased intracellular concentration of cAMP with a simultaneous increase of Ca^{2+} influx via slow channels. In the myocardium, this leads to enhanced contractility and, in vascular smooth, muscle to vasodilatation [51].

Furthermore, cAMP also affects diastolic heart function through the regulation of phospholamban, the regulatory subunit of the Ca^{2+} pump of the SR. As a result PDIs also enhance the rate of Ca^{2+} re-sequestration rate and hence improve diastolic relaxation.

Thus, the hemodynamic properties of PDIs are characterized by positive inotropy and potent vasodilation, a combined effect that has been termed as "inodilation" [20,21,26]. SVR (afterload) and pulmonary vascular resistance (PVR) (preload) are reduced, while the effects of these agents on HR appear to be minimal. Diastolic relaxation is improved and this effect, termed lucitropy, may be beneficial in patients with reduced ventricular compliance or predominant diastolic failure [51].

Patients are less likely to develop tolerance to these medications because they are not dependent on adrenoreceptor activity. Moreover, PDIs may prove particularly useful if adrenoreceptors are downregulated or desensitized in the setting of chronic HF, or after chronic β-agonist administration.

Due to their pharmacokinetic profile, titration of PDIs is markedly different from catecholamines. Drug half-lives may be prolonged, while the time of onset and offset are longer requiring a loading dose. Excretion of PDIs is predominantly renal and therefore they have the potential to accumulate in renal failure.

PDIs that have been used in clinical practice include the bipyridine derivatives amrinone and milrinone and the imidazolones enoximone and piroximone [20,21,26]. The cardiovascular effects are similar. These agents are administered by a continuous infusion possibly preceded by a bolus dose in patients with stable BP.

Milrinone is the PDI most commonly used for cardiovascular indications. Loading doses of 20-50 μg/kg are typically given, followed by an infusion of 0.2-0.75 μg/kg/min. Enoximone is more rapidly metabolised, but the metabolite is active and its cardiovascular effects persist for some hours. It is typically used in doses of 0.5-1.5 mg/kg followed by an infusion of 5-10 μg/kg per min. Amrinone is typically given as a loading dose of 0.75-1.5 mg/kg, followed by an infusion rate of 10 μg/kg/min. The oral form of amrinone is no longer used clinically due to a high incidence of thrombocytopenia, gastrointestinal and neurological side-effects.

PDIs are beneficial in cases of cardiac pump failure and may facilitate weaning from the cardiopulmonary bypass machine after cardiac surgery [20,21,26]. Vasodilation is a prominent feature of their use, and, in hypotensive or volume depleted patients, can reduce both CO and MAP.

Therefore PDIs should be used only where BP and pulmonary capillary wedge pressure (PCWP) can be monitored, while concomitant administration of a vasoconstrictor such as norepinephrine or phenylephrine is often required. PDIs are considered as less likely than catecholamines to cause adverse effects known to be associated with adrenoreceptor activity (e.g., tachycardia, myocardial ischemia). However, the incidence of tachyarrhythmias is greater with PDIs compared to dobutamine. Although PDIs are associated with less increased myocardial oxygen demand than catecholamine inotropes, they should be administered with caution in patients with coronary artery disease, because a possible increase in medium-term mortality. A main disadvantage of these agents is their long half life so that dose titration takes longer and adverse haemodynamic effects may persist for longer. These features can render the PDIs clinically less practical.

Moreover, amrinone and enoximone are used less often because of important side effects, which include dose-related thrombocytopenia [52,53].

Calcium-Sensitizing Agents

Levosimendan

Levosimendan is the most well known representative of Ca^{2+} sensitizers, a recently developed class of “inodilators” [54]. The positive inotropic action of levosimendan is due to its binding to troponin C which facilitates the interaction between actin and myosine filaments without changes in intracellular Ca^{2+} ion concentrations [55]. In addition, the drug produces peripheral and coronary vasodilation by opening ATP-sensitive potassium channels [55]. The combination of positive and vasodilation may favorably impact myocardial performance and energetics without relevant changes in oxygen requirements [56] and may confer a degree of myocardial protection during ischemia by the reduction of post-ischemic stunning [57,58]. Moreover, the combined inodilating effects may relieve pulmonary congestion and improve organ perfusion, including renal blood flow and GFR. Levosimendan has been also shown to have potentially beneficial effects not only on neurohormones, but also on inflammatory cytokines and apoptosis mediators in HF [59].

Levosimendan may be particularly beneficial during acute and decompensated chronic HF states, and represents an alternative for patients on β-blocker therapy [60]. There are also some new possible indications for levosimendan treatment, such as repetitive administration in patients with advanced HF [61,62], post-operative myocardial dysfunction following cardiac surgery [63,64], or right ventricular failure [65]. Two large trials have demonstrated improved haemodynamic function compared to dobutamine in cardiogenic shock and myocardial infarction, and improved short-term mortality [60,66] although definitive outcome-based results in critically ill patients are awaited.

Levosimendan may be administered as a bolus dose (3-24 μg/kg) during 10 min followed by a continuous infusion (0.05-2.0 μg/kg/min) for 24 h. However, before starting an infusion, it is essential to exclude and correct a hypovolemia due to preceding high dose IV diuretics or vasodilators, otherwise arterial hypotension may occur. A loading dose of levosimendan can be omitted in many patients, especially if the initial systolic BP is <100 mmHg. Low serum potassium should also be corrected to avoid proarrhythmic effects. Major side-effects of levosimendan include tachycardia, enhanced atrioventricular (AV) conduction and hypotension. A prolonged infusion (>24 hours) is not recommended, since the slowly formed active metabolites maintain the hemodynamic effects for several days and longer treatments lead to drug accumulation with tachycardia and hypotension [65].

Clinical Aspects

General Measures - Monitoring

Early goal-directed post-resuscitation care aims at optimization of preload, arterial oxygen content, afterload, contractility, and systemic oxygen utilization [2,10]. This approach has been proven to reduce mortality in sepsis [7], a condition that shares several common features with post-resuscitation syndrome [15,16]. Time is of the essence and, therefore, patients must be attended to early on and resuscitated adequately as soon as possible, to prevent extreme morbidity and mortality. The general management of post-cardiac arrest patients should follow the standards of care for most critically ill patients in the ICU setting [2]. Likewise, close monitoring is necessary for patients requiring treatment with inotropes and vasopressors for the titration of therapy and because of the potential for development of life-threatening side-effects (hypotension, arrhythmias, etc). General monitoring of such patients should include complete blood count (CBC), arterial blood gases (ABGs), saturation of peripheral oxygen (SpO_2) by pulse oximetry, arterial line for continuous BP assessment, continuous electrocardiogram (ECG), central venous pressure (CVP), central venous oxygen saturation ($ScvO_2$), temperature (bladder, esophagus), urine output, chest radiograph, and blood chemistries, including electrolytes, glucose, blood urea nitrogen (BUN), creatinine, serum lactate, and cardiac markers. Furthermore, current and previous drug therapy of the patient should be reviewed.

Depending on the status of the patient and local resources and experience, advanced hemodynamic monitoring including echocardiography, cardiac output monitoring either noninvasive or pulmonary artery catheter (PAC) as well as cerebral monitoring (electroencephalogram - EEG - on indication or continuously, computed tomography /magnetic resonance imaging - CT/MRI -) may be required [2]. Echocardiographic evaluation within the first 24 hours after arrest is helpful to determine the cause of hemodynamic instability and guide further treatment [67,68]. Echocardiographic/doppler imaging can be used to evaluate and monitor regional and global left and right ventricular systolic function, diastolic function, valvular structure and function, pericardial pathology or mechanical complications of acute myocardial infarction (AMI). For example, right ventricular infarction characteristically requires higher filling pressures to maintain CO, while evidence of papillary muscle rupture or ventricular septal defect may need surgical intervention. Advanced CO monitoring may be necessary to measure BP accurately and to determine the most appropriate combination of medications to optimize blood flow and distribution. If a PAC or some form of noninvasive CO monitor is being used, therapy can be further guided by CI and SVR. However, no evidence exists that the use of a PAC improves outcome after cardiac arrest [69-71]. Supplemental oxygen by face mask should be provided [2,72]. In severe shock or if ventilation is inadequate, airway intubation with mechanical ventilation is necessary. Hyperventilation should be avoided in the post-cardiac arrest period and ventilation should be monitored by regular measurement of ABG values in order to achieve normocarbia. Providers should determine volume status, adequacy of systemic perfusion and the contribution of precipitating factors and/or comorbidities. Infusion of fluids may be required to increase right heart filling pressures or, conversely, diuretics and vasodilators may be needed to treat left ventricular failure [2,72]. Correction of arterial hypotension and hypoperfusion increases oxygen delivery to tissues and improves the prognosis of patients [73]. Therefore, early and aggressive fluid loading is recommended, supplemented, if indicated, by the administration of inotropic or vasopressor agents. The provider should titrate volume administration and vasoactive (e.g. norepinephrine), inotropic (e.g. dobutamine), and inodilator (e.g. milrinone) drugs as needed to support BP, CI, and systemic perfusion. Most importantly, if an underlying condition caused or contributed to this crisis of cardiovascular dysregulation, it should be addressed [2,72]. If there is evidence of coronary occlusion, immediate revascularisation by percutaneous coronary intervention (PCI) or thrombolysis may be required. Electrolytes (especially potassium and magnesium) should be monitored and replaced, if needed, to reduce the likelihood of dysrhythmias. Dysrhythmias can be treated by the use of standard drug and electrical therapies.

Selection of Appropriate Agent

If the patient's condition is hemodynamically unstable, volume status, ventricular function and organ perfusion should be assessed and ensured to an adequate level [2,72]. If hypotension or hypoperfusion persists, despite an adequate or optimized preload, inotropic and/or vasopressor therapy should be initiated soon through a central line via an infusion pump that is known to be reliable. The choice of inotropic or vasopressor support can be guided by BP, HR, echocardiographic estimates of myocardial dysfunction, and surrogate measures of tissue oxygen delivery such as ScvO2, lactate clearance, and urine output [2]. Clinicians should not use a specific BP value, which might or might not mean hypotension, to dictate the necessity for inotropic agents. Rather, a depressed BP, signs of poor CO or hypoperfusion (e.g., cold clammy skin, cool extremities, decreased urine output, altered mentation) should prompt a consideration for more aggressive IV therapy. A simplistic view would be that where the heart is failing, and the peripheral vasculature appears to be in good order, an agent with predominant β-effect (especially a β_1 selective inotrope) would be preferable [20,21]. On the other hand, if there is vasodilatation, perhaps an agent with alpha agonism should be chosen, while the combination of failing heart and dilated peripheral vasculature points towards an agent with mixed effect, or a combination of agents with alpha and beta effects. Treatment with a combined inotrope/vasopressor therapy including norepinephrine or dopamine is frequently required if CO is not measured. When the capability exists for monitoring CO in addition to BP, specific agents may be used separately to target specific levels of MAP and CO. Insufficient data exist to allow selection of a specific inotropic agent in preference over another in the treatment of post-cardiac hemodynamic instability and controversy rages about this topic. Multicentre randomized controlled trials focusing on clinical rather than physiological outcomes are needed. Thus, clinical judgement should be used in combination with existing limited data. In the absence of definitive data, the following suggestions can be made.

Haemodynamic instability after cardiac arrest commonly manifests as hypotension, low CI and arrhythmias [2]. Underlying mechanisms include intravascular volume depletion, impaired vasoregulation, and myocardial dysfunction [6,13,14]. The post-cardiac arrest ischemia/reperfusion response causes intravascular volume depletion, relatively soon, after the heart is restarted, and volume expansion is usually required. Therefore, the first-line intervention for post-resuscitation hypotension is to optimize right-heart filling pressures by use of IV fluids [2,72]. In patients with low MAP, and low CVP or pulmonary artery occlusion pressure (PAOP), a fluid challenge technique is indicated with reassessment of pressures and CO. No evidence-based data exists to support a difference between crystalloid and colloid fluid resuscitation [74]. Fluid must be titrated according to the patient's specific needs, rather than blindly relying on formulae. If there is no reason for a discrepancy between left and right-sided cardiac function, fluid replacement can be titrated according to CVP. Fluid resuscitation should initially target a CVP of at least 8 mm Hg (12 mm Hg in mechanically ventilated patients) and be continued as long as the hemodynamic improvement (e.g., arterial pressure, HR, urine output) progresses. The rate of fluid administration should be reduced substantially when cardiac filling pressures (CVP or PAOP) increase without concurrent hemodynamic improvement.

Adequate fluid resuscitation is vital, but may not be enough, especially if there have been delays. Inotropes and vasopressors should be considered if hypotension or hyporperfusion persists despite optimized preload [2,72]. Post-cardiac arrest myocardial dysfunction and impaired vasoregulation are generally reversible and responsive to inotropes and vasopressors [6,18,19]. No individual drug or combination of drugs has been demonstrated to be superior in the treatment of post-cardiac arrest cardiovascular dysfunction. Although speculative, some assumptions could be extrapolarated from sepsis since post-resuscitation period manifests as a sepsis-like syndrome characterized by multi-organ ischemic injury, microcirculatory dysfunction and the activation of inflammatory and coagulation cascades [15,16]. Moreover, goal-directed therapy with volume and vasoactive drug administration has been effective in improving survival from sepsis [7]. The greatest survival benefit is due to a decreased incidence of acute hemodynamic collapse, a challenge also seen in the post-resuscitation setting.

Inotropic therapy is indicated in case of post-cardiac arrest myocardial dysfunction as suggested by low measured or suspected CO and elevated or optimized cardiac filling pressures (CVP/PAOP) [2,72]. In situations with moderately low MAP (70 to 80 mm Hg) with evidence of tissue hypoperfusion (such as low urine output or elevated lactic acid) dobutamine, started at 2-5 μg/kg/min, is considered as the preferable agent [18,75]. Guidelines for the treatment of sepsis published by the American College of Critical Care Medicine (ACCM) [76] recommend that dobutamine should be used as the first choice for patients with an adequate MAP and low CI and/or low venous saturation following adequate fluid resuscitation. In swine, dobutamine infusions of 5 to 10 μg/kg/min dramatically improve systolic (left ventricular ejection fraction) and diastolic (isovolumic relaxation of left ventricle) dysfunction after cardiac arrest [18]. The use of doses of 2 to 7.5 μg/kg/min is associated with the appearance of tachycardia, but myocardial oxygen consumption is affected significantly only at higher doses (7.5 μg/kg/min) [77]. However, because it may also cause vasodilation, dobutamine may need to be utilized in combination with vasoconstrictors to maintain blood pressure. The combination of dobutamine and noradrenaline stimulates both α and β adrenergic receptors and it is recommended as first-line treatment in hypotensive septic patients with a persistently low CO and SvcO2 [78]. However, vasopressors should be titrated carefully as the increase in afterload can decrease CI.

PDIs, such as milrinone, represent possible alternative choices for inotropic support in the setting of myocardial dysfunction [75,79]. Direct randomized comparisons of PDIs and dobutamine have been small and have demonstrated similar clinical outcomes in the setting of heart failure or post-operative support after cardiac surgery [80-86]. The results of comparative trials between dobutamine and PDIs can be summarized as follows: dobutamine is a pure β-adrenergic agonist with direct inotropic effects and at low to medium doses modestly increases contractility and CO with usually mild systemic vasodilation. PDIs generally have an equal effect on increasing the CI, but demonstrate a greater effect on decreasing PCWP and SVR than dobutamine. However, PDIs can cause severe systemic hypotension and often require the coadministration of vasoconstrictors. Although it has the most desirable side-effect profile of the β-agonists, dobutamine can augment myocardial oxygen demand, whereas PDIs have no effect on myocardial oxygen consumption. However, dobutamine also increases myocardial oxygen delivery, which counterbalances the effect on consumption. Accordingly, there have been no clinically significant differences demonstrated between the PDIs and dobutamine in terms of inducing myocardial ischemia. Studies generally show that the PDIs have the same or less effect on increasing HR. Dobutamine requires the beta-receptor for its inotropic effects, while milrinone does not. This may be a significant consideration for patients already maintained on beta-blocking drugs, while β-adrenergic receptor responses are often blunted in the failing human heart due to desensitization, as well as decreased density of the receptors [28]. On the other hand, PDIs such as milrinone, acting through a non-β-adrenergic mechanism, are not associated with diminished efficacy (tolerance) with prolonged use. Nevertheless, tolerance to dobutamine does not occur until 48 to 72 hours of administration and inotropic support should be a short-term treatment until more definitive therapy or mechanical support (e.g., a ventricular assist device) can be provided. A potential disadvantage is the long half-life of the PDIs as compared with that of dobutamine, as adverse reactions such as tachyarrhythmias may take longer to dissipate with the PDIs after discontinuation. Several studies have shown that PDIs can have additive effects when combined with dobutamine [87-89] and, therefore, these agents may be used in combination when an adequate CI cannot be obtained with either agent alone.

Levosimendan, a nonadrenergic inotropic Ca^{2+} sensitizer, can improve myocardial contractility without increasing oxygen requirements and produce peripheral and coronary vasodilation. In animal studies, levosimendan has the potential of improving post-resuscitation myocardial function and has been suggested as an alternative to dobutamine for management of post-resuscitation myocardial dysfunction [19,90]. An experimental study in pigs investigated the effects of levosimendan in comparison with adrenergic dobutamine for the management of post-resuscitation myocardial dysfunction. Levosimendan (loading dose of 20 mcg/kg over 10 min followed by an infusion of 0.4 mcg/kg/min) and dobutamine (infusion of 5 mcg/kg/min) produced comparable increases in CO. However, levosimendan produced significantly greater left ventricular ejection fraction and fractional area changes compared with dobutamine and saline placebo [19]. In rats, levosimendan (loading dose of 12 mcg/kg over 10 min, followed by infusion of 0.3 mcg/kg/min) and dobutamine (infusion at a dosage of 3 mcg/kg/min) produced comparable increases in CO and rate of left-ventricular pressure increase [90]. However, administration of levosimendan resulted in lower HR and lesser increases in left ventricular diastolic pressure compared with both dobutamine and placebo, while the duration of post-resuscitation survival was significantly greater with levosimendan.

Post-resuscitation myocardial dysfunction is often superimposed by excessive vasodilation that contributes to the maintenance of hypotension and may require the administration of vasopressors after volume replacement. In case of a particularly low MAP or if hypotension or hypoperfusion persists, combined inotropic/vasopressor effect may become necessary to maintain systemic perfusion and preserve end-organ performance [75]. Dopamine is usually the first choice in view of its mixed vasopressor/inotropic effects. In refractory cases, noradrenaline may be needed for its vasopressor effects to maintain vital organ perfusion. Either is recommended as a first choice vasopressor agent to correct hypotension in sepsis according to guidelines published by the ACCM [76] and the Surviving Sepsis Campaign [78]. Dopamine increases MAP and CO, primarily due to an increase in stroke volume and HR, but causes more tachycardia and may be more arrhythmogenic [91]. Norepinephrine increases MAP due to its vasoconstrictive effects, with little change in HR and less increase in stroke volume compared with dopamine. Alternatives include epinephrine and the peripheral vasoconstrictor phenylephrine. Epinephrine is considered as equally efficacious, but it may be associated with disadvantageous effects (tachycardia as well as reduction of splanchnic flow and hyperlactemia). Epinephrine is recommended as the first chosen alternative agent in septic shock that is poorly responsive to norepinephrine or dopamine [78]. Finally, phenylephrine, administered separately, is the adrenergic agent least likely to produce tachycardia, but, as a pure vasopressor, it would be expected to decrease stroke volume.

Inadequate vasopressin levels have been proposed as partly responsible for hypotension in sepsis [92]. Similarly, the importance of vasopressin in cardiac arrest was first recognised in studies of out-of-hospital cardiac arrest patients, where vasopressin levels were found to be higher in successfully resuscitated patients [93]. Therefore, and also because it works by a different mechanism, vasopressin represents another possible choice for patients who remain unresponsive to sympathomimetic amines. In the setting of norepinephrine refractory septic shock low-dose vasopressin (0.01-0.04 units/min) may be added to norepinephrine with anticipation of an effect equivalent to norepinephrine alone [78]. Higher doses of vasopressin are not recommended since they have been associated with cardiac, digital, and splanchnic ischemia [94]. A retrospective study examined the effects of supplementary arginine vasopressin (AVP) infusion (4 IU/h) in 23 patients with post-cardiac arrest cardiovascular failure unresponsive to standard haemodynamic therapy [95]. AVP significantly increased MAP and successfully reversed cardiovascular failure that was unresponsive to standard therapy in >90% of patients. Furthermore, AVP decreased norepinephrine, epinephrine, and milrinone requirements.

In situations where post-resuscitation assessment reveals evidence of left ventricular failure with volume overload (high cardiac filling pressures CVP/PAOP) manifested by pulmonary and/or systemic congestion, the administration of IV loop diuretics is required [72]. Urine output and signs and symptoms of congestion should be serially assessed, and diuretic dose should be titrated accordingly to relieve symptoms and to reduce extracellular fluid volume excess. In patients with ongoing congestion not sufficiently responsive to diuretics, IV vasodilators such as nitroprusside or nitroglycerin may be added to the treatment regimen in the absence of systemic hypotension. Vasodilators (e.g., nitroprusside, nitroglycerin) reduce the myocardial workload and may increase CO in patients without severe hypotension by increasing venous capacitance or lower systemic vascular resistance. There is no evidence of benefit for routine use of inotropic support in patients presenting with acute HF due to congestion only [96-99]. However, the American College of Cardiology Foundation (ACCF)/AHA Guidelines for the Diagnosis and Management of Heart Failure in Adults [100] point out that inotropic or vasopressor drugs such as dopamine, dobutamine, and milrinone should be administered in an appropriate clinical setting of low CO associated with elevated cardiac filling pressures (e.g., elevated CVP/PAOP) and evidence of decreased organ perfusion with or without congestion. Inotropes are of greatest value in patients with relative hypotension and intolerance or no response to vasodilators and diuretics. Thus, if signs of low CO with peripheral vasoconstriction and oliguria persist despite correction or exclusion of a hypovolemia and patients do not respond to vasodilators and diuretics, inotropes might be needed to maintain systemic perfusion and preserve end-organ performance while more definitive therapy is considered. Vasopressors (noradrenaline) are not recommended as first-line agents and are only indicated in cardiogenic shock when the combination of an inotropic agent and fluid challenge fails to restore systolic BP >90 mmHg with inadequate organ perfusion, despite an improvement in CO. Levosimendan may be effective in patients with decompensated chronic HF or post-operative myocardial dysfunction following cardiac surgery and represents an alternative for patients on β-blocker therapy. It may be administered as a bolus dose (3-12 μg/kg) during 10 min followed by a continuous infusion (0.05-2.0 μg/kg/min for 24 h).

Coronary artery disease (CAD) is present in the majority of out-of-hospital cardiac arrest patients and AMI is the most common cause of sudden cardiac death [101-103]. If there is evidence of coronary occlusion in patients resuscitated from cardiac arres,t immediate coronary angiography, with subsequent PCI, should be considered [2,72]. If PCI is not available, thrombolytic therapy is an appropriate alternative for post-cardiac arrest management of ST-elevation myocardial infarction. Inotropes and vasopressors are used routinely in the setting of critical hypotension complicating AMI. This practice is based on the notion that hemodynamic benefits usually outweigh specific risks of inotropic therapy when used as a bridge to more definitive treatment measures. Definitive evidence supporting use of specific agents in this setting is lacking. In cardiogenic shock complicating AMI, current guidelines of the ACCF/AHA, based on expert opinion, recommend dopamine or dobutamine as first-line agents with moderate hypotension (systolic BP 70 to 100 mm Hg) and norepinephrine as the preferred therapy for severe hypotension (systolic BP <70 mm Hg) [104]. Moderate doses dopamine or dobutamine are considered to maximize inotropy and avoid excessive α_1-adrenergic stimulation that can result in end-organ ischemia. Interestingly, moderate doses (7.5 μg/kg/min) of combinations of medications may potentially be more effective and limit important side effects compared with either individual agent administered at maximal doses (15 μg/kg/min) of any individual agent [105]. Dobutamine may also improve myocardial performance after excessive fluid administration in the setting of low CO due to significant right ventricular free-wall ischemia [106]. With an antithrombotic effect in addition to its pressor qualities, norepinephrine may be the optimal choice in patients with severe hypotention or refractory to a medium dose of dopamine or dopamine/dobutamine. Norepinephrine is preferred to epinephrine, which can exacerbate lactic acidosis and promote thrombosis in coronary vasculature [107]. Vasopressin is another promising agent, since in a study examining vasopressin use in cardiogenic shock after AMI, this agent was found to increase MAP without adversely impacting CI and wedge pressure [108]. Further studies to validate the use of vasopressin in this setting are needed.

If volume expansion and treatment with vasoactive and inotropic drugs do not restore adequate organ perfusion, mechanical circulatory assistance should be considered [109]. This treatment can support circulation in the period of transient severe myocardial dysfunction that often occurs for 24 to 48 hours after ROSC [6]. The intra-aortic balloon pump is the most readily available device to augment myocardial perfusion during low-output circulatory states refractory to drugs [10,110]. If additional cardiac support is needed, more invasive treatments such as percutaneous cardiopulmonary bypass, extracorporeal membrane oxygenation (ECMO), or transthoracic ventricular assist devices can be considered [111,112].

Owing to their chronotropic effects, β-adrenergic agonists can be useful for transient emergency treatment of bradyarrhythmias if atropine is ineffective [36]. The use of adrenaline, dopamine, dobutamine, or isoproterenol can stabilize the patient to allow time for a temporary pacemaker to be inserted [72]. Isoproterenol (1-4 µg/min) is also useful under the same circumstances to treat bradycardia-induced torsade des pointes. Finally, isoproterenol has also been used to suppress the trigger for ventricular fibrillation in patients with the Brugada syndrome who do not wish to have cardioverter-defibrillator implantation to prevent sudden cardiac death [113]. However, isoproterenol is not advised in patients with myocardial ischemia due to CAD.

Resuscitative End-Points of Inotropic and Vasopressor Treatment

Although the benefit of early hemodynamic optimization has not been studied in randomized prospective clinical trials, it has been hypothesized that this approach might improve the outcome of post-cardiac arrest patients [2]. The key to the success of this approach is initiation of monitoring and therapy as early as possible and achievement of goals within hours of presentation. However, little evidence is available about the optimal goals in post-cardiac arrest resuscitation. On the basis of the limited available evidence, reasonable goals for post-cardiac arrest syndrome include an MAP of 65 to 100 mm Hg (taking into consideration the patient's normal BP, cause of arrest, and severity of any myocardial dysfunction), CVP of 8 to 12 mm Hg, $ScvO_2$ >70%, urine output >1 ml/kg/h, and a normal or decreasing serum or blood lactate level [2]. Goals for hemoglobin concentration during post-cardiac arrest care remain to be defined. Goals of treatment may need to be adjusted according to the clinical situation; peculiarities of the particular patient and inter-individual variation and pre-existing disease (especially hypertension) should be taken into consideration.

The primary therapeutic tools of hemodynamic optimization are IV fluids, inotropes, vasopressors, and blood transfusion [2,72]. The initiation of these therapeutic modalities aims at providing an adequate perfusion pressure that will ensure blood flow to vital organs, as well as an adequate level of oxygen delivery to tissues. Available markers of microvascular perfusion and oxygen delivery include mixed venous oxygen saturation, hourly urine output, lactate levels and biochemical markers of renal function. Nevertheless, the use of inotropes and vasopressors has not been shown in randomized, controlled studies to ultimately lead to improved patient outcomes, at least in part because no clinical trials have been conducted with study size and power adequate to test their effect on improving survival. In the absence of such data, the definitive goals of post-resuscitative care must be considered of primary importance, and the role of inotropic and vasopressor therapy should be kept in a supportive context to allow treatment of the underlying disorder.

Measurement of CVP is currently the most readily obtainable target for fluid resuscitation. An important consideration is the potential for persistent precipitating pathology that could cause elevated CVP independent of volume status, such as cardiac tamponade, right-sided AMI, pulmonary embolism, and tension pneumothorax or any disease that impairs myocardial compliance. Elevated CVPs may also be seen with pre-existing clinically significant pulmonary artery hypertension. A risk also exists of precipitating pulmonary edema in the presence of post-cardiac arrest myocardial dysfunction. Adequate fluid resuscitation is a fundamental aspect of the hemodynamic management of patients, and should, ideally, be achieved before vasopressors and inotropes are used, but using these agents early as an emergency measure is frequently necessary. It has been suggested that vasopressors and inotropes should be titrated separately to different goals [76,78]. Vasopressors are titrated to maintain an adequate MAP, while inotropes are titrated to the desired effect on oxygen delivery.

Vasopressor therapy is initiated to maintain perfusion in the face of life-threatening post-ROSC hypotension that is a predictor of in-hospital death, and is associated with diminished functional status among survivors [73]. An elevated MAP after ROSC could theoretically increase cerebral oxygen delivery and positively affect neurological outcome [114]. However, post-resuscitation circulatory support is characterized by the simultaneous need to perfuse the postischemic brain adequately without putting unnecessary strain on the postischemic heart. Thus, a patient with an evolving AMI or severe myocardial dysfunction might benefit from the lowest target MAP that will ensure adequate cerebral oxygen delivery. The optimal MAP for post- cardiac arrest patients has not been defined by prospective clinical trials [9,10]. Pre-existing comorbidities should be considered as to most appropriate MAP target [2]. For example, a MAP of 65 mm Hg might be too low in a patient with severe uncontrolled hypertension, and in a young previously normotensive, a lower MAP might be adequate. If the patient's "normal" (pre-arrest) BP is unknown, estimates should take into account the possibility of patient derived from a population or age group where hypertension is prevalent, or evidence of hypertension, such as funduscopic changes, or left ventricular hypertrophy. Furthermore, the optimal MAP in the post-cardiac arrest period might be dependent on the duration of cardiac arrest, with higher pressures needed to overcome the potential no-reflow phenomenon observed with >15 minutes of untreated cardiac arrest [115-117]. In general, MAP should be maintained > 80 mm Hg in older adults, or > 60 mm Hg in younger and previously healthy patients. In patients known to be hypertensive, a reasonable target is systolic BP 30 mm Hg below pre-arrest level [2]. Supplementing end points such as BP with assessment of regional and global perfusion, such as blood lactate concentrations and urine output, is important.

In the absence of definitive data, titration of inotropic therapy should be guided by the adequacy of end-organ perfusion and oxygen delivery. The balance between systemic oxygen delivery and consumption can be monitored indirectly with mixed SvO2 [2]. An important caveat is that a subset of post-cardiac arrest patients have elevated central or mixed venous oxygen saturations despite inadequate tissue oxygen delivery, a phenomenon that is more common in patients given high doses of epinephrine during CPR [118]. This phenomenon, termed "venous hyperoxia," can be attributed to impaired tissue oxygen utilization caused by microcirculatory failure or mitochondrial failure. Additional surrogates for oxygen delivery include urine output and lactate clearance [2]. The usefulness of urine output could be limited in the presence of acute or chronic renal insufficiency. A single measurement of serum or blood lactate level during early hemodynamic optimization is of poor value because lactate concentrations are elevated early after ROSC due to the total-body ischemia of cardiac arrest. Lactate clearance has been associated with outcome in patients with ROSC after out-of-hospital cardiac arrest [119,120]. However, lactate clearance can be impaired by convulsive seizures, excessive motor activity, hepatic insufficiency, and hypothermia.

If a pulmonary artery catheter or some form of noninvasive CO monitor is being used, vasoactive and inotropic therapy can be further guided by CI and SVR [2,72]. However, consensus on PAC use during treatment with inotropic therapy is lacking. Although this tool can be helpful diagnostically, its routine use has never been shown to improve outcomes [69-71,121]. This may reflect an absence of effective evidence-based therapies to be used in response to PAC data in the treatment of critically ill patients [122]. Inotropic titration with PAC data in isolation can result in inappropriate stimulation of CO, thus negatively impacting prognosis in heterogeneous ICU patient populations [123]. This reinforces the concept that right heart catheterization is best reserved for those situations where a specific clinical or therapeutic question needs to be addressed. According to ACCF/AHA Guidelines for the Diagnosis and Management of Heart Failure in Adults [100], hemodynamic monitoring should be strongly considered in patients who are refractory to initial therapy and there is uncertainty regarding relative contributions of elevated filling pressures, hypoperfusion, and vascular tone. Patients with clinically significant hypotension and/or worsening renal function during initial treatment requiring escalating pressor therapy might also benefit. Finally, patients being considered for cardiac transplantation or placement of a mechanical circulatory support device are also candidates for complete right heart catheterization, a necessary part of the initial evaluation.

Careful and frequent serial evaluation of the patient is important primarily to assess volume status and adequacy of circulatory support [2,72]. Continuous BP monitoring with an arterial line is essential both to accurately titrate therapy and because inotropes and vasopressors have the potential to induce life-threatening hypo- or hypertension. Laboratory parameters are likewise necessary to judge efficacy of treatment. Once the target pressure is achieved and there is evidence of substantial improvement in metabolic status great effort should be directed to weaning inotropes and vasopressors with continuing fluid resuscitation, but without permitting autoregulatory failure to become re-established. Persistence of reversible vasopressor dependency has been reported for up to 72 hours after out-of hospital cardiac arrest despite preload optimization and reversal of global myocardial dysfunction [6]. Despite improving hemodynamic values, the effect on survival of inotropes and vasopressors in the post-cardiac arrest phase has not been studied in humans. The administration of these agents is associated with serious side-effects and therefore they should be used in the minimal dose necessary to achieve low-normal MAP and adequate systematic perfusion.

Conclusions

In conclusion, inotropes and vasopressors play an essential role in the supportive care of post-cardiac arrest patients. To date, the impact on clinical outcomes of these agents has yet to be demonstrated in randomized prospective clinical trials, despite their widespread use in cardiovascular illness. Therefore, the definitive goals of post-resuscitative care must be considered of primary importance, and the role of inotropic therapy should be kept in a supportive context to allow treatment of the underlying disorder. A better understanding of the physiology and important adverse effects of these medications should lead to directed clinical use, with realistic therapeutic goals. Smaller combined doses of inotropes and vasopressors may be advantageous over a single agent used at higher doses to avoid dose-related adverse effects. Large randomized trials focusing on clinical outcomes are needed to better assess the clinical efficacy of these agents in the setting of post resuscitation care.

References

[1] Negovsky VA. The second step in resuscitation: the treatment of the "post–resuscitation disease." *Resuscitation* 1972;1:1–7.

[2] Neumar RW, Nolan JP, Adrie C, Aibiki M, Berg RA, Böttiger BW, Callaway C, Clark RS, Geocadin RG, Jauch EC, Kern KB, Laurent I, Longstreth WT Jr, Merchant RM, Morley P, Morrison LJ, Nadkarni V, Peberdy MA, Rivers EP, Rodriguez–Nunez A, Sellke FW, Spaulding C, Sunde K, Vanden Hoek T. Post–cardiac arrest syndrome: epidemiology pathophysiology treatment and prognostication. A consensus statement from the International Liaison Committee on Resuscitation (American Heart Association Australian and New Zealand Council on Resuscitation, European Resuscitation Council Heart and Stroke Foundation of Canada, InterAmerican Heart Foundation Resuscitation Council of Asia and the Resuscitation Council of Southern Africa), the American Heart Association Emergency Cardiovascular Care Committee, the Council on Cardiovascular Surgery and Anesthesia, the Council on Cardiopulmonary Perioperative and Critical Care, the Council on Clinical Cardiology, and the Stroke Council. *Circulation* 2008;118:2452-2483.

[3] Nolan JP, Laver SR, Welch CA, Harrison DA, Gupta V, Rowan K. Outcome following admission to UK intensive care units after cardiac arrest: a secondary analysis of the ICNARC Case Mix Programme Database. *Anaesthesia* 2007;62:1207-1216.

[4] Langhelle A, Tyvold SS, Lexow K, Hapnes SA, Sunde K, Steen PA. In–hospital factors associated with improved outcome after out–of–hospital cardiac arrest: a comparison between four regions in Norway. *Resuscitation* 2003;56:247-263.

[5] Herlitz J, Engdahl J, Svensson L, Angquist KA, Silfverstolpe J, Holmberg S. Major differences in 1–month survival between hospitals in Sweden among initial survivors of out–of–hospital cardiac arrest. *Resuscitation* 2006;70:404-409.

[6] Laurent I, Monchi M, Chiche JD, Joly LM, Spaulding C, Bourgeois B, Cariou A, Rozenberg A, Carli P, Weber S, Dhainaut JF. Reversible myocardial dysfunction in survivors of out–of–hospital cardiac arrest. *J. Am. Coll. Cardiol.* 2002;40:2110-2116.

[7] Rivers E, Nguyen B, Havstad S, Ressler J, Muzzin A, Knoblich B, Peterson E, Tomlanovich M; Early Goal–Directed Therapy Collaborative Group. Early goal–directed therapy in the treatment of severe sepsis and septic shock. *N. Engl. J. Med.* 2001;345:1368-1377.

[8] Busch M, Soreide E, Lossius HM, Lexow K, Dickstein K. Rapid implementation of therapeutic hypothermia in comatose out–of–hospital cardiac arrest survivors. *Acta Anaesthesiol. Scand.* 2006;50:1277-1283.

[9] Oddo M, Schaller MD, Feihl F, Ribordy V, Liaudet L. From evidence to clinical practice: effective implementation of therapeutic hypothermia to improve patient outcome after cardiac arrest. *Crit. Care Med.* 2006;34:1865-1873.

[10] Sunde K, Pytte M, Jacobsen D, Mangschau A, Jensen LP, Smedsrud C, Draegni T, Steen PA. Implementation of a standardised treatment protocol for post resuscitation care after out–of–hospital cardiac arrest. *Resuscitation* 2007;73:29-39.
[11] Ruiz–Bailén M, Aguayo de Hoyos E, Ruiz–Navarro S, Díaz–Castellanos MA, Rucabado–Aguilar L, Gómez–Jiménez FJ, Martínez–Escobar S, Moreno RM, Fierro–Rosón J. Reversible myocardial dysfunction after cardiopulmonary resuscitation. *Resuscitation* 2005;66:175-181.
[12] Kern KB, Hilwig RW, Rhee KH, Berg RA. Myocardial dysfunction after resuscitation from cardiac arrest: an example of global myocardial stunning. *J. Am. Coll. Cardiol.* 1996;28:232-240.
[13] Karimova A, Pinsky DJ. The endothelial response to oxygen deprivation: biology and clinical implications. *Intensive Care Med.* 2001;27:19-31.
[14] Adams JA. Endothelium and cardiopulmonary resuscitation. *Crit. Care Med.* 2006;34:S458-465.
[15] Adrie C, Adib–Conquy M, Laurent I, Monchi M, Vinsonneau C, Fitting C, Fraisse F, Dinh–Xuan AT, Carli P, Spaulding C, Dhainaut JF, Cavaillon JM. Successful cardiopulmonary resuscitation after cardiac arrest as a "sepsis–like" syndrome. *Circulation* 2002;106:562-568.
[16] Adrie C, Laurent I, Monchi M, Cariou A, Dhainaou JF, Spaulding C. Post–resuscitation disease after cardiac arrest: a sepsis–like syndrome? *Curr. Opin. Crit. Care* 2004;10:208-212.
[17] Cerchiari EL, Safar P, Klein E, Diven W. Visceral hematologic and bacteriologic changes and neurologic outcome after cardiac arrest in dogs: the visceral post–resuscitation syndrome. *Resuscitation* 1993;25:119-136.
[18] Kern KB, Hilwig RW, Berg RA, Rhee KH, Sanders AB, Otto CW, Ewy GA. Post–resuscitation left ventricular systolic and diastolic dysfunction. Treatment with dobutamine. *Circulation* 1997;95:2610-2613.
[19] Huang L, Weil MH, Tang W, Sun S, Wang J. Comparison between dobutamine and levosimendan for management of post–resuscitation myocardial dysfunction. *Crit. Care Med.* 2005;33:487-491.
[20] Cooper BE. Review and update on inotropes and vasopressors. *AACN Adv. Crit. Care* 2008;19:5-13.
[21] Myburgh JA. *Inotropes and vasopressors*. In: Oh's Intensive Care Manual. London: Butterworth–Heinemann Ltd, 2008. p. 921–934.
[22] Hein L. Adrenoceptors and signal transduction in neurons. *Cell Tissue Res.* 2006;326:541-551.
[23] Hieble JP. Subclassification and nomenclature of alpha– and beta–adrenoceptors. *Curr. Top. Med. Chem.* 2007;7:129-134.
[24] Abel JJ, Taveau RD. On the decomposition products of epinephrine hydrate. *J. Biol. Chem.* 1905;1:1-32.
[25] Barger G, Dale HH. Chemical structure and sympathomimetic action of amines. *J. Physiol.* 1910;41:19-59.
[26] Overgaard CB, Dzavík V. Inotropes and vasopressors: review of physiology and clinical use in cardiovascular disease. *Circulation* 2008;118:1047-1056.
[27] Magder S, Rastepagarnah M. Role of neurosympathetic pathways in the vascular response to sepsis. *J Crit. Care.* 1998;13:169-176.

[28] Tilley DG, Rockman HA. Role of beta–adrenergic receptor signaling and desensitization in heart failure: new concepts and prospects for treatment. *Expert Rev. Cardiovasc. Ther*. 2006;4:417-432.

[29] Li HT, Long CS, Rokosh DG, Honbo NY, Karliner JS. Chronic hypoxia differentially regulates $_{\alpha 1}$–adrenergic receptor subtype mRNAs and inhibits $_{\alpha 1}$–adrenergic receptor–stimulated cardiac hypertrophy and signaling. *Circulation* 1995;92:918-925.

[30] Modest VE, Butterworth JF 4th. Effect of pH and lidocaine on beta–adrenergic receptor binding: interaction during resuscitation? *Chest* 1995;108:1373-1379.

[31] Stamm C, Friehs I, Cowan DB, Cao–Danh H, Choi YH, Duebener LF, McGowan FX, del Nido PJ. Dopamine treatment of post–ischemic contractile dysfunction rapidly induces calcium–dependent pro–apoptotic signaling. *Circulation* 2002;106:I290-298.

[32] Myburgh JA. Driving cerebral perfusion pressure with pressors: how which when? *Crit. Care Resus.* 2005;7:200-205.

[33] Day NP, Phu NH, Bethell DP, Mai NT, Chau TT, Hien TT, White NJ. The effects of dopamine and adrenaline infusions on acid–base balance and systemic haemodynamics in severe infection. *Lancet* 1996;348:219-223.

[34] Jones CJ, DeFily DV, Patterson JL, Chilian WM. Endothelium–dependent relaxation competes with alpha 1– and alpha 2–adrenergic constriction in the canine epicardial coronary microcirculation. *Circulation* 1993;87:1264-1274.

[35] Singh K, Xiao L, Remondino A, Sawyer DB, Colucci WS. Adrenergic regulation of cardiac myocyte apoptosis. *J. Cell Physiol.* 2001;189:257-265.

[36] ECC Committee Subcommittees and Task Forces of the American Heart Association. 2005 American Heart Association Guidelines for Cardiopulmonary Resuscitation and Emergency Cardiovascular Care. *Circulation* 2005;112:IV1–203.

[37] Tune JD, Richmond KN, Gorman MW, Feigl EO. Control of coronary blood flow during exercise. *Exp. Biol. Med. (Maywood)* 2002;227:238-250.

[38] Communal C, Singh K, Pimentel DR, Colucci WS. Norepinephrine stimulates apoptosis in adult rat ventricular myocytes by activation of the β–adrenergic pathway. *Circulation* 1998;98:1329-1334.

[39] Denton MD, Chertow GM, Brady HR. "Renal–dose" dopamine for the treatment of acute renal failure: scientific rationale experimental studies and clinical trials. *Kidney Int.* 1996;50:4-14.

[40] Bellomo R, Chapman M, Finfer S, Hickling K, Myburgh J; Australian and New Zealand Intensive Care Society (ANZICS) Clinical Trials Group. Low–dose dopamine in patients with early renal dysfunction: a placebo–controlled randomised trial. *Lancet* 2000;356:2139-2143.

[41] Kellum J, Decker J. Use of dopamine in acute renal failure: a meta–analysis. *Crit. Care Med.* 2001;29:1526-1531.

[42] Ruffolo RR Jr. The pharmacology of dobutamine. *Am. J. Med. Sci.* 1987;294:244-248.

[43] Unverferth DA, Blanford M, Kates RE, Leier CV. Tolerance to dobutamine after a 72 hour continuous infusion. *Am. J. Med.* 1980;69:262-266.

[44] Hupf H, Grimm D, Riegger GA, Schunkert H. Evidence for a vasopressin system in the rat heart. *Circ. Res.* 1999;84:365-370.

[45] Guillon G, Grazzini E, Andrez M, Breton C, Trueba M, Serradeil–LeGal C, Boccara G, Derick S, Chouinard L, Gallo–Payet N. Vasopressin: a potent autocrine/paracrine regulator of mammal adrenal functions. *Endocr. Res.* 1998;24:703-710.

[46] Salzman AL, Vromen A, Denenberg A, Szabo C. K(ATP)–channel inhibition improves hemodynamics and cellular energetics in hemorrhagic shock. *Am. J. Physiol.* 1997;272:H688—694.

[47] Kusano E, Tian S, Umino T, Tetsuka T, Ando Y, Asano Y. Arginine vasopressin inhibits interleukin–1 beta–stimulated nitric oxide and cyclic guanosine monophosphate production via the V1 receptor in cultured rat vascular smooth muscle cells. *J. Hypertens.* 1997;15:627-632.

[48] Hamu Y, Kanmura Y, Tsuneyoshi I, Yoshimura N. The effects of vasopressin on endotoxin–induced attenuation of contractile responses in human gastroepiploic arteries in vitro. *Anesth. Analg.* 1999;88:542-548.

[49] Okamura T, Ayajiki K, Fujioka H, Toda N. Mechanisms underlying arginine vasopressin–induced relaxation in monkey isolated coronary arteries. *J. Hypertens.* 1999;17:673-678.

[50] Dunser MW, Mayr AJ, Ulmer H, Knotzer H, Sumann G, Pajk W, Friesenecker B, Hasibeder WR. Arginine vasopressin in advanced vasodilatory shock: a prospective, randomized, controlled study. *Circulation.* 2003;107:2313-9.

[51] Erhardt L. An emerging role for calcium sensitisation in the treatment of heart failure. *Expert Opin. Investig. Drugs.* 2005;14:659-670.

[52] Ansell J, Tiarks C, McCue J, Parrilla N, Benotti JR: Amrinone–induced thrombocytopenia. *Arch. Intern. Med.* 1984;144:949-952.

[53] Gunnicker M, Hess W: Preliminary results with amrinone in perioperative low cardiac output syndrome. *Thorac. Cardiovasc. Surg.* 1987;35:219-225.

[54] Follath F. Newer treatments for decompensated heart failure: focus on levosimendan. *Drug. Des. Devel. Ther.* 2009;3:73-78.

[55] Haikala H, Kaivola J, Nissinen E, Wall P, Levijoki J, Lindén IB. Cardiac troponin C as a target protein for a novel calcium sensitizing drug, levosimendan. *J. Mol. Cell Cardiol.* 1995;27:1859-1866.

[56] Ukkonen H, Saraste M, Akkila J, Knuuti J, Karanko M, Iida H, Lehikoinen P, Någren K, Lehtonen L, Voipio–Pulkki LM. Myocardial efficiency during levosimendan infusion in congestive heart failure. *Clin. Pharmacol. Ther.* 2000;68:522-531.

[57] Jamali IN, Kersten JR, Pagel PS, Hettrick DA, Warltier DC. Intracoronary levosimendan enhances contractile function of stunned myocardium. *Anaesth. Analg.* 1997;85:23-29.

[58] Sonntag S, Sudberg S, Lehtonen LH, Kleber FX. The calcium sensitizer levosimendan improves the function of stunned myocardium after percutaneous transluminal coronary angioplasty in acute myocardial ischemia. *J. Am. Coll. Cardiol.* 2004;43:2177-2182.

[59] Trikas A, Antoniades C, Latsios G, Vasiliadou K, Karamitros I, Tousoulis D, Tentolouris C, Stefanadis C. Log–term effects of levosimendan infusion on inflammatory processes and sFAS in patients with severe heart failure. *Eur. J. Heart Fail.* 2006;8:804-809.

[60] Follath F, Cleland JG, Just H, Papp JG, Scholz H, Peuhkurinen K, Harjola VP, Mitrovic V, Abdalla M, Sandell EP, Lehtonen L, Steering Committee and Investigators of the Levosimendan Infusion versus Dobutamine (LIDO) Study. Efficacy and safety of intravenous levosimendan compared with dobutamine in severe low–output heart failure (the LIDO study): a randomised double–blind trial. *Lancet* 2002;360:196-202.

[61] Nanas JN, Papazoglou P, Tsagalou EP, Ntalianis A, Tsolakis E, Terrovitis JV, Kanakakis J, Nanas SN, Alexopoulos GP, Anastasiou–Nana MI. Efficacy and safety of intermittent long–term concomitant dobutamine and levosimendan infusions in severe heart failure refractory to dobutamine alone. *Am. J. Cardiol.* 2005;95:768-771.

[62] Berger R, Moertl D, Huelsmann M, Bojic A, Ahmadi R, Heissenberger I, Pacher R. Levosimendan and prostaglandin E1 for uptitration of beta–blockade in patients with advanced chronic heart failure. *Eur. J. Heart Fail.* 2007;9:202-908.

[63] Labriola C, Siro–Brigiani M, Carrata F, Santangelo E, Amantea B. Hemodynamic effects of levosimendan in patients with low–output heart failure after cardiac surgery. *Int. J. Clin. Pharmacol. Ther.* 2004;42:204-211.

[64] De Hert SG, Losomradee S, Cromheecke S, Van der Linden PJ. The effects of levosimendan in cardiac surgery patiens with poor left ventricular function. *Anaesth. Analg.* 2007;104:766-773.

[65] Poelzl G, Zwick RH, Grander W, Metzler B, Jonetzko P, Frick M, Ulmer H, Pachinger O, Roithinger FX. Safety and effectiveness of levosimndan in patients with predominant right heart failure. *Herz* 2008;33:368-373.

[66] Moiseyev VS, Põder P, Andrejevs N, Ruda MY, Golikov AP, Lazebnik LB, Kobalava ZD, Lehtonen LA, Laine T, Nieminen MS, Lie KI. Safety and efficacy of a novel calcium sensitizer, levosimendan, in patients with left ventricular failure due to an acute myocardial infarction. A randomized, placebo–controlled, double–blind study (RUSSLAN). *Eur. Heart J.* 2002;23:1422-1432.

[67] Spaulding CM, Joly LM, Rosenberg A, Monchi M, Weber SN, Dhainaut JF, Carli P. Immediate coronary angiography in survivors of out–of–hospital cardiac arrest. *N. Engl. J. Med.* 1997;336:1629-1633.

[68] Bunch TJ, White RD, Gersh BJ, Meverden RA, Hodge DO, Ballman KV, Hammill SC, Shen WK, Packer DL. Long–term outcomes of out–of–hospital cardiac arrest after successful early defibrillation. *N. Engl. J. Med.* 2003;348:2626-2633.

[69] Mimoz O, Rauss A, Rekik N, Brun–Buisson C, Lemaire F, Brochard L. Pulmonary artery catheterization in critically ill patients: a prospective analysis of outcome changes associated with catheter–prompted changes in therapy. *Crit. Care Med.* 1994;22:573-579.

[70] Vincent JL, Dhainaut JF, Perret C, Suter P. Is the pulmonary artery catheter misused? A European view. *Crit. Care Med.* 1998;26:1283-1287.

[71] Bernard GR, Sopko G, Cerra F, Demling R, Edmunds H, Kaplan S, Kessler L, Masur H, Parsons P, Shure D, Webb C, Weidemann H, Weinmann G, Williams D. Pulmonary artery catheterization and clinical outcomes: National Heart Lung and Blood Institute and Food and Drug Administration workshop report. *JAMA* 2000;283:2568-2572.

[72] Nolan JP, Deakin CD, Soar J, Böttiger BW, Smith G; European Resuscitation Council. European Resuscitation Council guidelines for resuscitation 2005. Section 4. Adult advanced life support. *Resuscitation* 2005;67:S39-86.

[73] Trzeciak S, Jones AE, Kilgannon JH, Milcarek B, Hunter K, Shapiro NI, Hollenberg SM, Dellinger P, Parrillo JE. Significance of arterial hypotension after resuscitation from cardiac arrest. *Crit. Care Med.* 2009;37:2895-2903.

[74] Finfer S, Bellomo R, Boyce N, French J, Myburgh J, Norton R; SAFE Study Investigators. A comparison of albumin and saline for fluid resuscitation in the intensive care unit. *N. Engl. J. Med.* 2004;350:2247-2256.

[75] American Heart Association in collaboration with International Liaison Committee on Resuscitation. Guidelines 2000 for Cardiopulmonary Resuscitation and Emergency Cardiovascular Care: International Consensus on Science. Part 6. Advanced Cardiovascular Life Support: Section 6. Pharmacology II: Agents to Optimize Cardiac Output and Blood Pressure. *Circulation* 2000;102:I129-135.

[76] Hollenberg SM, Ahrens TS, Annane D, Astiz ME, Chalfin DB, Dasta JF, Heard SO, Martin C, Napolitano LM, Susla GM, Totaro R, Vincent JL, Zanotti–Cavazzoni S. Practice parameters for hemodynamic support of sepsis in adult patients: 2004 update. *Crit. Care Med.* 2004;32:1928-1948.

[77] Vasquez A, Kern KB, Hilwig RW, Heidenreich J, Berg RA, Ewy GA. Optimal dosing of dobutamine for treating post–resuscitation left ventricular dysfunction. *Resuscitation* 2004;61:199-207.

[78] Dellinger RP, Levy MM, Carlet JM, Bion J, Parker MM, Jaeschke R, Reinhart K, Angus DC, Brun–Buisson C, Beale R, Calandra T, Dhainaut JF, Gerlach H, Harvey M, Marini JJ, Marshall JC, Ranieri M, Ramsay G, Sevransky J, Thompson BT, Townsend S, Vender JS, Zimmerman JL, Vincent JL. Surviving Sepsis Campaign: International guidelines for management of severe sepsis and septic shock: 2008. *Intensive Care Med.* 2008;34:17-60.

[79] Niemann JT, Garner D, Khaleeli E, Lewis RJ. Milrinone facilitates resuscitation from cardiac arrest and attenuates postresuscitation myocardial dysfunction. *Circulation* 2003;108:3031-3035.

[80] Grose R, Strain J, Greenberg M, LeJemtel TH. Systemic and coronary effects of intravenous milrinone and dobutamine in congestive heart failure. *J. Am. Coll. Cardiol.* 1986;7:1107-1113.

[81] Monrad ES, Baim DS, Smith HS, Lanoue AS. Milrinone dobutamine and nitroprusside: comparative effects on hemodynamics and myocardial energetics in patients with severe congestive heart failure. *Circulation* 1986;73:S168-174.

[82] Biddle TL, Benotti JR, Creager MA, Faxon DP, Firth BG, Fitzpatrick PG, Konstam MA, Krebs C, Walton L, Kershner RP, Jacobsen J, Luczkowec CA, Montenaro MJ, Tandon PK, Fitzpatrick S, Schwarz RP Jr. Comparison of intravenous milrinone and dobutamine for congestive heart failure secondary to either ischemic or dilated cardiomyopathy. *Am. J. Cardiol.* 1987;59:1345-1350.

[83] Marcus RH, Raw K, Patel J, Mitha A, Sareli P. Comparison of intravenous amrinone and dobutamine in congestive heart failure due to idiopathic dilated cardiomyopathy. *Am. J. Cardiol.* 1990;66:1107-1112.

[84] Mager G, Klocke RK, Kux A, Höpp HW, Hilger HH. Phosphodiesterase III inhibition or adrenoreceptor stimulation: milrinone as an alternative to dobutamine in the treatment of severe heart failure. *Am. Heart J.* 1991;121:1974-1983.

[85] Karlsberg RP, DeWood MA, DeMaria AN, Berk MR, Lasher KP; Milrinone–Dobutamine Study Group. Comparative efficacy of short–term intravenous infusions of milrinone and dobutamine in acute congestive heart failure following acute myocardial infarction. *Clin. Cardiol.* 1996;19:21-30.

[86] Aranda JM Jr, Schofield RS, Pauly DF, Cleeton TS, Walker TC, Monroe VS Jr, Leach D, Lopez LM, Hill JA. Comparison of dobutamine versus milrinone therapy in hospitalized patients awaiting cardiac transplantation: a prospective randomized trial. *Am. Heart J.* 2003;145:324-329.

[87] Gage J, Rutman H, Lucido D, LeJemtel TH. Additive effects of dobutamine and amrinone on myocardial contractility and ventricular performance in patients with severe heart failure. *Circulation* 1986;74:367-373.

[88] Uretsky BF, Lawless CE, Verbalis JG, Valdes AM, Kolesar JA, Reddy PS. Combined therapy with dobutamine and amrinone in severe heart failure. *Chest* 1987;92:657-662.

[89] Sundram P, Reddy HK, McElroy PA, Janicki JS, Weber KT. Myocardial energetics and efficiency in patients with idiopathic cardiomyopathy: response to dobutamine and amrinone. *Am. Hear J.* 1990;119:891-898.

[90] Huang L, Weil MH, Sun S, Cammarata G, Cao L, Tang W. Levosimendan improves post–resuscitation outcomes in a rat model of CPR. *J. Lab. Clin. Med.* 2005;146:256-261.

[91] Regnier B, Rapin M, Gory G, Lemaire F, Teisseire B, Harari A. Haemodynamic effects of dopamine in septic shock. *Intensive Care Med.* 1977;3:47-53.

[92] Sharshar T, Carlier R, Blanchard A, Feydy A, Gray F, Paillard M, Raphael JC, Gajdos P, Annane D. Depletion of neurohypophyseal content of vasopressin in septic shock. *Crit. Care Med.* 2002;30:497-500.

[93] Lindner KH, Haak T, Keller A, Bothner U, Lurie KG. Release of endogenous vasopressors during and after cardiopulmonary resuscitation. *Heart* 1996;75:145-150.

[94] Dunser MW, Mayr AJ, Tur A, Pajk W, Barbara F, Knotzer H, Ulmer H, Hasibeder WR. Ischemic skin lesions as a complication of continuous vasopressin infusion in catecholamine–resistant vasodilatory shock: incidence and risk factors. *Crit. Care Med.* 2003;31:1394-1398.

[95] Mayr V, Luckner G, Jochberger S, Wenzel V, Ulmer H, Pajk W, Knotzer H, Friesenecker B, Lindner K, Hasibeder W, Dünser M. Arginine vasopressin in advanced cardiovascular failure during the post–resuscitation phase after cardiac arrest. *Resuscitation* 2007;72:35-44.

[96] O'Connor CM, Gattis WA, Uretsky BF, Adams KF Jr, McNulty SE, Grossman SH, McKenna WJ, Zannad F, Swedberg K, Gheorghiade M, Califf RM. Continuous intravenous dobutamine is associated with an increased risk of death in patients with advanced heart failure: insights from the Flolan International Randomized Survival Trial (FIRST). *Am. Heart J.* 1999;138:78-86.

[97] Cuffe MS, Califf RM, Adams KF Jr, Benza R, Bourge R, Colucci WS, Massie BM, O'Connor CM, Pina I, Quigg R, Silver MA, Gheorghiade M; Outcomes of a Prospective Trial of Intravenous Milrinone for Exacerbations of Chronic Heart Failure (OPTIME–CHF) Investigators. Short–term intravenous milrinone for acute exacerbation of chronic heart failure: a randomized controlled trial. *JAMA* 2002;287:1541-1547.

[98] Abraham WT, Adams KF, Fonarow GC, Costanzo MR, Berkowitz RL, LeJemtel TH, Cheng ML, Wynne J; ADHERE Scientific Advisory Committee and Investigators, ADHERE Study Group. In–hospital mortality in patients with acute decompensated heart failure requiring intravenous vasoactive medications: an analysis from the Acute Decompensated Heart Failure National Registry (ADHERE). *J. Am. Coll. Cardiol.* 2005;46:57-64.

[99] Elkayam U, Tasissa G, Binanay C, Stevenson LW, Gheorghiade M, Warnica JW, Young JB, Rayburn BK, Rogers JG, DeMarco T, Leier CV. Use and impact of

inotropes and vasodilator therapy in hospitalized patients with severe heart failure. *Am. Heart J.* 2007;153:98-104.

[100] Hunt SA, Abraham WT, Chin MH, Feldman AM, Francis GS, Ganiats TG, Jessup M, Konstam MA, Mancini DM, Michl K, Oates JA, Rahko PS, Silver MA, Stevenson LW, Yancy CW. 2009 focused update incorporated into the ACC/AHA 2005 Guidelines for the Diagnosis and Management of Heart Failure in Adults: a report of the American College of Cardiology Foundation/American Heart Association Task Force on Practice Guidelines: developed in collaboration with the International Society for Heart and Lung Transplantation. *Circulation* 2009;119:e391-479.

[101] Huikuri HV, Castellanos A, Myerburg RJ. Sudden death due to cardiac arrhythmias. *N. Engl. J. Med.* 2001;345:1473-1482.

[102] Zheng ZJ Croft JB, Giles WH, Mensah GA. Sudden cardiac death in the United States 1989 to 1998. *Circulation*2001;104:2158–2163.

[103] Pell JP, Sirel JM, Marsden AK, Ford I, Walker NL, Cobbe SM. Presentation management and outcome of out of hospital cardiopulmonary arrest: comparison by underlying aetiology. *Heart* 2003;89:839-842.

[104] Antman EM, Anbe DT, Armstrong PW, Bates ER, Green LA, Hand M, Hochman JS, Krumholz HM, Kushner FG, Lamas GA, Mullany CJ, Ornato JP, Pearle DL, Sloan MA, Smith SC Jr, Alpert JS, Anderson JL, Faxon DP, Fuster V, Gibbons RJ, Gregoratos G, Halperin JL, Hiratzka LF, Hunt SA, Jacobs AK, Ornato JP. ACC/AHA guidelines for the management of patients with ST–elevation myocardial infarction: a report of the American College of Cardiology/American Heart Association Task Force on Practice Guidelines (Committee to Revise the 1999 Guidelines for the Management of Patients With Acute Myocardial Infarction). *J. Am. Coll. Cardiol.* 2004;44:E1-211.

[105] Richard C, Ricome JL, Rimailho A, Bottineau G, Auzepy P. Combined hemodynamic effects of dopamine and dobutamine in cardiogenic shock. *Circulation* 1983;67:620-626.

[106] Ferrario M, Poli A, Previtali M, Lanzarini L, Fetiveau R, Diotallevi P, Mussini A, Montemartini C. Hemodynamics of volume loading compared with dobutamine in severe right ventricular infarction. *Am. J. Cardiol.* 1994;74:329-333.

[107] Lin H, Young DB. Opposing effects of plasma epinephrine and norepinephrine on coronary thrombosis in vivo. *Circulation* 1995;91;1135-1142.

[108] Jolly S, Newton G, Horlick E, Seidelin PH, Ross HJ, Husain M, Dzavik V. Effect of vasopressin on hemodynamics in patients with refractory cardiogenic shock complicating acute myocardial infarction. *Am. J. Cardiol.* 2005;96:1617-1620.

[109] Massetti M, Tasle M, Le Page O, Deredec R, Babatasi G, Buklas D, Thuaudet S, Charbonneau P, Hamon M, Grollier G, Gerard JL, Khayat A. Back from irreversibility: extracorporeal life support for prolonged cardiac arrest. *Ann. Thorac. Surg.* 2005;79:178-183.

[110] Hovdenes J, Laake JH, Aaberge L, Haugaa H, Bugge JF. Therapeutic hypothermia after out–of–hospital cardiac arrest: experiences with patients treated with percutaneous coronary intervention and cardiogenic shock. *Acta Anaesthesiol. Scand.* 2007;51:137-142.

[111] Nichol G, Karmy–Jones R, Salerno C, Cantore L, Becker L. Systematic review of percutaneous cardiopulmonary bypass for cardiac arrest or cardiogenic shock states. *Resuscitation* 2006;70:381-394.

[112] Sung K, Lee YT, Park PW, Park KH, Jun TG, Yang JH, Ha YK. Improved survival after cardiac arrest using emergent autopriming percutaneous cardiopulmonary support. *Ann. Thorac. Surg.* 2006;82:651-656.

[113] Marquez MF, Salica G, Hermosillo AG, Pastelin G, Cardenas M. Drug therapy in Brugada syndrome. *Curr. Drug Targets Cardiovasc. Haematol. Disord.* 2005;5:409-417.

[114] Müllner M, Sterz F, Binder M, Hellwagner K, Meron G, Herkner H, Laggner AN. Arterial blood pressure after human cardiac arrest and neurological recovery. *Stroke* 1996;27:59-62.

[115] Ames A 3rd, Wright RL, Kowada M, Thurston JM, Majno G. Cerebral ischemia. II. The no–reflow phenomenon. *Am. J. Pathol.* 1968;52:437-453.

[116] Wolfson SK Jr, Safar P, Reich H, Clark JM, Gur D, Stezoski W, Cook EE, Krupper MA. Dynamic heterogeneity of cerebral hypoperfusion after prolonged cardiac arrest in dogs measured by the stable xenon/CT technique: a preliminary study. *Resuscitation* 1992;23:1-20.

[117] Shaffner DH, Eleff SM, Brambrink AM, Sugimoto H, Izuta M, Koehler RC, Traystman RJ. Effect of arrest time and cerebral perfusion pressure during cardiopulmonary resuscitation on cerebral blood flow metabolism adenosine triphosphate recovery and pH in dogs. *Crit. Care Med.* 1999;27:1335-1342.

[118] Rivers EP, Rady MY, Martin GB, Fenn NM, Smithline HA, Alexander ME, Nowak RM. Venous hyperoxia after cardiac arrest: characterization of a defect in systemic oxygen utilization. *Chest* 1992;102:1787-1793.

[119] Kliegel A, Losert H, Sterz F, Holzer M, Zeiner A, Havel C, Laggner AN. Serial lactate determinations for prediction of outcome after cardiac arrest. *Medicine (Baltimore)* 2004;83:274-279.

[120] Donnino MW, Miller J, Goyal N, Loomba M, Sankey SS, Dolcourt B, Sherwin R, Otero R, Wira C. Effective lactate clearance is associated with improved outcome in post–cardiac arrest patients. *Resuscitation* 2007;75:229-234.

[121] Summerhill EM, Baram M. Principles of pulmonary artery catheterization in the critically ill. *Lung* 2005;183:209-219.

[122] Shah MR, Hasselblad V, Stevenson LW, Binanay C, O'Connor CM, Sopko G, Califf RM. Impact of the pulmonary artery catheter in critically ill patients: meta–analysis of randomized clinical trials. *JAMA* 2005;294:1664-1670.

[123] Hayes MA, Timmins AC, Yau EH, Palazzo M, Hinds CJ, Watson D. Elevation of systemic oxygen delivery in the treatment of critically ill patients. *N. Engl. J. Med.* 1994;330:1717-1722.

In: Drugs in Cardiopulmonary Resuscitation
Editor: Theodoros Xanthos

ISBN: 978-1-61122-512-9

Chapter 12

Drugs in Neonatal Resuscitation

Nicoletta Iacovidou, Filippia Aroni and Angeliki Syggelou

Abstract

Current guidelines for neonatal resuscitation at birth stress the importance of temperature control, airway management and support of circulation for the majority of neonates who require help at birth. For the minority of neonates in which the basic steps of resuscitation fail to reverse an adverse situation, medications are justifiable. The 2005 International Liaison Committee on Resuscitation (ILCOR) guidelines state: "*Medications are rarely needed in neonatal resuscitation. Those that may be used include epinephrine and fluids. Very rarely, a narcotic antagonist, sodium bicarbonate, or vasopressors may be useful after resuscitation*". Even though medications have been in use in neonatal resuscitation for many years, their doses, order and route of administration have been the source of an ongoing debate among neonatologists. Existing data are mainly extrapolated from animal studies or studies on adults. This chapter will focus on the evidence behind the medications that are currently used in neonatal resuscitation.

Introduction

In 1897, DeLee mentioned that 'there are three grand principles governing treatment of asphyxia neonatorum: first maintain the body heat, second free the air passage form obstructions and third stimulate respiration, or supply air to the lungs for oxygenation of the blood" [1].

The majority of newborns require little assistance for their stabilization in the delivery room and for adaptation to extrauterine life. For those neonates in need for more extensive help, securing the airway and effectively ventilating their lungs, remains, in most cases, the key to a successful resuscitation. Cardiopulmonary resuscitation (CPR) and/or drug administration, following failure of ventilation and chest compressions to reverse the condition, is rarely needed (1.2 per 1000 live births) [2]. These neonates typically suffer from severe asphyxia, with resulting increased mortality and long-term morbidity with neurologic deficits [3-5].

Although existing evidence regarding drug administration in neonatal resuscitation is not conclusive, it remains one of the steps that are included in the 2005 ILCOR guidelines for management of neonates at birth [6]. Medication is necessary in less than 0.1% of live births [7,8]. The role of medication in neonatal resuscitation as well as the appropriate doses, order and route of administration, are all controversial and remain an ongoing issue of debate among neonatologists [9]. The existing data on medication used in newborn resuscitation, mostly derive from studies on adults and animal models rather than from pediatric or neonatal clinical trials. The main reason for this is the difficulty in obtaining informed consent in order to conduct clinical trials. Furthermore, administering an unknown drug or a drug of uncertain benefit to human is not ethically acceptable.

Therefore, optimization of the neonatal resuscitation regimen is necessary and more research is needed to shed light on the necessity and prospects of medication in neonatal resuscitation.

Medication

Epinephrine

Epinephrine is an adrenergic agonist that binds strongly to a1, a2, β1, β2 adrenergic receptors [9]. Crile [10,11], and Crile and Dolley in the early 1900's showed that epinephrine was beneficial when added to ventilation and cardiac massage in resuscitating asphyxiated dogs [10-12]. Later studies by Redding and Pearson [13] (using an animal model of asphyxia-induced ventricular fibrillation) showed that epinephrine, administered intravenously (IV) during CPR, was successful in returning of spontaneous circulation in these animals. This action was showed to be mediated via its a-agonist-mediated vasoconstriction and not via its β-agonist mediated increased myocardial contractility and cardiac rate, results that were verified by Otto and colleagues in later studies [14].

When epinephrine is administered in cardiac arrest, its vasoconstrictive action causes increase of the aortic to right atrial pressure gradient during the relaxation phase of CPR [8,15]. Coronary artery perfusion and return of circulation are increased, resulting in an effective myocardial blood flow [16].

Although the majority of data come from animal and adult models, the use of epinephrine is justifiable in neonatal resuscitation if effective ventilation and chest compressions fail to reverse the situation. The 2005 ILCOR guidelines for Neonatal Resuscitation recommend: "*Despite the lack of human data, it is reasonable to continue to use epinephrine when adequate ventilation and chest compressions have failed to increase the heart rate to >60 beats per minute. Use the IV route for epinephrine as soon as venous access is established. The recommended IV dose is 0.01 to 0.03 mg/kg. If the tracheal route is used, give a higher dose (up to 0.1mg/kg). The safety of these higher tracheal doses has not been studied. Do not give high doses of IV epinephrine*" [6,9]. Therefore, in clinical practice, in cases of a) persistent bradycardia (heart rate < 60 beats per minute), despite efficient ventilation of the lungs and chest compressions (minimum duration of 30 sec) and hypotension (defined as a mean blood pressure below the 10th percentile for a given gestation) [17] or b) asystole, epinephrine can be administered IV at a dose of 0.1-0.3 ml/kg of 1:10 000 (0.01-0.03mg/kg) repeated every 3 to 5 minutes, as required [9].

Concerning dosing regimen, despite the long history of epinephrine use, studies to determine appropriate dosing are lacking for all age groups. In the initial experiments of Crile and Dolley, 1 mg of the drug was used, i.e. 0.1 mg/kg for an average 10-kg dog. Subsequent studies in adults, used the same dose of epinephrine of 1 mg, but when adjusted for weight it resulted in a 10-fold lower dose (0.01 mg/kg). This dose was extrapolated to paediatric patients, but soon this was questioned as to its efficacy; the use of higher dosing regimen started to appear in the literature. The higher dose of IV epinephrine has never been adopted in neonatal resuscitation, but there are case series of higher epinephrine dose administered via the endotracheal tube (ETT) in neonatal resuscitation, reporting successful return of spontaneous circulation. Randomized, though, comparisons do not exist [18-20]. However, a recent, multi-centre, randomized, double-blind trial compared high-dose (0.1 mg/kg) versus standard-dose epinephrine (0.01 mg/kg) in children with cardiac arrest and showed a lower 24-hour survival for the high-dose group. If the cardiac arrest had been precipitated by asphyxia, there was a markedly reduced survival in the group of children that were treated with the high-dose adrenaline [21].

There are animal studies in asphyxiated newborn piglets, comparing the high-dose versus the standard-dose epinephrine showing no better outcome at 24 hours [22]. The high-dose epinephrine was also associated with tachycardia and hypertension, side effects that could worsen the condition of the myocardium during the asphyxial episode. If this would occur in a premature infant, it could increase the risk of intraventricular hemorrhage [23].

Regarding the endotracheal route of epinephrine administration, despite its widespread use in resuscitation, there are no placebo controlled neonatal studies to evaluate this. There are animal studies showing that when epinephrine is given via the ETT, considerably higher doses than the currently recommended need to be administered, in order to have a positive effect, but then concerns about its safety arise [24-26].

Chen *et al.*, reported that epinephrine delivered via a catheter through the laryngeal mask has similar effect, as when administered via an ETT, in terms of plasma epinephrine levels, heart rate elevation and mean arterial blood pressure change [27]. This provides an alternative way of administering the drug, when intubation or catheterization of the umbilical vein might not be possible, depending on the experience of the person who performs the resuscitation [28].

Sodium Carbonate

Asphyxia results in anaerobic metabolism, which contributes to metabolic and respiratory acidosis during cardiopulmonary arrest. During an acute episode of asphyxia, there is redistribution of blood flow and oxygen delivery to heart, brain and adrenals. Reduced circulation to other organs results in tissue hypoxia and intravascular or intracellular acidosis. The intracardiac and brain acidosis lead to dysfunction of these organs, thus contributing to further deterioration of the clinical status of the asphyxiated neonate [29]. Metabolic acidosis has adverse effects and increases the risk of death [30].

According to the equation $H^+ + HCO_3 \leftarrow H_2CO \leftarrow CO_2 + H_2O$, sodium bicarbonate buffers the acid by reacting with H^+ ions to form H_2O and CO_2. This has positive effects if CO_2 can be easily transported to and cleared by the lungs. It is therefore necessary to establish effective inflation and ventilation of the lungs prior to the administration of sodium bicarbonate [29].

Treatment of metabolic acidosis includes the use of alkalies such as sodium bicarbonate and tromethamine. Dawes *et al.*, in their initial experiments on neonatal asphyxia in mammals, showed that infusions of alkali during the period of asphyxia prolonged the time to last gasp, made easier the resuscitation of the animals, and seemed to protect the brain from some of the damage caused by asphyxia [31]. When metabolic acidosis is reversed, pulmonary vascular resistance is decreased, whereas contractility of the myocardium, hemodynamic responses to resuscitation with epinephrine and oxygen, and survival are increased [32-35].

The use of bicarbonate in neonatal resuscitation remains controversial. There are a few neonatal or animal studies examining the role of sodium bicarbonate in resuscitation at birth. Animal studies showed that the decrease in blood flow may lead to accumulation of CO_2 at tissue level. In neonates, hyperosmolar solutions are associated with decrease in cerebral blood flow and intraventricular haemorrhage [9,36].

The use of sodium bicarbonate is not recommended during brief CPR due to the numerous adverse effects combined with a profound lack of compelling supporting evidence for beneficial effects in neonatal resuscitation. It is recommended only for use during prolonged arrests, which do not respond to other therapy, and only after securing adequate ventilation and circulation. If administered, a dose of 1 to 2 mEq/kg of a 0.5 mEq/mL (4.2%) solution of bicarbonate may be given. The administration should be IV, in a slow infusion over at least 2 min [9]. Sodium bicarbonate must never be given down the ETT.

Volume Expansion: Crystalloids and Colloids

Very rarely, bradycardia not responding to ventilation of the lungs, chest compressions and drug administration, may be due to hypovolemia. The history and clinical condition of the baby will usually be indicative of acute perinatal blood loss. Clinical situations in which blood loss may occur are feto-maternal hemorrhage, vasa previa, placenta previa, incision of the placenta at cesarean section, and tight nuchal cord [37,38]. Loss of blood out of the fetal - placental unit may also occur. Clinical signs raising suspicion that blood loss has occurred are pallor, poor perfusion and weak pulses. The newborn may be bradycardic or tachycardic[8]. In case of bradycardia, resuscitation efforts will not be effective unless the blood pressure of the neonate is raised above a critical level [39]. Transfusion of O Rh negative packed red blood cells, at a dose of 10-15 ml/Kg, is the most appropriate fluid to be administered, but if not available immediately, a bolus of NaCl 0.9% may be given while waiting for the blood to arrive in the delivery suite.

On certain occasions, normovolemic asphyxiated infants may have the same clinical presentation as in hypovolemic shock and distinguishing them is often problematic in the delivery suite [40]. If there is no evidence of blood loss, bradycardia in the newborn may be due to myocardial dysfunction. In this case fluids should be administered very cautiously, as fluid overload may further disable myocardial function [3,8,38,41].

Concerning the choice of crystalloid or colloid solutions and the appropriate doses of these volume expanders, So *et al.* reported that isotonic saline is as effective as 5% albumin for treating hypotension in preterm infants, and it has the additional advantage of causing less fluid retention in the first 48 hours [42]. Two more randomized trials in neonates have shown that isotonic crystalloid is as effective as albumin in treating hypotension [43,44].

The current 2005 ILCOR guidelines for neonatal resuscitation at birth recommend: "*In consideration of cost and theoretical risks, an isotonic crystalloid solution rather than albumin should be the fluid of choice for volume expansion in neonatal resuscitation*".[6]

If required, administration of 10 ml/kg of normal saline or Ringer's lactate is considered as the ideal therapy for volume expansion, IV over 5 to 10 min, which can be repeated as required [9]. Large volumes (more than 40 ml/Kg) of 0.9% NaCl may exacerbate metabolic acidosis through hyperchloremia and should be avoided [45].

Dextrose

In utero, the fetus is totally dependent on the mother for glucose. Heart and brain use glucose, either aerobically or anaerobically, as the source of energy for their function. Glycogen stores in fetal liver increase with progressing gestation, especially from 36 weeks of gestation onwards, during which time it is deposited in other fetal tissues as well, such as skeletal and myocardial muscle [46]. Under normal conditions, hormonal changes occurring during delivery induce mobilization of the hepatic glycogen.

Any asphyxia insult accelerates the use of glycogen and as a consequence liver stores are depleted and brain metabolic demands cannot be met. Administration of glucose during resuscitation might be necessary in premature babies (gestational age less than 36 weeks), in SGA neonates (small for gestational age, birth weight below the 5th centile), in IUGR (intrauterine growth restriction) neonates requiring prolonged resuscitation and in cases of unresponsive bradycardia and asystole [47]. In all these circumstances, newborns have either reduced or depleted stores of glycogen and they are prone to hypoglycemia. Blood glucose < 40 - 45 mg/dl in a term or preterm neonate requires exogenous glucose administration [48].

There are some data in experimental models of newborn hypoxia in animals suggesting that glucose administration prior to hypoxia may improve survival and neurological outcome [48,49]. On the other hand, there are conflicting reports on the neurological effect of post-hypoxia glucose administration. Hattori *et al.* [50] reported that post-hypoxic glucose administration reduces hypoxic-ischemic brain damage in the neonatal rat, addressing thus the important role of glucose in the development of neonatal hypoxic-ischemic encephalopathy, whereas Sheldon *et al.* [51] reported opposite results, questioning the protective role of normoglycaemia in the development of neonatal hypoxic-ischemic encephalopathy. However, the existing evidence in humans does not suggest the same [48].

The current 2005 ILCOR guidelines for neonatal resuscitation recommend: "*Based on available evidence, the optimal range of blood glucose concentration to minimize brain injury following asphyxia and resuscitation cannot be defined. Infants requiring resuscitation should be monitored and treated to maintain glucose in the normal range*" [6].

If the plasma glucose concentration is less than 40 mg/dL (2.2 mmol/L), glucose has to be administered IV, via a catheter sited in the umbilical vein [52]. The recommended dose is 2 ml/kg of Dextrose 10% in a bolus administration over one minute. If this fails to correct hypoglycemia, the same dose can be repeated. A glucose infusion at 8 mg/kg/min may be necessary in order to ensure normoglycaemia [53]. The low concentration glucose infusion avoids hyperglycemia, rebound secretion of insulin and possible prolongation of hypoglycaemia. A blood glucose concentration 20 minutes after the bolus infusion is measured and the infusion rate or dextrose concentration is adjusted as required to maintain plasma glucose concentration greater than 45 mg/dL; although there are controversies as to the appropriate level of plasma glucose to justify hypoglycaemia, this therapeutic objective allows a margin of safety.

Naloxone Hydrochloride

Naloxone is a pure opioid antagonist without respiratory depressant activity, specifically indicated for respiratory depression due to narcotics exposure [54]. It acts directly to the central nervous system and it's half - life time is 1-1.5 hours. Herschel *et al.* provide a comprehensive history of the drug's introduction and summarise much of the subsequent literature [55].

Despite its frequent use in neonatal resuscitation, there are no significant data on the impact of naloxone on clinically important outcomes and in particular on its safety. Administration of the drug is justifiable in neonates with apnoea or respiratory depression, whose mothers have had repeated doses of opiate narcotics less than 3 hours apart or had received doses of an opioid IV rather than intramuscularly (IM) or had received narcotics within four hours of delivery [54].

If a neonate is apnoeic due to maternal opioid use, the standard steps of neonatal resuscitation are required. Inflation and ventilation of the lungs and good heart rate have to be established, prior to considering naloxone administration as it is not an emergency drug and there is evidence that its use may in fact delay the administration of adequate ventilatory support, thereby increasing the risk of postpartum anoxia [56].

The 2005 ILCOR guidelines recommend: "*the appropriate dose Naloxone is not recommended as part of the initial resuscitation of newborns with respiratory depression in the delivery room. Before naloxone is given, providers should restore heart rate and color by supporting ventilation. The preferred route should be IV or intramuscular. Tracheal administration is not recommended. There is no evidence to support or refute the current dose of 0.1 mg/kg*" [6].

The recommended dose is 0.1 mg/kg of a 0.4 mg/ml or 1.0 mg/ml solution, given IV via an umbilical vein catheter [8]. Naloxone peaks in the plasma at 5 to 40 min if given IV. It may be administered IM or subcutaneously if perfusion is adequate. Naloxone given IM, peaks at 30 min to 2 h with onset of action in 15 min and prolonged duration of action [54,57]. Continuous assessment of the respiratory function is essential, since the duration of narcotics may exceed that of naloxone (the effect of pethidine may last for more than 24 hrs in newborn) therefore, repeated doses of naloxone may be required in order to prevent recurrent apnoeic episodes [58]. Naloxone has minimal toxic effects [59]. Cardiac arrest has been reported in a neonate after naloxone administration [60]. Furthermore, it should not be given to newborns whose mothers are suspected of abusing other narcotics, such as heroin because it may precipitate abrupt withdrawal symptoms in these neonates [61]. There is a report that naloxone given to an infant born to an opioid-addicted mother was associated with seizures [62].

*Other Drugs

There is no proven place for any other drug for neonatal resuscitation at birth [47].

*Order of Administration

The 2005 ILCOR guidelines recommend adrenaline to be given first. There are reports in the literature demonstrating that a mixture of alkali and glucose could cause a rapid rise in heart rate and blood pressure in terminal apnoea [63]. If adrenaline has no effect, a dose of bicarbonate followed by another dose of adrenaline may be appropriate.

Route of Administration

If drugs are to be administered in a neonate whose heart has not respond to effective lung ventilation and chest compressions, they have to be delivered as close to the heart as possible, since the circulation is not functioning. Therefore, venous access must be achieved and the most easily and quickly accessible vein in a collapsed neonate, is the umbilical vein in the ligated cord stump. It is always better to practice on preparations of umbilical cord prior to attempting a catheterization in a real-time situation.

The equipment required should always be sterile and available to be used, at any time necessity arises in the delivery room. A basic pack should contain: a scalpel with a large blade, a proper-sized umbilical catheter, a 3-way tap, syringes, artery forceps, one umbilical vein probe, sterile gauzes and a cord tape.

The procedure, if not emergent, has to be performed under aseptic conditions. In an urgent situation, the umbilical vein catheterization has to be performed as aseptic as possible, but this should not be a priority under such circumstances.

A size 5.0 F catheter for preterms and 8.0 F for term infants is used. Feeding tubes should not be used, except as last resort. As to the position of the catheter for resuscitation purposes, 4-6 cm of the catheter should be inserted to achieve blood return. When no longer needed, it should be removed. If the catheter is to remain *in situ*, it should be secured with tape and sutures [64].

An alternative route for drugs administration is the intraoosseous one. It provides immediate access to the intravascular space when the IV access cannot be established quickly, during CPR [65]. There are few reports in the literature on the successful use of the intraosseous access to newborns [66,67]. Medications, volume expanders, blood and glucose can be given intraosseously. The doses of drugs or fluids administered intraosseously are the same as in IV administration [68].

The technique to establish an intraosseous access in young infants and children is easy to learn, requires little equipment and has been described extensively in the literature [69,70]. The proximal tibia (1 cm below the tibial tuberosity and medially located on the tibial plateau) is the most commonly preferred site for intraosseous access in infants. Several needles for intaosseous access, containing a stylet to prevent plugging, are commercially available [71]. If not available, a large-gauge needle with a stylet can be used, but plugging with bone spicules can be a problem. Local anaesthesia is given to the patient, prior to introducing the needle nearly perpendicular on the bone with a twisting motion [70]. It should be directed away from the knee joint. When the needle is into the marrow space, decreased resistance is felt, and aspiration of blood or bone marrow usually confirms the placement. Practicing on manikins is required prior to using the technique in real-time situations.

Conclusion

Current guidelines call for the use of adrenaline (0.1 ml/kg of 1:10000 solution repeated every 3-5 minutes if required), sodium bicarbonate (1-2 ml/kg of 4.2% solution), glucose (2ml/kg of 10% solution), and 0.9% NaCl as volume expander (10 ml/kg) in neonatal resuscitation. Very rarely an opioid antagonist, such as naloxone (of 0.1 mg/kg), may be required to reverse respiratory depression in neonates exposed to narcotics. The use of drugs in neonatal resuscitation is only justified if the lungs of a depressed neonate have been efficiently ventilated and the circulation has been supported.

The evidence behind the recommended medications most commonly used in neonatal resuscitation is poor: The efficacy of the medications, the dosages, the routes of administration and outcome need to be tested in future studies in neonatal models of asphyxia.

References

[1] De Lee JB, Asphyxia Neonatorum: causation and treatment. *Medicine* (Detroit) 1897;3:643-660.

[2] Perlman JM, Risser R. Cardiopulmonary resuscitation in the delivery room. Associated clinical events. *Arch. Pediatr. Adolesc. Med.* 1995;149:20–25.

[3] Wyckoff MH, Perlman JM, Laptook AR. Use of volume expansion during delivery room resuscitation in near-term and term infants. *Pediatrics.* 2005;115:950–955.

[4] Haddad B, Mercer BM, Livingston JC, Talati A, Sibai BM. Outcome after successful resuscitation of babies born with apgar scores of 0 at both 1 and 5 minutes. *Am. J. Obstet. Gynecol.* 2000;182:1210–1214.

[5] Patel H, Beeby PJ. Resuscitation beyond 10 minutes of term babies born without signs of life. *J. Paediatr. Child Health.* 2004;40:136–138.

[6] The International Liaison Committee on Resuscitation (ILCOR) Consensus on science with treatment recommendations for pediatric and neonatal patients: neonatal resuscitation. *Pediatrics* 2006;117:e978-88.

[7] Perlman JM, Risser R. Cardiopulmonary resuscitation in the delivery room: associated clinical events. *Arch. Pediatr. Adolesc. Med.* 1995;149:20-25.

[8] Wyllie J, Niermeyer S. The role of resuscitation drugs and placental transfusion in the delivery room management of newborn infants. *Semin. Fetal Neonatal. Med.* 2008;13:416-23.

[9] Wyckoff MH, Perlman J, Niermeyer S. Medications during resuscitation – what is the evidence? *Semin. Neonatol.* 2001;6:251–259.

[10] Crile GW: Preliminary note on a method of resuscitation of apparently dead animals. *Cleveland Medical Journal* 1903;2:35.

[11] Crile GW: Resuscitation of animals apparently dead. *St. Louis Medical Surgical Journal* 1903;84:299-302.

[12] Crile GW, Dolley DH: An experimental research into the resuscitation of dogs killed by anesthetics and asphyxia. *Journal of Experimental Medicine* 1906;8:713-724.

[13] Redding JS, Pearson JW: Evaluation of drugs for cardiac resuscitation. *Anesthesiology* 1963;24:203-207.

[14] Otto CW, Yakatis RW, Blitt CD. Mechanism of action of epinephrine in resuscitation from asphyxial arrest. *Crit. Care Med.* 1981;9:321-324.

[15] Michael JR, Guerci AD, Koehler RC, Shi AY, Tsitlik J, Chandra N, Niedermeyer E, Rogers MC, Traystman RJ, Weisfeldt ML. Mechanisms by which epinephrine augments cerebral and myocardial perfusion during cardiopulmonary resuscitation in dogs. *Circulation* 1984;69:822-35.

[16] Paradis NA, Martin GB, Rivers EP, Goetting MG, Appleton TJ, Feingold M, Nowak RM. Coronary perfusion pressure and the return of spontaneous circulation in human cardiopulmonary resuscitation. *JAMA* 1990;263:1106;1113.

[17] Campbell ME, Byrne PJ. Cardiopulmonary resuscitation and epinephrine infusion in extremely low birth weight infants in the neonatal intensive care unit. *J. Perinatol.* 2004;24:691-695.

[18] Wyckoff MH, Perlmann JM. Use of high-dose epinephrine and Sodium Bicarbonate during neonatal resuscitation: is there proven benefit? *Clin Perinatol* 2006;33:141-151. 19. Schwab KO, von Stockhausen HB. Plasma catecholamines after endotracheal administration of adrenaline during postnatal resuscitation. *Arch. Dis. Child Fetal. Neonatal. Ed.* 1994;70F:213-217.

[19] O' Donnell AI, Gray PH, Rogers YM. Mortality and neurodevelopmental outcome for infants receiving adrenaline in neonatal resuscitation. *J. Paediatr. Child Health* 1998;34:551-556.

[20] Perondi MB, Reis AG, Paiva EF, Nadkarni VM, Berg RA. A comparison of high-dose and standard-dose epinephrine in children with cardiac arrest. *N. Engl. J. Med.* 2004;350:1722-1730.

[21] Berg RA, Otto CW, Kern KB, et al. A randomized blinded trial of high-dose epinephrine versus standard-dose epinephrine in a swine model of pediatric asphyxial cardiac arrest. *Crit. Care Med.* 1996;24:1695-1700.

[22] Pasternak JF, Groothuis DR, Fischer JM, Fischer DP. Regional cerebral blood flow in the beagle puppy model of neonatal intaventricular hemorrhage: studies in systemic hypertension. *Neurology* 1983;33:559-566.

[23] Ralston SH, Voorhees WD, Babbs CF. Intrapulmonary epinephrine during prolonged cardiopulmonary resuscitation: improved regional blood flow and resuscitation in dogs. *Ann. Emerg. Med.* 1984;13:79–86.

[24] Ralston SH, Tacker WA, Showen L, Carter A, Babbs CF. Endotracheal versus intravenous epinephrine during electromechanical dissociation with CPR in dogs. *Ann. Emerg. Med.*1985;14:1044–1048.
[25] Redding JS, Asuncion JS, Pearson JW. Effective routes of drug administration during cardiac arrest. *Anesth. Analg.* 1967;46:253–258.
[26] Chen KT, Lin HJ, Guo HR, Lin MT, Lin CC. Feasibility study of epinephrine administration via laryngeal mask airway using a porcine model. *Resuscitation* 2006;69:503-507.
[27] Barber CA, Wyckoff MH. Use and efficacy of endotracheal versus intravenous epinephrine during neonatal cardiopulmonary resuscitation in the delivery room. *Pediatrics* 2006;118:1028-1034.
[28] Aschner JL, Poland RL. Sodium bicarbonate: basically useless therapy. *Pediatrics* 2008;122:831-835.
[29] Goldaber KB, Gilstrap LC, Leveno KJ. Pathologic fetal acidemia. *Obstet. Gynecol.* 1991;78:1103–1107.
[30] Dawes GS, Hibbard E, Windle WF. The effect of alkali and glucose infusion on permanent brain damage in rhesus monkeys asphyxiated at birth. *J. Pediatr.* 1964;65:801–806.
[31] Preziosi MP, Roig JC, Hargrove N, Burchfield DJ. Metabolic acidemia with hypoxia attenuates the hemodynamic responses to epinephrine during resuscitation in lambs. *Crit. Care Med.* 1993;21:1901–1907.
[32] Anderson MN, Mouritzen CV. Effect of acute respiratory and metabolic acidosis on cardiac output and peripheral resistance. *Ann. Surg.* 1966;163:161–168.
[33] Nakanishi T, Seguchi M, Tsuchiya T, Yasukouchi S, Takao A. Effect of acidosis on intracellular pH and calcium concentration in the newborn and adult rabbit myocardium. *Circ. Res.* 1990;67:111–123.
[34] Rudolph AM, Yuan S. Response of pulmonary vasculature to hypoxia and H^+ ion concentration changes. *J. Clin. Invest.* 1966;45:399–411.
[35] Hein HA. The use of sodium bicarbonate in neonatal resuscitation: help or harm? *Pediatrics* 1993;91;496-497.
[36] Keenan WJ. Neonatal resuscitation: what role for volume expansion? *Pediatrics* 2005;115;1072-1073.
[37] Vanhaesebrouck P, Vanneste K, de Praeder C, Van Trappen Y, Thiery M. Tight nuchal cord and neonatal hypovolaemic shock. *Arch. Dis. Child* 1987;62:1276–1277.
[38] Dawes GS, Jacobson HN, Mott JC, Shelley HJ, Stafford A. The treatment of asphyxiated mature foetal lambs and rhesus monkeys with intravenous glucose and sodium carbonate. *J. Physiol.* 1963;169:167-184.
[39] Anderson PAW, Kleinman CS, Lister G, Talner NS. Cardiovascular function during normal fetal and neonatal development and with hypoxic stress. In: Polin RA, Fox WW, eds. *Fetal and Neonatal Physiology*. Philadelphia, PA: W.B Saunders; 1998:861–865.
[40] Yao AC, Lind J. Blood volume in the asphyxiated term neonate. *Biol. Neonate.* 1972;21:199-209.
[41] So KW, Fok TF, Ng PC, Wong WW, Cheung KL. Randomised controlled trial of colloid or crystalloid in hypotensive preterm infants. *Arch. Dis. Child Fetal. Neonatal. Ed.* 1997; 76:F43–F46.

[42] Oca MJ, Nelson M, Donn SM. Randomized trial of normal saline versus 5% albumin for the treatment of neonatal hypotension. *J. Perinatol.* 2003;23:473-476.

[43] Emery EF, Greenough A, Gamsu HR. Randomised controlled trial of colloid infusions in hypotensive preterm infants. *Arch. Dis. Child* 1992;67:1185-1188.

[44] Skellett S, Mayer A, Durward A, Tibby SM, Murdoch IA. Chasing the base deficit: hyperchloraemic acidosis following 0.9% saline fluid resuscitation *Arch. Dis. Child.* 2000;83:514-516.

[45] Shelley HJ, Neligan GA. Neonatal hypoglycaemia. *Br. Med. Bull.* 1966;22:34-39.

[46] Richmond S, Drugs in Resuscitation at Birth-The Newborn Life Support Provider Manual. Publ Resuscitation Council, UK, London 2006.

[47] Voorhies TM, Rawlinson D, Vannucci RC. Glucose and perinatal hypoxic-ischemic brain damage in the rat. *Neurology* 1986;36:1115-1118.

[48] Holowach-Thurston J, Hauhart RE, Jones EM. Anoxia in mice: reduced glucose in brain with normal or elevated glucose in plasma and increased survival after glucose treatment. *Pediatr. Res.* 1974;8:238-243.

[49] Hattori H, Wasterlain CG. Posthypoxic glucose supplement reduces hypoxic-ischemic brain damage in the neonatal rat. *Ann. Neurol.* 1990;28:122-128.

[50] Sheldon RA, Partridge JC, Ferriero DM. Postischemic hyperglycemia is not protective to the neonatal rat brain. *Pediatr. Res.* 1992;32:489-493.

[51] Hay WW, Levin M., Sondheimer JM, Deterding RR. Hypoglycemia. Mc Graw Hill. Current Diagnosis and Treatment in Pediatrics, 18th edition.

[52] Lilien LD, Pildes RS, Srinivasan G, Voora S, Yeh TF. Treatment of neonatal hypoglycemia with minibolus and intravenous glucose infusion. *J. Pediatr.* 1980;97:295-298.

[53] Gill AW, Colvin J. Use of naloxone during neonatal resuscitation in Australia: compliance with published guidelines. *J. Paediatr. Child Health.* 2007;43:795-798.

[54] Herschel M, Khoshnood B, Lass NA. Role of naloxone in newborn resuscitation. *Pediatrics* 2000;106:831–834.

[55] Mitchell A, Niday P, Boulton J, Chance G, Dulberg C. A prospective clinical audit of neonatal resuscitation practices in Canada. *Adv. Neonatal. Care* 2002;2:316-326.

[56] Moreland TA, Brice JE, Walker CH, Parija AC. Naloxone pharmacokinetics in the newborn. *Br. J. Clin. Pharmacol.* 1980;9:609-612.

[57] Etherington J, Christenson J, Innes G, Grafstein E, Pennington S, Spinelli JJ, Gao M, Lahiffe B, Wanger K, Fernandes C. Is early discharge safe after naloxone reversal of presumed opioid overdose. *CJEM.* 2000; 2:156-162.

[58] Handal KA, Schauben JL, Salamone FR. Naloxone. *Ann. Emerg. Med.* 1983;12:438-445.

[59] Deshpande G, Gill A. Cardiac arrest following naloxone in an extremely preterm neonate. *Eur. J. Pediatr.* 2009;168:115-117.

[60] Roberts RJ. Fetal and infant intoxication. In: Drug therapy in infants; pharmacologic principles and clinical experiences. Philadelphia: Saunders;1984.p 322-383.

[61] Gibbs J, Newson T, Williams J, Davidson DC. Naloxone hazard in infant of opioid abuser. *Lancet* 1989;2:159-160.

[62] Daniel SS, Dawes GS, James LS, Ross BB. Analeptics and the resuscitation of asphyxiated monkeys. *Br. Med. J.* 1966;2:562-563.

[63] Feick HJ, Donn SM: Vascular access and blood sampling. In Donn SM, Faix RG (ed): Neonatal Emergencies. Mt Kisco, NY Futura Publishing, 1991, pp31-50.
[64] Engle WA: Intraosseous access for administration of medications in neonates. *Clin. Perinatol.* 2006;33:161-168.
[65] Ellemunter H, Simma B, Trawoeger R, Maurer H. Intraosseous lines in preterm and full term neonates. *Arch. Dis. Child Fetal. Neonatal. Ed.* 1999;80:F74-75.
[66] Kelsall AWR. Resuscitation with intraosseous lines in neonatal units. *Arch. Dis. Child* 1993;68:324-325.
[67] Jaimovich DG, Kecskes S. Intraosseous infusion: a re-discovered procedure as an alternative for pediatric vascular access. *Indian. J. Pediatr.* 1991;58:329-334.
[68] Rosetti VA, Thompson BM, Miller J, Mateer JR, Aprahamian C. Intraosseous infusion: an alternative route of pediatric intravascular access. *Ann. Emerg. Med.* 1985; 14:885-888,
[69] LaRocco BG, Wang HE. Intraosseous infusion. *Prehosp. Emerg. Care,* 2003;7:280-285.
[70] Orlowski JP. Emergency alternatives to intraosseous access. Intraosseous, intratracheal, sublingual and other-site drug administration. *Pediatr. Clin. North Am.* 1994;41:1183-1199.

Index

C

D

E

I

J

K

L

M

T